Health Psychology

An Introduction for Nurses and other Health Care Professionals

Neil Niven BSc PhD CPsychol AFBPsS

Lecturer in Health Psychology, Faculties of Medicine and Dentistry, University of Newcastle upon Tyne, UK

SECOND EDITION

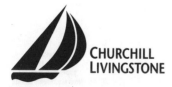
CHURCHILL
LIVINGSTONE

EDINBURGH LONDON MADRID MELBOURNE NEW YORK AND TOKYO 1994

CHURCHILL LIVINGSTONE
Medical Division of Pearson Professional Ltd.

Distributed in the United States of America by Churchill Livingstone Inc., 650 Avenue of the Americas, New York, N.Y. 10011, and by associated companies, branches and representatives throughout the world.

© Longman Group Limited 1989, 1994
© Pearson Professional Ltd 1996

First edition 1989
Second edition 1994
   Reprinted 1995
   Reprinted 1996

ISBN 0 443 04810 X

British Library Cataloguing in Publication Data
A catalogue record for this book is available from the British Library.

Library of Congress Cataloging in Publication Data
Niven, Neil
   Health psychology: an introduction for nurses and other health care professionals/Neil Niven. — 2nd ed.
      p.   cm.
   Includes bibliographical references and index.
   ISBN 0-443-04810-X
   1. Clinical health psychology. 2. Nursing. I. Title.
   [DNLM: 1. Attitude to Health. 2. Health Promotion.
3. Stress, Psychological–psychology. 4. Pain-psychology.
5. Professional–Patient Relations.   W 85 N734h 1994]
R726.7.N58   1994
613'.01'9—dc20
DNLM/DLC
for Library of Congress   94-8465

The publisher's policy is to use **paper manufactured from sustainable forests**

Produced by Longman Singapore Publishers (Pte) Limited
Printed in Singapore

Contents

Preface to the second edition

It is encouraging that interest in the area of health psychology continues to grow. Perhaps more significant is the increased involvement of health professionals in the teaching and research of the subject. The main aim of the second edition of this book is to continue to provide a basic introduction to the subject but at the same time to include some more recent studies and highlight a few new developments.

The new edition contains a section after each chapter on recommended reading. It is important for an introductory text to provide the readers with the opportunity to pursue their interests in different areas. Thus each chapter ends with a selection of recent texts that have been annotated in order to give a clearer indication of their relevance and content.

Another feature of the book is the inclusion of some new topics such as the role of framing in making decisions, new models of health behaviour and cultural determinants of health. The structure of the book remains the same and I hope the format continues to provide a useful framework for understanding health psychology.

Finally, thanks to all who provided comments on the first edition. I have certainly attempted to incorporate as many of the suggestions as was possible in this edition. However, as I have said before, the subject is new and continues to grow; therefore I hope that further comments will help inform future editions.

Hexham, Northumberland 1994   N.N.

Preface to the first edition

Health psychology is a new subject. The Division of Health Psychology of the American Psychological Association was established in 1982 and the Section of Health Psychology in the British Psychological Society was established as recently as December 1986. Yet it is incorrect to say that psychologists have just discovered the health system and are the last of the social and behavioural sciences to do so. Psychologists have been writing, teaching and researching on problems of physical as well as mental health since the beginning of the century. Watson, in 1912, joined with others to investigate how psychology could contribute to medical education and practice. One reason for the apparent misconception is a disproportionate emphasis on the role of the psychologist in the treatment of mental illness with a comparative disregard for those psychologists working with health professionals to improve the quality of health care and to help prevent illness and disease. Over the last decade there has been a growing realisation that psychology has a significant role to play in the provision of health care and this is reflected in the inclusion of the subject in a large proportion of health courses at the basic and post basic levels.

Unfortunately there is still some confusion regarding the nature of health psychology. Firstly, it is not psychiatry, clinical or abnormal psychology. It is the study of normal human behaviour. Secondly, the emphasis is not on illness or treatment but on health. The concerns of the health psychologist are with the stresses and strains of everyday life, effective communication with patients and establishing why some people do not comply with medical advice and others do. This is not to say that psychology has no role to play in the treatment of stroke patients, diabetes, rheumatoid arthritis and other such conditions. Many clinical psychologists have contributed a great deal to an analysis of the psychological factors associated with illness, disease and handicap, but the emphasis of health psychology is on developing preventive programmes of health care, improving the quality of life and developing in individuals the competence to adapt to 'life crises' and cope with common problems of pain, stress and depression.

Health psychology is not the exclusive domain of professional psychologists. Miller (1969) in his presidential address to the American Psychological Association said of psychology:

The techniques involved are not some esoteric branch of witchcraft that must be reserved for those with PhD degrees in psychology. When the ideas are made sufficiently concrete and explicit, the foundations of psychology can be grasped by sixth-grade children.

He goes on to suggest that psychology is a subject that should be studied by everyone. In this he is perfectly correct. Similarly, health psychology should be the domain of the practitioners of health care rather than the sole concern of the professional psychologist. Thus this book is aimed at those individuals who wish to know about health psychology and those who wish to use it in their everyday practice.

The structure of the book was guided by developments in the area of health psychology itself. Stone (1979) was one of the first to propose that health psychology should not be structured along the lines of an introductory psychology text, but should reflect the needs of health professionals. Indeed, he goes further and says that health psychology should not consist of those aspects of psychology that can be applied to health care, but a psychology of health. Niven (1984) proposed a structure based on similar views, which emphasised a psychological perspective that emanated from the health professional. The content of health psychology should be 'driven' by health professionals with a knowledge of psychology as well as professional psychologists.

The book is structured into three sections: process, content and models. The first section of the book investigates how psychology informs the process of interacting with patients, facilitating the delivery of health care. The practical nature of this process has sometimes been described as 'hands on' experience. Throughout this section there are a number of practical exercises. It is hoped that the reader will be encouraged to take part in the exercises as they are designed to give insight into the psychological substrates of interpersonal communication.

Most individuals would admit to having experienced some degree of stress and pain in their lives and to having felt 'a bit down' or depressed at times. The second section deals with the psychological components of such basic experiences. Pain and stress management throughout the life span and some of the basic features of health behaviour are among the issues discussed in the section.

The third section of the book is entitled models. Up until now it has been assumed that the subjects of health psychology are adults, who live in the same environment, come from the same culture and are treated by highly motivated health professionals. This section concentrates on the differences in behaviour that occur as a result of age, on the effect of the environment and culture on behaviour and the stresses and strains of working in an organisational setting.

The emphasis of the book is on the psychology of prevention and not treatment. It is concerned with the problems that confront normal people during the course of their everyday lives and not with treating abnormal behaviour or mental illness. It is hoped that readers will be suitably stimulated to 'delve deeper' into those areas that interest them. Health psychology is in its infancy. I hope that it continues to develop into a most exciting fusion of human behaviour and health care.

I would like to thank my colleagues, the health professionals whom I have taught over the years and the fieldwork and practical teachers, all of whom provided constructive criticism that led me to reformulate a number of ideas. Further thanks to Sandy Wolfson who helped with a number of the exercises on interpersonal skills and to Chris Dracup for his help with the exercise on individual decision making. I would also like to thank the staff at Churchill Livingstone for their help and encouragement.

However, the most praise must go to my wife, Josephine. Writing a book in one's spare time is only possible if one has the time to spare. She made it possible for me to spend time working on the book when I could have spent more time with my family. The book is as much a product of her helpful support as it is of my writing.

N.N.

REFERENCES

Miller G A 1969 Psychology as a means of promoting human welfare. American Psychologist 24: 1063–1075
Niven N 1982 Health psychology. Nursing Times 78: 417–419
Stone G C 1979 Psychology and the health system. In: Stone G C, Cohen F, Adler N E (eds) Health psychology: a handbook. Jossey Bass, San Francisco

Acknowledgements

I am grateful to the following publishers for permission to use previously published material:

Academic Press, Orlando, Florida for Tables II and IX from Wolkind S, Zajicek (eds) 1981 Pregnancy: a psychological and social study.
Plenum Publishing Corporation, New York for the flow charts of stress inoculation training from Meichenbaum D, Jaremko M F (eds) 1983 Stress reduction and prevention. Coping response strategies from Billings A G, Moos R H 1981 Journal of Behavioural Medicine 4: 139–157
Pergamon Press for the social readjustment scale from Holmes T H, Rahe R H 1967 Journal of Psychosomatic Research 11: 213–218

and to Beatrice Sofaer and Joan Eland for permission to use extracts from their contributions to Copp L A (ed) 1984 Perspectives on pain. Churchill Livingstone, Edinburgh.

The author and publishers have made every effort to trace the copyright holders for borrowed material. If they have inadvertently overlooked any, they will be pleased to make the necessary arrangements at the first opportunity.

Process

1

Interpersonal skills

The purpose of this chapter is to provide information concerning the process by which people interact with each other and to give an opportunity to practise the skills used in interpersonal interaction. Thus, topics such as nonverbal communication, questioning techniques, personality, self-disclosure and social skills are discussed in a psychological context with a view to providing a practical and conceptual aid to the improvement of social and helping skills.

What do we mean by interpersonal skills? In what skills are health care professionals most interested? A number of psychologists have limited their definitions to behaviour that can be experimentally verified and reliably taught. However, a major development in the field of interpersonal skills was the finding that there existed specific elements of behaviour that made up the repertoire of skilful health professionals. Until that time, it had been assumed that proficiency at interpersonal skills, like the bedside manner of the 'caring nurse' or the warmth and concern of the 'trusted doctor', was a skill with which one was born or developed slowly after years of experience. It was thought that these essential interpersonal skills could not possibly be taught by any training programme. But it soon became established that interpersonal skills could be taught to anybody and when this became accepted, the necessary first step in developing ways of teaching these skills was achieved.

Kagan (1979)

It is not enough, however, to be a competent technician at interpersonal skills; it is important to understand how patients defend and distort as well as how interpersonal communication can be improved. This is not to suggest that the

3

health professional should become an expert in social psychology, personality theory or psychotherapy, but without some additional cognitive framework for understanding how people behave in specific ways, the ability to help patients may be limited.

NONVERBAL COMMUNICATION

In the last decade there has been a great upsurge of interest in the process of nonverbal communication between health professional and patient. This is not surprising as Birdwhistell (1970) estimated that only 30–35% of the social meaning of a conversation is carried by words alone. Other features of speech such as tone of voice, inflection, rate of speaking, duration and pauses all convey meaning. A variety of meanings are also conveyed by nonvocal, nonverbal behaviours such as gestures, dress, physical proximity, facial expressions, posture and orientation. It is thus important to distinguish between nonvocal and nonverbal behaviours (Table 1.1). Verbal communication is based on a language of some kind and is usually characterised by everyday speech. However there are languages that are not spoken (nonvocal) such as morse code and sign language. Nonverbal communication does not utilise words, but is concerned with behaviours such as body contact, facial expression and gestures (nonvocal); and voice tone, pitch and volume (vocal). Nonverbal communication serves a number of functions:

- *Communicating emotions and attitudes.* In many circumstances feelings are communicated not by what is said but by facial expressions.

Similarly, relationships between individuals are often assessed by looking at the nonverbal communication that occurs between them.

- *Synchronising conversation.* An individual wishing to start a conversation may hope to 'catch a person's eye' in order to indicate to the other person that he wishes to say something. Similarly, conversations may be terminated using nonverbal channels. The 'flow' of the conversation is regulated by glancing away from the speaker or nodding agreement to her, thus providing feedback.
- *Supplementing speech.* When a speaker puts more stress on certain words than others, or pauses between words, or varies the tone and speed of his speech, he is supplementing the conversation nonverbally. In some circumstances the speaker may even contradict what he is saying verbally by his nonverbal expressions.

Exercise 1.1

This exercise may be done in a group or in pairs.

As a group
Count the number of people in the group. On the same number of cards, or pieces of paper, write an emotion, e.g. Fear, Disbelief, Sadness, Dominance, Boredom, Disgust, Interest, Shame, Anger, Surprise, Love, Embarrassment, Admiration, Happiness etc. Distribute the cards to the members of the group face down. Give the following instructions:

On the card in front of you is written an emotion. You have to stand up in front of the group and communicate this emotion nonverbally, that is you must not use any words. You can communicate vocally by altering such things as the pitch, tone and volume of your voice by counting from 1 to 5 whilst using any other nonverbal channel. Other members of the group write down the emotion they think is being demonstrated as each member takes his turn.

In pairs
Take turns to demonstrate the emotions to each other, writing down what you think they are.

Table 1.1 Communication systems

	Nonverbal	Verbal
Vocal	Volume Tone Pitch	Everyday speech
Nonvocal	Gesture Eye contact Proximity Posture	Morse code Sign language

Exercise 1.1 illustrates that there are large individual differences in the ability to transmit and to interpret emotions nonverbally. Why should this be? One explanation is that it is difficult for most people to 'turn on an emotion'

as they would a light switch. Some people are better actors than others and thus find it easier to transmit emotions without actually feeling them. Further, emotions occur in a particular context, and it is this context that gives cues and clues to the sort of emotion to expect. Given these difficulties, it is useful to think about the problems of trying to communicate confidence and assuredness when feeling nervous and unsure of oneself. Are patients able to detect true emotions through a disguise? This important problem of 'leakage' will be discussed in greater detail later on in the chapter, but for the moment it is necessary to investigate the different forms of nonverbal communication and the functions they perform.

Facial expressions

Emotions that are most easily recognised via the face are happiness, sadness, surprise, fear, anger and disgust. (In Exercise 1.1 you might have noted that these emotions were easier to transmit and decipher than some of the others.) These facial expressions tend to be universal, i.e. people all over the world smile when they are happy and frown when they are sad (Ekman & Friesen 1975). Similarly there is evidence that facial expressions tend to have a universality of meaning, i.e. smiles are recognised as a sign of happiness and frowns are recognised as a sign of sadness all over the world (Ekman & Friesen 1975).

An important issue in the field of interpersonal skills is the extent to which facial expressions can actually make people feel differently. Can smiling a lot actually make people happy? The answer is a tentative 'yes'. Zuckerman et al (1981) divided males and females into three groups. The first group were shown a film of a pleasant scene. The second group were shown a film of a neutral scene. The third group were shown a film of a nasty scene. Within each of these groups, a third of the people were asked to suppress their facial reactions, a third were told to exaggerate them, and a third were not asked to do anything at all. The subjects' physiological arousal was

recorded during the films and they rated their emotional reactions to the scenes after the films had finished. Those people who were asked to exaggerate their facial expressions showed higher levels of arousal to both the pleasant and unpleasant scenes and also reported stronger positive and negative emotional reactions than individuals asked to suppress their facial expressions. Thus exaggerating one's facial expressions seems to increase one's feelings, whether positive or negative and suppressing facial expressions decreases feelings. Although this study has been criticised on methodological grounds, recent support for the facial feedback hypothesis has come from McCanne & Anderson (1987). Two implications of this research for health professionals are:

- making patients smile more may actually make them feel better
- learning to suppress facial expressions in times of stress may decrease the emotional experience of the stress itself.

Eye contact

Generally speaking, eye contact can be equated with friendliness. If one were to measure the amount of eye contact between couples in a restaurant and obtain a measure of their friendliness towards each other, there would be a correlation between the two. Therefore, engaging in eye contact usually signifies that a person wishes to appear friendly. However, if he goes too far and starts to stare, this has the opposite effect. Most people become nervous when stared at. This is partly due to an uneasiness about the intentions of the person staring and partly due to an innate apprehension of danger. For instance, animals stare before they are about to attack.

Another function of eye contact is to signify that a person wishes to engage in some form of interaction. It is very hard to avoid contact with somebody wishing to sell something in a street once they have 'caught your eye'.

Finally, when a person has something difficult to say, or is lying, he will often look away from the listener. It is hard to look someone straight in the eye and lie, though practised liars are often capable of such deception.

Bodily contact

Not surprisingly, families and intimate friends engage in more bodily contact than strangers and the meaning of bodily contact varies according to the length of contact, the part of the anatomy touched and the relationship between the individuals. However, there are two research findings of particular importance. The first is concerned with the large cultural differences in bodily contact and touching. Some cultures touch each other much more often than others.

Jourard (1966) surveyed who is touched by whom and where. He observed pairs of people engaged in conversation in coffee shops in San Juan (Puerto Rico), London and Paris. He counted the number of times one person touched the other during a 1-hour period. The scores were: San Juan, 180; Paris, 110; and London, 0. The British tend to shy away from a great deal of touching.

Davitz & Davitz (1985) report that American patients' perceptions of British nurses might be influenced by different cultural norms:

The expression of a range of emotions on the part of American patients, in many situations, often made the British nurses uncomfortable and even more reserved. It is interesting to note that a number of patients whom we interviewed judged this discomfort as dislike, insensitive, and hard boiled. 'They're efficient,' noted one patient, 'but they're not sympathetic.'

A reluctance to respond to patients' emotions and to engage in bodily contact might contribute to this view of British nurses.

A second piece of research highlights the status differences involved in touching. Whitcher & Fisher (1979) arranged for nurses to either touch or not touch patients while providing them with information about impending operations. The nurses in the 'touch condition' touched the patients on the hand whilst showing them a booklet describing the operation, whereas those in the 'no touch' condition did not touch the patients at all. All the nurses were female. The patients were asked for their views about the hospital and the prospective operation.

After the operation, the patients' blood pressure was measured. Female patients touched by nurses reported lower anxiety, more positive feelings to the hospital and had lower blood pressure after the operation than those not touched. On the other hand, male patients who were touched reported greater anxiety, more negative feelings and higher blood pressure after the operation than those who were not touched. Whitcher & Fisher (1979) suggest that one explanation for these results stems from status differences. Higher status individuals are at liberty to touch lower status individuals, but not vice versa. Thus females perceived the touching as a sign of caring and warmth; males perceived it as a threatening gesture which communicated the nurses' superior status in the hospital setting.

Physical proximity

Conducting a conversation too close to a person causes him to become nervous and apprehensive. The normal degree of physical proximity varies between cultures. Similarly, there are individual differences in interpersonal distance. Problems arise when individuals from different cultures cannot agree on the 'correct' interpersonal distance—one person is unable to get close enough because the other keeps moving back. Health professionals should be aware of cultural and individual differences in physical proximity because speaking too close to somebody will appear intrusive; speaking too far away appears cold and impersonal. There is one condition in which an invasion of personal space can prove productive. Baron (1978) found that if a person's need for help is great and she is able to convince the potential helper of this fact, then an invasion of personal space will result in more offers of help than standing at a distance.

Orientation

This refers to the angle at which people sit or stand in relation to each other. People may sit or stand face to face, side by side or at an angle. If person A is sitting at a table, then person B can come and sit in several different places. If person B is asked to cooperate with person A, then she would probably sit next to her. If she were asked to compete or bargain with person A, then she would probably station herself opposite person A. If she were asked to have a discussion or conversation with person A, then she might position herself at right angles to the table. Whenever there is the opportunity to vary the orientation of tables, chairs etc., one should consider the sorts of nonverbal information that are to be conveyed.

Postures, gestures and nods

The way people stand, sit and lie conveys a variety of social meanings. Standing erect, with head held back and hands on hips is a dominant posture. Crouching, with head held low, looking upwards is a submissive posture. Emotional state may be signalled by specific postures. Extreme depression may be signalled by a drooping, listless pose, while extreme anxiety can be seen in a tense, stiff, upright person. Status differences are also communicated via posture. High status individuals tend to adopt a more relaxed position when they are seated, whereas low status individuals sit more upright and rigid in their chairs. People who lean forward in their chairs usually have a more positive attitude towards a subject than those people who tend to lean backwards.

Gestures may be used to supplant and replace speech. It is very difficult to communicate with someone without using gestures of some sort. One has only to observe people using a telephone to see that, even though the person on the other end of the phone cannot see them, they still adopt a wide range of nonverbal behaviours. In many circumstances individuals are not aware of the gestures they use, therefore it is important to examine in some detail one's nonverbal repertoire in order to gain insight into the sorts of messages that are being transmitted unknowingly to others. Further, 'leakage' via gestures may indicate 'true' emotional state in people trying to hide their feelings, e.g. face-touching—anxiety; scratching—self-blame; forehead wiping—tiredness etc.

Head nods have two distinct roles in nonverbal communication. The first role concerns the provision of reinforcement. Head nods can be used to reward and encourage behaviours or conversation. They can be used to encourage a person to talk more about a certain topic and often they signify to the speaker that the listener is 'actively' attending to what he is saying. A second role of head nods is the synchronisation of speech. A nod gives the other person permission to carry on talking, whilst a rapid succession of nods indicates that the nodder wants to speak himself.

Appearance

The clothes one chooses to wear, the type of hairstyle, the use of make-up or perfume, sporting a beard etc. all convey nonverbal messages. Usually there is some choice as to one's appearance and thus the sort of message one wants to communicate, but there is only a limited amount one can do to improve physical attractiveness. In some situations physical attractiveness can be important, for instance, Esses & Webster (1988) presented subjects with photographs of adults who had been identified as sex offenders. The least attractive offenders were rated as more dangerous and more likely to commit a further crime than were attractive and average looking offenders. Indeed, because people are influenced by the appearance of a person, a certain degree of caution should be exercised before assuming too much about someone's character and behaviour. In comparison to other features of nonverbal communication, perhaps too much attention is paid to appearance at the expense of more reliable indications of character.

Voice quality

There are six main voice qualities: volume, tone, pitch, clarity, pace and speech disturbances. Variations in volume carry the following meanings: soft—sadness, affection; moderate—pleasantness, happiness; loud—dominance, confidence. The resonance of the voice or tone can be pleasant (resonant) or unpleasant (thin, nasal, raucous). Resonance can indicate sadness, dominance or affection, whilst negative tones indicate the following: sharp voice—complaining, helpless; flat voice—sickly, depressed; breathy voice—anxious; and thin voice—submissiveness.

Pitch often varies with volume so that high pitch, low volume may indicate submissiveness and grief whereas high pitch, high volume indicates activity and anger. Similarly, low pitch, low volume indicates boredom and sadness; low pitch, high volume indicates dominance. Clarity refers to clipping on the one hand and drawl on the other. Clipped speech—upper class, anger, impatience; drawl—lower class, sadness, boredom. Pace varies on a continuum from fast to slow. Fast speech may mean anger, surprise and animation; slow speech may mean sadness, boredom and disgust.

Finally, speech disturbances may be classified into 'pause fillers' such as 'ums' and 'ers' and stutterings, repetitions and omissions. Too many pause fillers can be interpreted as boredom, and too few, as anger or contempt. Leaving words out or sentences unfinished is often a sign of anxiety.

Nonverbal communication should always be interpreted within the context in which it appears. It should not be viewed in isolation. If health professionals are able to interpret the nonverbal signals of patients as well as to reflect on their own nonverbal skills, the chances of misinterpretations and misunderstandings are significantly reduced. Hargie et al (1981) state:

A knowledge of the various facets of nonverbal communication, and of their effects in social interaction, can therefore enable us to improve both our ability to interpret the cues which are emitted by others and our ability to control the impressions which we are conveying to others.

Exercise 1.2

This exercise allows the person with access to a video recorder to assess his or her nonverbal skills during a real or simulated interview. Circle the answers which best apply to you. The ratings should be carefully considered and suggestions for improvement made.

1. **Gaze**—the amount of time spent looking directly at the person being interviewed:

   Far too little
   Not enough
   About right
   A bit too much
   Far too much

2. **Facial expression**—the kinds of expression used:

   Smile, Frown, Neutral
   Sympathetic, Inquiring, Hostile
   Interested, Bored, Tired
   Acceptance, Disbelief

3. **Posture**—the kinds of posture adopted:

   Alert?
   Encouraging?
   Neutral?
   Threatening?

4. **Gesture**—the kinds of hand, arm, leg and foot movement:

   Always the same?
   Varied?
   Any irritating or obvious mannerisms (touching face or hair, fiddling with rubber bands, etc.)?

5. **Voice**—tone, pitch, clarity, etc.:

   Dull . . . . . Lively
   Slow . . . . . Fast
   Low . . . . . High
   Unclear . . . . . Clear
   Confident . . . . . Stuttering

6. **Position**

   Proximity:
     too near
     about right
     too far
   Orientation:
     side-by-side
     right-angle
     head-on

(Add others as appropriate)

QUESTIONING

As a communication skill, questioning is far harder to study and describe than to acquire and practise.

Dillon (1986)

Before investigating the different types of questions that may be used in interpersonal communication, there are a few general points to be made about the overall use of questions themselves.

- *The most important part of questioning is listening.* Many people are too involved constructing their next question instead of listening to the answers.
- *Determine the reasons for asking the questions.* Be sure it is known what is to be gained by asking questions.
- *Do not ask too many questions,* sometimes they are better rephrased as statements. Benjamin (1981) says:

I feel certain that we ask too many questions, often meaningless ones. We ask questions that confuse the interviewee, that interrupt him. We ask questions the interviewee cannot possibly answer. We even ask questions we don't want the answer to, and, consequently, we do not hear the answers when forthcoming.

There are a number of different types of question that can be used depending on the context. The most basic distinction is between the open and closed question.

Closed questions

These questions afford the questioner control over the conversation in that there are a fixed and limited number of responses. They are usually quite simple such as 'Are you Scottish?', 'Do you prefer milk or cream?' and 'How old are you?' Apart from providing useful factual information, they can be used at the beginning of an interview to break the ice. If a person is particularly anxious or nervous, being able to answer a simple question can reduce tension. Too many closed questions can cause problems. Health professionals who ask closed questions to which the patient responds with one-word answers find themselves asking more and more questions and paying less and less time listening to the answers.

As an exercise, try asking a friend a series of purely closed questions for as long as possible and observe (a) how difficult it is, and (b) how stilted it sounds.

Open questions

The use of open questions gives the respondents the opportunity to respond in any way they wish. There is very often no correct answer and individuals can elaborate at length on any topic. The advantages of this type of question are that it leaves the respondent free to discuss the sorts of things he wants to or the sorts of things he feels relevant and lets the questioner adopt an active listening role. A disadvantage lies in having to curtail rambling irrelevancies, though the use of well-timed closed questions can bring a wandering conversation back to the issue at hand.

Open and closed questions can be used in sequences that enable the respondent to predict the 'direction' of the conversation. Beginning an interview with an open question and gradually becoming more specific has been termed 'funnelling' (Kahn & Cannell 1957). A sequence might begin: 'What would you do if you had more spare time?'; gradually becoming more specific 'What sorts of plants do you grow in the garden?'; to 'Do you prefer to grow vegetables or flowers?' There are other sorts of sequences: 'inverse funnel' (going from specific details to general topics) and the 'tunnel' (a series of closed questions). Neglecting to provide a sequence can disorientate people, since they are unable to predict what sort of question is coming next and consequently may become confused.

There has been some discussion concerning the use of open or closed questions in research interviews. Jesudason (1976) compared the efficacy of open and closed questions in eliciting what foods were taboo during lactation for Indian women. The sample consisted of 1151 women who were asked either to name the foods that were taboo (open) or were read out a list of 12 foods and asked whether they ate each food during lactation (closed). About 53% did not report any food taboos when given the question in open form. When these women were read the list of 12 foods, 32% considered 5 or more items taboo.

This finding suggests that health professionals should be extremely careful when asking what might seem simple questions to people from different cultures who may have difficulties understanding the purpose of the question. The most appropriate technique to adopt in these circumstances would be to present the women with a list of items and then to ask an open question concerning any other taboo foods not on the list.

Affective questions

These questions relate to feelings and emotions. 'How do you feel after your operation?' Individuals may be asked how they felt in the past, how they feel now and the reasons that underlie these feelings. In this way people are offered the opportunity to reflect on how they feel and the questioner is able to communicate concern and empathy by asking such questions. Not all the emotions expressed in an interview will be the ones directly concerned with the problem; anger may hide fear, happiness may hide guilt. It is through the process of asking individuals to examine their emotions that they themselves may be able to realise the true reasons for their true feelings. The most important feature of the affective question is the element of concern. All too often the question 'How do you feel?' is used as an opening introduction to a conversation. The questioner does not really care about how the person feels, but uses the question as a 'matter of fact opener'. Many patients detect that this sort of question is not the opportunity to divulge exactly how they feel and not surprisingly respond 'Oh, I'm fine.' If you are genuinely concerned with people's feelings, take the time to talk about them properly.

Probing questions

It is necessary at times to encourage or prompt patients into talking when they fail to do so spontaneously. Probes and prompts are verbal tactics for helping patients talk about themselves and define their situation more clearly. They need not necessarily be questions: 'I can see that you are angry, but I'm not sure what it is about.' Such statements make some demand on the patient to talk or be more specific. Another function of probing questions is to clarify the experiences that give rise to certain behaviours: 'I realise that you often get angry when your husband visits you, but I'm still not sure what he does that makes you angry.' Helping patients to describe their behaviour can help clarify a situation. 'When you were told that you had cancer, you said that you were both relieved and depressed. You've mentioned that life has been a bit chaotic since then. Tell me what you've been doing.'

Probes and prompts can be put in a subtle form. Hackney & Cormier (1979) suggest the use of the 'accent' and 'minimal' prompt. The accent is a short (one or two words) restatement that echoes and focuses a previous statement, e.g.:

Patient: Since my husband's accident we have had a fairly good relationship, even though I'm not *entirely* satisfied.
Doctor: Not *entirely* satisfied?
Patient: Well, perhaps I should say . . .

Patient: In the evening what with the children, the baby, tea to get ready, making sure the house is tidy, I'm absolutely exhausted.
Nurse: Exhausted?
Patient: Tired, angry, hurt, my husband does absolutely nothing . . .

The use of minimal prompts is based on a large number of nonverbal responses. It includes 'uh-huh', 'mmm', 'ah', and 'yes, I see.'

Patient: There are a lot of things that I hate about this hospital. (Pause)
Nurse: Uh-huh.
Patient: For instance . . .

Patient: I don't know whether I should be telling you this. I haven't told anyone before.
Doctor maintains good eye contact and leans forward slightly.
Patient: Well, I . . .

Using accent and echo prompts as well as nonverbal prompts helps patients to use their own initiative to clarify what they mean. Both prompts and probes can be overused. The conversation can turn into an interrogation. Therefore once a probe has been used, let the patient take the initiative, for if it has been effective, the information produced by the patient needs to be listened to and understood.

Leading questions

Even the most simple, seemingly innocuous, question can lead people to respond in a prescribed fashion. There are three main types of leading question:

Conversational lead. This leads people to reflect common opinion or views they already hold. It is sometimes called the conversational lead as it suggests the answer the respondents would have given if they had been given the opportunity to do so. Examples are: 'Isn't she a marvellous cook?' or 'Have you ever seen him looking so well?' If the conversational lead accurately reflects a person's thoughts or feelings, it can be used to convey the impression of friendliness and that the listener is attending carefully to what is being said.

Pressurised agreement. The next type of leading question puts pressure on people to agree with the questioner. 'You do, of course, brush your teeth every day?'; 'Aren't prescription charges too high?' Blatantly incorrect leading questions can serve to stimulate a response in an otherwise uncommunicative person. 'Isn't it the case that nurses get paid far too much for the work they do?' Sometimes the leading question uses implication to make people justify their views. 'Like all good politicians, wouldn't you agree that deception is iniquitous?' or 'Anyone who really cared for his country would never allow the National Health Service to fall into decline, so don't you think we should spend more money on it?' Disagreement with these sorts of questions implies that you are not a very good politician or do not care enough. Television interviewers often use these

types of questions because disagreement implies some form of justification on the part of the respondent. In general, the use of leading questions is to be discouraged since they encourage invalid responses.

Hidden subtleties. A final category of question 'leads' the respondent without their knowledge. Loftus (1975) interviewed 40 people about headaches and headache products, ostensibly for market research. They were asked either 'Do you get headaches frequently, and if so, how often?' or 'Do you get headaches occasionally, and if so, how often?' The subjects in the 'frequently' group reported an average of 2.2 headaches a week; the subjects in the 'occasionally' group reported an average of 0.7 headaches a week. There is no reason to suppose that the two groups should differ in the number of actual headaches they get each week.

The subjects were also asked how many products they had tried for their headaches. One group was given a choice of 1, 2, or 3; another the choice of 1, 5, or 10. The first group's average was 3.3, the second's 5.2. Again, there is no reason to suppose that there was a difference between the two groups in the number of products they took for their headaches; however, manipulating the choices caused the subjects to respond differently.

Further research has indicated that similar results can be obtained when short and tall are contrasted and even when the definite article 'the' is used instead of the indefinite article 'a'. The question 'Did you see the broken headlight?' produced fewer uncertain responses than Did you see a broken headlight? (Loftus & Zanni 1975). The research on subtle leading questions suggests that one must be very careful about how questions are phrased, as even the slightest manipulation can cause people to respond in significantly different ways.

There are other sorts of question such as multiple questions, rhetorical questions and consensus questions. There are also differences in the frequency, rate and sequence of questions asked. The aspects of questioning that have been discussed above are an introduction to a large and, as yet, little-researched area. The skilful use of questions is much more difficult than it seems at first sight.

In conclusion there are two pieces of advice with regard to asking questions:

- If you have to ask too many questions, they are not the right ones.
- Prepare 'dummy' answers to some of your questions beforehand and see if they form the sort of knowledge wanted. Dillon (1986) advises: 'Dummy answers are clever; they can tell us what we want to know and also how to ask for it. So: make a dummy of the answer before the answer makes a dummy out of you.'

PERSONALITY

Assessment

The ability to communicate effectively with patients is determined to a certain extent by one's personality. One feature of improving interpersonal communication is a fuller knowledge of oneself. Try the next exercise before reading further.

Exercise 1.3

Listed below are a number of statements. Each represents a commonly held point of view and there are no right or wrong answers. You will disagree with some items and agree with others. Read each statement carefully and indicate the extent to which you agree or disagree by circling the corresponding alternative.

Disagree strongly	1
Disagree somewhat	2
Disagree slightly	3
Neutral	4
Agree slightly	5
Agree somewhat	6
Agree strongly	7

Read each statement and decide if you agree or disagree and the strength of your opinion. Mark only one item on the answer sheet. Read each item carefully, but work as fast as you can. Please give your opinion on every statement. If you find that the choices given do not correspond to your views, circle the one that is closest.

1. Child murderers must be insane.
   1 2 3 4 5 6 7

2. Everybody has a part of them that is nasty and it will emerge if given the chance.
   1 2 3 4 5 6 7

3. If people are to benefit from training, they have to be given detailed information.
   1 2 3 4 5 6 7

4. Women do not have the same job opportunities as men
   1 2 3 4 5 6 7

5. The greatest difference between most prisoners and others is that the prisoners are daft enough to get caught.
   1 2 3 4 5 6 7

6. Most health professionals do more than is required of them.
   1 2 3 4 5 6 7

7. There is no excuse for lying to a patient.
   1 2 3 4 5 6 7

8. If you keep on trying you will be rewarded in the end.
   1 2 3 4 5 6 7

9. You should act only when sure it is morally right to do so.
   1 2 3 4 5 6 7

10. The most effective way of dealing with patients and colleagues is to tell them what they want to hear.
    1 2 3 4 5 6 7

11. Many people do not realise the degree to which their lives are controlled by secret plans.
    1 2 3 4 5 6 7

12. Politics, not human nature, causes wars.
    1 2 3 4 5 6 7

13. It is wrong to say that there is a fool born every minute.
    1 2 3 4 5 6 7

14. The majority of people are good and kind deep down inside.
    1 2 3 4 5 6 7

15. Young people produce the most original ideas.
    1 2 3 4 5 6 7

16. Never tell a patient, or anyone else, the real reason for your actions unless you think it useful to do so.
    1 2 3 4 5 6 7

17. It is better to live for the present and not the future.
    1 2 3 4 5 6 7

18. It is best always to be honest.
    1 2 3 4 5 6 7

19. In general, men will not work hard unless forced to do so.
    1 2 3 4 5 6 7

20. It is better to be unassuming and genuine rather than important and dishonest.
    1 2 3 4 5 6 7

21. It is important for health professionals to get on well with their families.
    1 2 3 4 5 6 7

22. It is possible to be good in all aspects of life.
1 2 3 4 5 6 7

23. If you place your complete trust in someone else, you are asking for trouble.
1 2 3 4 5 6 7

24. Parents should provide their children with an authoritative upbringing.
1 2 3 4 5 6 7

25. Most people in an emergency will show bravery.
1 2 3 4 5 6 7

26. Most politicians are not really interested in the average man or woman.
1 2 3 4 5 6 7

27. It would help us all if we were able to have complete faith in God.
1 2 3 4 5 6 7

28. It is a good idea to flatter one's superiors and other important people.
1 2 3 4 5 6 7

29. Health is the most important feature of life.
1 2 3 4 5 6 7

30. The people who succeed in life lead clean, moral lives.
1 2 3 4 5 6 7

31. It is easier for a man to forget the death of his father than the loss of all his property.
1 2 3 4 5 6 7

32. In today's world, it's the way that you make money that is more important than how much you make.

1 2 3 4 5 6 7

33. We are better off today than we ever were.
1 2 3 4 5 6 7

34. You cannot get on in life without cutting corners now and then.
1 2 3 4 5 6 7

35. Some day science may prove all our beliefs wrong.
1 2 3 4 5 6 7

36. It is always best to give the real reasons for wanting something.
1 2 3 4 5 6 7

37. Most people will do what you want if the reward is great enough.
1 2 3 4 5 6 7

38. Patients suffering from a terminal illness should have the right to chose whether to live or die.
1 2 3 4 5 6 7

39. People do not always do what they say they will do.
1 2 3 4 5 6 7

40. Concern is essentially a feminine characteristic.
1 2 3 4 5 6 7

Scoring the scale

The scale consists of 40 items. For each statement you should have circled a number from 1 to 7 which best indicates your agreement with the statement.

For the purposes of scoring the scale, we are only interested in certain statements.

Step 1
- Add together the numbers you circled on the following statements: 2 5 10 16 19 23 28 31 34 38
- Your score should be between 10 and 70.

Step 2
- Add together the numbers you circled on the following statements: 7 9 13 14 18 20 22 25 30 36
- Subtract the total from 100.
- The result should be between 90 and 30.

Step 3
- Add the score you obtained in Step 1 to the score you obtained in Step 2.
- This is your final score.

The exercise you have just completed should give you an indication of the extent to which you agree with the writings of the political theorist Machiavelli. His writings contend that people are selfish, untrustworthy and flawed. People with high scores (High Machs) tend to hold a cynical outlook about humanity and attempt to manipulate and take advantage of other people, whereas low scorers (Low Machs) are more positive and sympathetic about mankind. High Machs are also known to interact more coldly and impersonally than Low Machs. The average scores on the scale tend to be around 95, with males scoring slightly higher than females. Extreme scores are those lower than 80 (Low Machs) and higher than 110 (High Machs). As with all tests there is a margin for error, thus you should not take your score as a fixed integer. Rather, you should view your score as giving a general indication of whether you tend towards High Mach (closer to 110) or Low Mach (closer to 80). How does this relate to interpersonal skills and health care?

Implications for communication

Communicating effectively with patients requires a certain degree of empathy and the ability to see things from their point of view. If health professionals have a cynical, cold, impersonal outlook on life it can make it very difficult for them to empathise with patients. Therefore individuals who score high on the scale should perhaps look at their communication style to see whether they can make it a bit 'warmer'. Low scorers on the scale should have little trouble appearing sympathetic to patients but they may lack a degree of firmness in their interview style and be more open to manipulation by High Mach patients. Whatever score has been obtained, it is only an indication of the direction one should take in improving one's communication style.

Another issue relates to the persistence of the Machiavellian character. Are individuals born high or low on the scale? Does this persist through life? Do people select jobs to suit their character? The answer to all three of these questions is 'probably not'. Firstly there is evidence that parents who are High Mach tend to have children who are Low Mach and vice versa (Christie & Geis 1970). This tends to rule out genetic transmission of the characteristic. Secondly there is some evidence that children scoring highly on the Mach Scale score highly when they become adults. This would imply that 'the job picks the man'. However, the author has administered this scale to many health professionals and has found significant differences between the scores of individuals who have just joined the profession and those who have been in it a long time (Niven unpublished). Indeed, the problem of 'burnout' or negative attitude change has become widespread in the health professions (see Ch. 9). Further Niven & Wolfson (unpublished) have administered the scale to large numbers of police detectives and noted similar differences between officers new to the job and officers of long-standing service.

It seems that there is something about certain professions that causes some individuals to become more detached and impersonal. One element of the health profession that contributes to this detachment is stress. In order to deal with continuous levels of stress caused by particular circumstances individuals tend to cope by distancing themselves from the stressful event

(Ch. 5). If this detachment persists, it can lead to the development of a more cynical view of patients and human nature in general. Not all experienced health professionals are disillusioned or cynical but the nature of the work transpires to make the maintenance of empathy and sympathy very difficult.

SELF-DISCLOSURE

In its simplest form, self-disclosure refers to the ways in which people let details of themselves be known to others. However, it is important to consider the self-disclosure of the health professional on the one hand and the self-disclosure of the patient on the other. Disclosing aspects of oneself or one's experiences can help develop a sense of empathy between individuals. Jourard (1971) proposed that self-disclosure is an important social skill. He suggested that if one person makes an initial self-disclosure this will encourage the other to do likewise. Thus one way to encourage other people to talk about themselves is to lead off with a short 'self-statement'. For example, a GP may say to a woman who has just experienced a miscarriage: 'I had a miscarriage the first time I became pregnant, but now I have three children.' This self-statement can lead to a discussion of the particular problems experienced by the woman. Whilst short, pertinent disclosures are useful in many different contexts, care must be taken not to overuse the technique. Patients do not want to hear prolonged oratory about the trials and tribulations of the health professional.

Johari windows

Luft & Ingham (1955) encapsulate the notion of overt and covert communication in their 'Johari window' (Box 1.1). The word 'Johari' is derived from a combination of the Christian names of Joe Loft and Harry Ingham. There are four aspects of the self. There is the 'open self' which consists of details that we know about ourselves and which others know too. The 'blind self' is unknown to us but known to others. The 'hidden self' is known to us but is not revealed

Box 1.1 The Johari window	
Open self known to self known to others	**Blind self** unknown to self known to others
Hidden self known to self unknown to others	**Unknown self** unknown to self unknown to others

to other people. Finally, there is the 'unknown self' that consists of details unknown to us and unknown to everybody else as well. The last category, the unknown self, has led some people to ask 'How do we know it exists if we don't know about it and nobody else does either?' This is a fair question. However, as the unknown self consists of unconscious motives and desires that may affect us without our knowledge, we are not always aware of the reasons why we behave in particular ways and thus are unable to communicate this aspect of ourselves.

The effect of self-disclosure is to increase the size of the open self at the expense of the other three. The increase in this segment causes both parties in an interview to become more aware of the 'self'. Therefore it may be argued that self-disclosure not only gives others more information about ourselves but also gives individuals themselves valuable insight into their own thoughts, feelings and behaviour.

Features of self-disclosure

Ivey & Authier (1978) list four main features of self-disclosure:

1. *The use of I.* The use of the personal pronoun 'I' or 'my' or 'mine' identifies the statement, unambiguously, as a self-disclosure. To say 'Having a baby can be quite stressful' is not the same as 'I find having a baby quite stressful'.

2. *Fact or feelings.* Usually when two people meet for the first time they exchange basic facts about themselves, their names, what they do for a living etc. They very rarely divulge details of their innermost feelings, indeed comments about feelings are usually kept at a superficial level. Thus asking people early on in a conversation to divulge 'deep feelings' or even divulging one's own 'deep feelings' can result in embarrassment. As people get to know each other better they are able to talk about more facts and deeper feelings, but initially this can prove very difficult. Even if one person has a great desire to confide in the other he may decide that to do so is too risky and places him in a vulnerable position. In certain circumstances strangers may talk about very intimate features of their lives. Sometimes people who have just suffered the death of a loved one find it easier to talk to a 'stranger' than members of their own family; similarly if two people realise that there is little or no chance of them seeing each other again, they might be tempted to disclose personal thoughts and feelings. Disclosure of feelings involves an element of discomfort between two individuals, thus it is necessary to employ self-disclosure techniques carefully to help patients overcome initial embarrassment and feel 'comfortable' with the conversation.

3. *Reacting to the other person.* When somebody says 'I just couldn't cope with the pain and nobody seemed to care at all, they all thought I was play-acting' there are two sorts of self-disclosure response. One can react to the person's feelings by saying 'I can see that being taken for a play actor must have made the pain very difficult to cope with'; or 'That happened to me too, and it was awful'. The first response conveys concern and directs attention towards the individual encouraging her to disclose more fully. The second demonstrates that she is not alone in her feelings and takes the focus away from her onto the health professional. Both responses are appropriate in different contexts.

4. *Past, present and future.* Self-disclosures can be couched: *in the past*—'I felt desolated when I lost my job'; *in the present*—'I'm very happy with life at the moment'; and *in the future*—'I think I'm going to hate going into hospital'. However, Galvin & Ivey (1986) stress that the 'here and now' immediate self-disclosure remains a controversial issue.

The self-disclosure of the health professional's personal experience to the patient should be approached with caution. Nelson-Jones (1983) mentions six positive features of self-disclosure to the patient:

1. *Modelling.* Some patients will have had little opportunity to practise self-disclosure themselves. They may not have learned how to do it or they may be afraid to do it. Self-disclosure by the health professional may signal to the patient both the opportunity to engage in this behaviour and also the manner in which it can be 'phrased'.

2. *Genuineness.* Whilst health professionals must illustrate a level of expertise that inspires confidence in the patient, it is sometimes beneficial to appear a 'real person' and not hide behind a distant, wooden persona.

3. *Sharing experiences.* An advantage of sharing experiences with patients is to provide them with a new perspective on their situation, which may lead to a different way of managing it. It is important that patients have the opportunity to accept or reject the relevance of such disclosures.

4. *Sharing feelings.* Sometimes it is appropriate to share feelings with patients. Wright (1986) says that many nurses are worried about the fact that they might cry when they have to break the news that someone has died. 'Many nurses will ask "But what if I cry?" believing that this shows some weakness or lack of professionalism. On the occasions I have seen this happen it has increased the feelings of caring and understanding.'

5. *Sharing opinions.* Sharing opinions is less revealing than sharing experiences or feelings. Also it keeps the focus on the patient. The distinction between sharing opinions and sharing experiences is similar to the distinction made by Ivey & Authier (1978) between their two ways of 'reacting to the other person'.

6. *Being assertive.* Self-disclosures can be used to 'stand up' to an aggressive patient. Being firm and setting limits can contribute to a relationship. Sometimes revealing displeasure or annoyance increases what Nelson-Jones (1983) calls 'therapeutic genuineness'.

Inappropriate self-disclosure

Inappropriate self-disclosures may result in the following:

- *Burdening the patient.* Patients have problems of their own without the burden of other people's. Further, whilst patients may appreciate the health professionals' skill, they may not be fascinated with them as people.

- *Seeming weak and unstable.* There is often a need for patients to perceive their carers as strong and competent. Too many self-disclosures can make the health professional appear maladjusted and weak. There has to be a consideration of the context; sometimes sharing feelings is appropriate, sometimes it isn't. Usually it is reasonably clear when to disclose in this manner and when not to. If there is any doubt, then the best solution is to adopt a 'patient focused' approach and use 'sharing opinions' disclosures rather than 'sharing feelings' disclosures'. If the communication is proceeding effectively, then patients will pick up the concern and empathy in the nonverbal behaviour.

- *Domination.* Too much self-disclosure can make patients feel dominated. Nelson-Jones (1983) cites Loughary & Ripley (1979) who mention four types of domination: the 'You think you've got a problem! Let me tell you about mine!' type; the 'Let me tell you what to do' type; the 'I understand because I had the same problem myself' type; and the 'I'll take charge and deal with it' type.

- *Doing it for yourself.* This is called counter transference in psychoanalysis, but simply refers to the situations where health professionals are self-disclosing for their own purposes. In other words the health professional may use self-disclosure to meet her own wishes for approval and affection at the expense of the patient. Warning signs include 'going well out of one's way' for a particular patient and reorganising one's time needlessly to become emotionally involved rather than professionally concerned.

It can be seen that self-disclosures on the part of the health professional are essential interpersonal skills if used wisely and sparingly. However, facilitating self-disclosure in the patient is equally useful.

Blocks to self-disclosure

Exercise 1.4

This exercise illustrates the difficulties in discriminating between people who are telling the truth and people who are lying.

Ask for three volunteers and sit them in front of the group. They are required to tell the group what they did on the previous Saturday. Two will tell the truth and one will lie. Take three pieces of paper and write L on one and T on the other two to indicate who will tell the truth and who will lie. Give the pieces of paper to the three volunteers. After they have given a brief résumé of their day, the rest of the group can ask questions to try to establish who is lying. When each of the volunteers has had a turn to talk and be questioned, the group vote on who they think was telling lies. The person who has lied stands up.

Points to illustrate

1. Ask the person who lied what technique they used. Did they use substitution (they talked about what they actually did on some other day) or invent a different set of circumstances entirely. Did the person who used substitution find lying easier than the person who used invention? Why?

2. Did the group notice any particular nonverbal behaviours of the volunteers? In particular, did the person who lied exhibit any specific nonverbal cues? Individuals who are not telling the truth have difficulty maintaining eye contact. They are least aware of controlling their feet, thus the person lying in the exercise may have exhibited more foot movements than the others.

3. Individuals using invention should find it more difficult to control their nonverbal behaviour since they are concentrating on constructing lies which takes more effort than substitution.

4. Did the volunteers feel pressured in any way by the questioning? Did those that were telling the truth find it difficult when people seemed to express disbelief at their stories?

5. Finally, what cues did the successful questioners use and what misled the others?

As can be seen from Exercise 1.4, it is not always easy to detect someone not telling the truth. The hidden self appears to succeed in misleading other people with relative ease. There are several blocks to self-disclosure which are perfectly normal given some of the situations in which people find themselves. The first is a fear of becoming too intense. Self-disclosures, by their very nature, lead to interpersonal communication becoming very personal. People do not always wish to reach this level of interaction in a very short period of time with a relative

stranger. A second block is the concern for confidentiality. Some patients find it incredibly difficult to trust anyone at all. A third refers to the fear of facing details of oneself that one wishes to remain hidden. Maintaining a facade is preferable to facing up to or exploring the potentially distasteful unknown self. Fourthly, some individuals are ashamed to talk about certain topics, particularly when these topics are directed towards themselves. Finally, blocks to self-disclosure can occur because people realise that they may have to change as a result of the sorts of things that they have to face up to about themselves.

These blocks are perfectly normal and in many cases necessary to maintain a certain degree of self-equilibrium. Getting people to discard their inhibitions, for whatever reason, is not the goal of the health professional. Realising why people have difficulties in self-disclosing, understanding some of these difficulties and creating an atmosphere that facilitates patient self-disclosure is, however, an important element of the health professional's repertoire of interpersonal skills.

The reluctant patient

All health professionals encounter, from time to time, the reluctant or resistant patient. This is not necessarily the person who wishes to have no degree of contact whatsoever or who will not cooperate no matter what is said or done to him. Maguire (1984) relates the case of the 53-year-old woman who noticed that she had a small lump in her breast and feared that it might be cancer. She did not want to waste the doctor's time so she waited until it had increased in size. She was worried that a small lump might seem an insufficient reason for a visit but was nevertheless convinced that she ought to go. She decided to make an appointment to see her doctor but felt it would be easier if she first mentioned that she had been suffering from bad headaches for some months since she had changed her job. This seemed an acceptable reason for making an appointment. When she arrived at the surgery it was very busy and the doctor appeared flustered. He quickly related the headaches to the pressure of the new job and prescribed a tranquilliser, asking her to come back and see him in a month's time. She felt unable to mention the lump and left.

This case illustrates the importance of allowing access to self-disclosure. Some patients are reluctant to talk about their real problems and need to be eased gently into talking about them. On the other hand there is evidence that people are likely to engage in high levels of self-disclosure if they are undergoing some form of stress, if they like the persons they are talking to and are not likely to interact with them again. Sometimes patients are too willing to talk about themselves and need to be tactfully discouraged.

Guidelines for appropriate self-disclosure

As with all interpersonal skills, there are no hard and fast rules that apply to all people in all situations, however Nelson-Jones (1983) suggests some general guidelines for appropriate self-disclosure:

- *Be direct.* If you decide to talk about yourself do not 'beat about the bush', speak clearly and honestly.
- *Be sensitive.* Try to realise when self-disclosures are helpful and when they are a burden. Intimate feeling disclosures might not be as appropriate as opinion disclosures, particularly at the beginning of a relationship.
- *Be relevant.* Do not wander from the main purpose of the interview. Keep closely to the patient's concerns.
- *Be non-possessive.* Do not press a patient to respond to you in a way that meets your needs and not theirs.
- *Be reasonably brief.* Not all patients have the stamina or willingness to engage in long, searching self-examinations.
- *Do not do it too often.* Talking about yourself too often not only keeps the focus on you but also raises doubts about the stability of your professional competence.

Faulkner (1992) relates the experience of a young nurse who had just found out that her patient's husband was having an affair with another woman and she was acompanying him at visiting time in the hospital. The nurse was shocked and annoyed at this behaviour and when the woman asked if she was being unreasonable by being annoyed at her husband the nurse replied, 'Hard on him? Hard on him? I'd go for the b****** with a bread knife.' Faulkner (1992) says that the response of the nurse enabled the patient to be much more open in discussing her fears and concerns.

Exercise 1.5

This exercise is best conducted in pairs. Toss a coin to decide who will play the role of the patient and who will play the role of the health professional. You can reverse roles later. The person in the role of the 'patient' should try to think of an actual patient she has met in the past who had some specific difficulty or 'problem' and reproduce it. As the patient relates a problem the health professional should try to introduce a personal experience which might help her. Talk for about 5 minutes and discuss how the interview went with each other. Repeat this procedure swapping roles and trying out feeling self-disclosures ('I feel ...') then opinion self-disclosures ('I get the impression ...'). At the end of the whole exercise concentrate on the appropriateness of the self-disclosures.

SOCIAL SKILLS

The skills involved in social interaction, like other skills, need to be practised. Having identified some features of interpersonal skills and discussed how they may be incorporated into the health professional's behavioural repertoire, it is necessary to amalgamate these 'microskills' into a working programme. The format adopted here is based on the skills training programme of Kagan (1979), who proposes that social skills are made up of the following:

- response modes
- interpersonal allergies
- knowing.

Response modes

There are four types of responses that can be made to a patient: exploratory responses, listening responses, feeling responses, and honest labelling. Before examining how these responses may be practised, it is necessary to describe and give examples of what is meant by these terms.

Exploratory responses are open questions that elicit further discussion of an issue. 'Can you tell me more about how the pain started?' is a question much more likely to elicit useful information than the question 'Did the pain come on quickly or slowly?' which confines the patient to a limited 'quickly/slowly' response.

Listening responses clarify, paraphrase and communicate back to the patient 'active listening'. They do not evaluate or interpret what has been said. Their function is to make clear to both parties the substance of the communication and illustrate to the speaker that the listener has been paying attention to what has been said. Thus a correct listening response to 'I'm not sure that my husband wants to visit me here. We had a big row recently,' would be 'You've just had a big argument' not 'Having a row doesn't mean he dislikes you.'

Feeling responses communicate emotion to the patient or comment on the feelings of the patient. 'You seem very tense whenever the operation is mentioned' is an example.

Honest labelling reveals honest thoughts about the patient or the patient's attitude such as 'I get the feeling you don't really think I'm very good at my job.'

Exercise 1.6

This exercise is designed to develop your paraphrasing skills and your feeling responses. Try to answer the questions on your own, then discuss your answers with a partner or in a group.

1.6A
Example: 'I used to be able to go out and enjoy myself. Now I really have to force myself to go out and I don't enjoy it at all. I have this continual feeling of not being part of the group and this really makes me feel rotten.'

Paraphrase: 'In the past you seem to have gone out and had fun. At the moment, though, you've lost your motivation and don't get much pleasure out of going out. To cap it all you feel left out and low in company.'

Restate or paraphrase the following statements:

1. 'My life is great now that I've got my health back. In the past, I just could not cope with four children, but now I

enjoy having them at home with me. I'm sure Bill and me can cope all right.'

2. 'It's over a year since my David was killed and I still find myself going into his room and crying. I miss him so much.'

3. 'Getting through the day was a real effort but I've made a lot of progress, really. I used to dread getting up in the morning. Now I don't get upset nearly so easily.'

1.6B
For each of the following statements:

a. Identify the words or phrases the person has used to describe how she feels.
b. Suggest other words or phrases to describe how she feels.
c. Produce a response that focuses and reflects the feelings expressed.

Example: 'I feel that I have very little time left on this earth, but you know, I've had a good life and I've loved my family, who mean more to me than the whole world put together. I don't want to die but I'm not afraid of it.'

Response:
a. Words used to describe feelings—'very little time left', 'loved', 'mean more to me', 'want to' and 'afraid of'.
b. Other words that could be used as replacements include—'not long to go', 'adored', 'most important of all', 'desire' and 'frightened'.
c. Possible reply—'You feel that your time is coming to an end. You give thanks for the joys of life, especially the time with your family. The prospect of death is unwelcome but doesn't frighten you.'

Statements:
1. 'I was absolutely devastated when I heard that I had an incurable disease. I still really haven't come to terms with it and I often feel very anxious and depressed.'
2. 'I'm glad I came to London, since I've got quite a good job and we had no money at all at home. I miss my family though. Also I felt everybody was much friendlier at home.'
3. 'I had a terrible set to with a relative of a patient the other day. I felt she was trying to put me down. Though I've noticed just recently that I very quickly become irritable with people.'

Interpersonal allergies

Kagan (1979) states: 'in listening to a person's concerns, we react physiologically, emotionally, intellectually and exhibit nonverbal behaviours, usually without being aware of them. The physician brings to each interaction a host of stereotypes and prejudices about such things as age, sex, body size and shape.' It is not suggested that health professionals should immediately discard all their 'prejudices', but that they seek to become more aware of them. Awareness of one's interpersonal allergies is a first, essential step in understanding and overcoming blocks to effective communication.

Exercise 1.7

After reading the following descriptions of people, write down your feelings about them. Try to identify how these feelings might interfere with the job of the health professional.

1. Joe is a 40-year-old Irishman who doesn't care about his clothes, swears a lot and is very rude. His looks are unkempt and he hasn't had a job for years.
2. Mary is a very prim and proper 35-year-old, upper middle-class woman. She continually refers to herself as 'one', tries to control her emotions and says that she is glad men are in control because she just cannot stand uncertainty. Her views are strongly right wing.
3. Susan is a 25-year-old married woman with a lot of problems in the home. She does not seem to get on with anyone, especially her husband, and she sees you as a potential ally. She blames everyone but herself.
4. Arthur is a young homosexual who has recently been rejected by his partner and feels like committing suicide. He sees you as a new friend and potential confidant.
5. Jane has taken her fourth drug overdose. This is the third time you have seen her. Each time she says that she will not do it again, but she still does. She is aggressive and says her life is none of your business.

Knowing

Knowing is made up of interpersonal involvement and self-protective thinking. There are four basic fears of interpersonal involvement: 'I will hurt you'; 'You will hurt me'; 'I will engulf you'; and 'You will engulf me'. If people become too involved with others they will experience anxiety; if they are too distant they will experience boredom or even loneliness. Knowing refers to the ability to establish the correct distance in the correct context. Self-protective thinking refers to the 'defence mechanisms' that are used to protect us from those aspects of our personality that we think should remain hidden. Knowing refers to the process of examining these defence mechanisms.

Exercises designed to assess self-protective thought and defence mechanisms suffer from 'unconscious determinism'. This simply means that if our defence mechanisms are working correctly then we are not aware of the threat because we are being protected from it. Many of the things we do, feel and think have their roots in the unconscious, which means that we do not have direct access to them. If we are not aware of the 'difficult areas' of our lives it is not easy to discuss them. Having said this, there are certain aspects of the self that can be explored.

Exercise 1.8

Imagine that you are with a specific person in whom you can trust and confide. Try to establish what topics would cause you to feel threatened if they were to be discussed. Threat involves the degree to which you might feel uncomfortable, embarrassed and be esteemed less as a result of your disclosures.

If you could not discuss the topic: score 5
You could discuss it but it is very threatening: score 4
Only moderately threatening: score 3
Slightly threatening: score 2
No problem at all: score 1

Topics
Politics
Intellectual ability
Homosexuality
Class background
Social and family relationships
Your body
Death
Sexual feelings and behaviour
Your work
Things that make you angry, happy, sad
Feelings of depression
Religion
Fears and anxieties

Look at the topics that carry the highest score and determine what it is about them that makes them threatening.

Explore what is being protected. What exactly are you afraid of? Determine how you protect yourself from the threat.

Patient feedback

An essential ingredient of effective communication is the ability to accept patient feedback. Interpersonal skills include responding to what the patient has to say in a way that he or she understands. Empathic responding shows patients that you can see things from their point of view and understand their needs and concerns.

Exercise 1.9

Much has been made of the use of empathy in social inter-action. Empathic responding involves being able to see things from the patients' point of view and illustrating this to them by communicating back an understanding in such a way that they can see that you have understood their 'frame of reference'.

Here are some statements with three responses to them. Assess the responses in terms of their empathy by allocating a score according to the following scale:

5	very good
4	good
3	moderate
2	slight
1	none

Example

Student: I can't decide whether to pack my course in or not. My father wants me to press on, as it will be worth it in the end. My mother says that there is no point in doing something that you hate. I can't please both of them and they can't both be right.

Tutor:
a. Well, I'm afraid it's your life and your decision.
b. I can see that you are a bit confused at the moment about what is right for you. You are under pressure from the family, but wonder whether they have the correct solution.
c. Let's explore why you would like to please your parents. One of them is going to be disappointed you know.

Suggested ratings and comments:
a. 1—external frame of reference and patronising
b. 4—shows good understanding
c. 2—leading, interpreting, only slightly in correct frame of reference.

Statements

Patient: I know this is stupid but I'm really worried about my operation. Will something go wrong? Will I be the same after? Will it hurt?

Doctor:
a. It's perfectly normal to worry, but worrying about it will not help much.
b. I'm sure you will be able to cope. It isn't going to hurt at all.
c. You feel foolish about the fact that you are worried about the operation and would like reassurance that it will not hurt and everything will be all right.

Wife: It's depressing to see one's parents grow old and gradually become unable to look after themselves. What are we going to do about Dad, now that Mum is in hospital?

Husband:
a. We'll manage somehow, dear.
b. Yes, your Dad never made any effort to look after himself. Now he's stranded.
c. You're sad seeing them both old and vulnerable and are wondering how best to handle Mum going into hospital.

Retiring nurse: I've always been a very active woman and retirement fills me with excitement and fear. It's a great opportunity to do anything I want, but every now and then I find myself getting anxious and waking up at night.

Supervisor:
a. Your retirement presents an exciting challenge because you will have the freedom to do the things you really want to do, but are naturally anxious concerning the unknown.
b. Well you like being busy, now you can be busy doing the things you like.
c. Anxiety and sleepless nights indicate that you need to plan for your retirement much more thoroughly.

Suggested ratings and comments
Doctor:
a. 2—advising and not responding to the patient as a person
b. 3—first part, patronising; second part, not too bad
c. 4—good understanding.

Husband:
a. 2—sympathy rather than empathy
b. 2—judgemental, internal frame of reference
c. 4—good attempt at understanding.

Supervisor:
a. 5—very good understanding
b. 2—starts off OK, then becomes leading
c. 1—awful.

It should be noted that these are suggestions for the most appropriate empathic responses. The circumstances described could well call for other types of responding as well.

CONCLUSION

An increased knowledge of the nature of communication should, hopefully, be followed by an increase in social competence. This competence encompasses an ability to perceive and interpret accurately the cues being emitted by others, and a capacity to behave skilfully in response to others. Therefore it is vital that the information presented is used by the reader, who should be prepared to experiment with various social techniques until the most effective response repertoire is developed in any particular situation. This is not a comprehensive review of all communication skills, and it should be recognised that this is a rapidly developing field of study. As knowledge increases, further skills and dimensions will be identified, and awareness of interpersonal communication expanded accordingly.

REFERENCES

Baron R A 1978 Invasions of personal space and helping: mediating effects of invaders' apparent need. Journal of Experimental Social Psychology 14: 304–312

Benjamin A 1981 The helping interview, 3rd edn. Houghton Mifflin, Boston

Birdwhistell R 1970 Kinesis and context. University of Pennsylvania Press, Philadelphia

Christie R, Geis F L 1970 (eds) Studies in Machiavellianism. Academic Press, New York

Davitz L L, Davitz J R 1985 Culture and nurses' inferences of suffering. In: Copp L A (ed) Perspectives on pain. Churchill Livingstone, Edinburgh

Dillon J 1986 Questioning. In: Hargie O (ed) A handbook of communication skills. Croom Helm, Beckenham

Ekman P, Friesen W V 1975 Unmasking the face. Prentice-Hall, Englewood Cliffs NJ

Esses V M, Webster C D 1988 Physical attractiveness, dangerousness, and the Canadian criminal code. Journal of Applied Social Psychology 18: 1017–1031

Faulkner A 1992 Effective interaction with patients. Churchill Livingstone, Edinburgh

Galvin M, Ivey A 1986 Self-disclosure in therapy. In: Hargie O (ed) A handbook of communication skills. Croom Helm, Beckenham

Hackney H, Cormier L 1979 Counselling strategies and objectives, 2nd edn. Prentice-Hall, Englewood Cliffs NJ

Hargie O, Saunders C, Dickson D 1981 Social skills in interpersonal communication. Croom Helm, Beckenham

Ivey A, Authier J 1978 Micro-counselling: innovations in interviewing, counselling, psychotherapy and psychoeducation. C C Thomas, Springfield, Illinois

Jesudason S V, 1976 Open-ended and closed-ended questions: are they complementary? Journal of Family Welfare 25: 66–68

Jourard S M 1966 An exploratory study of body-accessibility. British Journal of Social and Clinical Psychology 5: 221–231

Jourard S M 1971 Self-disclosure. Wiley, London

Kagan N 1979 Interpersonal skills and health care. In: Stone G C, Cohen F, Adler N E (eds) Health psychology. Jossey Bass, New York

Kahn R L, Cannell C F 1957 The dynamics of interviewing. Wiley, New York

Loftus E F 1975 Leading questions and the eyewitness report. Cognitive Psychology 17: 560–572

Loftus E F, Zanni G 1975 Eyewitness testimony: the influence of the wording of a question. Bulletin of the Psychonomic Society 5: 86–88

Loughary J W, Ripley T M 1979 Helping others to help themselves. McGraw Hill, New York

Luft J, Ingham H 1955 The Johari window: a graphic model for interpersonal relationships. University of California, Western Training Laboratory in Group Development

Maguire P 1984 Communication skills and patient care. In: Steptoe A, Mathews A (eds) Health care and human behaviour. Academic Press, London

McCanne T R, Anderson J A 1987 Emotional responding following experimental manipulation of facial electromyographic activity. Journal of Personality and Social Psychology 52: 759–768

Nelson-Jones R 1983 Practical counselling skills. Holt Rinehart Winston, Eastbourne

Stewart J E 1980 Defendant's attractiveness as a factor in the outcome of criminal trials: an observational study. Journal of Applied Social Psychology 10: 348–361

Whitcher S J, Fisher J D 1979 Multidimensional reaction to therapeutic touch in the hospital setting. Journal of Personality and Social Psychology 39: 87–96

Wright B 1986 Caring and crisis: a handbook of intervention skills for nurses. Churchill Livingstone, Edinburgh

Zuckerman M, Klorman R, Larrance D T, Spiegel N H 1981 Facial, autonomic, and subjective components of emotion: the facial feedback hypothesis versus the externalizer–internalizer distinction. Journal of Personality and Social Psychology 41: 929–944

RECOMMENDED READING

Argyle M 1988 Bodily communication, 2nd edn. Methuen, London
  This book contains a comprehensive analysis of nonverbal communication. It is well structured and written in a style that is easily understood.
Faulkner A 1992 Effective interaction with patients. Churchill Livingstone, Edinburgh
  Ann Faulkner has been involved in research and teaching in this field for many years. Here she presents a practical book based on her multidisciplinary workshops.
Kagan C 1987 A manual of interpersonal skills for nurses. Harper & Row, London
  An 'oldie but goldie' introduction to designing exercises in interpersonal skills for health professionals. If I were asked to produce a course in this area I would consult this book first.
Wright B 1992 Caring and crisis: a handbook of intervention skills for nurses, 2nd edn. Churchill Livingstone, Edinburgh
  Gives excellent guidelines of how to deal with people who are experiencing some form of crisis. The book is based on his experience in accident and emergency departments in this country and abroad.

Egan G 1986 The skilled helper, 3rd edn. Brooks/Cole, Monterey California
Hargie O (ed) 1986 A handbook of communication skills. Croom Helm, Beckenham

2

Attitudes and prejudice

Many of the problems that face people involved with health care relate to the attitudes of the patients or clients. This chapter seeks to give information concerning how attitudes are formed and measured, and most importantly, how they can be changed. Changing people's attitudes to health is an important stage in any health programme. Also, the attitudes of health personnel towards their clients are discussed, looking at labelling theory, 'blaming the patient', prejudice, stereotypes and ways of reducing prejudice. The exercises are designed to investigate our own prejudices and misattributions.

It might seem obvious to state that a person's attitude towards health is an important component of health behaviour, but this assumes that there is a direct link between attitudes and behaviour. A positive attitude to health may not necessarily result in a positive behavioural outcome; but a negative attitude to health will almost certainly result in a negative behavioural outcome. For instance, a belief that 'fatty foods' do not constitute a healthy diet will not always result in a person avoiding eating such foods. However, if people believe that such foods do not do any harm at all, they are likely to engage in their consumption with no self-recrimination whatsoever. At the time of writing there is no cure for AIDS. Changing people's attitudes to sex represents the first stage in the process of altering sexual behaviour and reducing the spread of the disease. Therefore it is important to consider how attitudes are formed, measured and, perhaps most important of all, changed.

When people continue to ignore medical advice, those people involved in the provision of health care are faced with a certain degree of frustration. A person may keep appearing with the same health problem despite frequent efforts to persuade him to alter his behaviour. 'Why doesn't the stupid man give up smoking? He knows it is killing him' and 'How can she allow herself to get pregnant again? She has six children and her husband has been out of work for 2 years' are two comments which criticise the behaviour of the individual concerned. In these circumstances it is assumed that it is the individual who is at fault and that the behaviour is due to some personality defect. However, the blame may have been attributed incorrectly. Circumstances outside the control of the individual could have determined the 'inappropriate behaviour' and not some aspect of the personality. Attribution theory seeks to explain the errors that are made when trying to determine the causes of behaviour.

Finally, the importance of realising one's prejudices has been emphasised in the previous chapter. Negative feelings, beliefs and behaviour toward a person, merely because he or she is a member of a particular group, constitute prejudice and can affect the quality of health care delivery. It is not just racial prejudice that needs to be examined, but negative attitudes towards any group of individuals, such as women, homosexuals, old people, the poor, the handicapped, the mentally ill, etc. In order to promote psychological well-being between groups of individuals, it is necessary to investigate the development of prejudice and ways in which it can be reduced.

ATTITUDES

Attitudes are made up of three main components:

- *The affective component.* This refers to feelings and emotions about someone or something. We may like or hate pizzas; we may like or hate the Prime Minister.
- *The cognitive component.* An attitude also comprises thoughts or beliefs about people and objects. We may think pizzas are fattening; we may believe or disbelieve the words of the Prime Minister.

- *The behavioural component.* Attitudes are made up of people's actions and behaviour. Thus, we may eat pizzas or avoid them; similarly if the Prime Minister appears on television we might switch it on or off.

Attitudes are not always extreme. Often, a subject will command neither love nor hate. The strength of an attitude is dependent on a number of variables, the most important being those factors which contribute to attitude formation.

Attitude formation

Children are not born into the world with a predisposition to view religion, politics and other cultures in a specific way. They acquire their views over a considerable period of time. The nature of this acquisition may be explained by instrumental conditioning, modelling and direct experience.

Instrumental conditioning

The key word to describe this process is reward. Put very simply, parents and others reward children for having the 'correct' attitude, and tend to criticise them for holding views which are at odds with their own. The reward itself need not be particularly large, in most cases a simple 'good' in response to something the child says is enough to ensure repetition. Over a period of years children gradually take on many of the attitudes of parents, older children, teachers and other significant people in their lives through continuous exposure to reinforcement and punishment schedules. A more detailed exposition of instrumental conditioning occurs in the next chapter.

Modelling

The keyword in this process is copying. Children are continually looking at adult behaviour for information. Not surprisingly, adults and older children exert a considerable influence on young children by their actions as well as their words. This influence often occurs without the 'model's' awareness. An example might be the family who have gone out for a drive in the car. Suddenly, a car swerves in front of them and the father says jokingly to the wife, 'I bet that was a woman driver.' This comment may have been interpreted as a joke by the wife, but the children may have failed to see it in the same way. They may genuinely believe that their father views female drivers as careless and may take on the same attitude themselves. The father may have been totally unaware of the influence he was exerting on his children. Modelling, or observational learning, is a powerful process of attitude formation.

Parents have an important role to play in the development of their children's attitudes towards health by giving rewards for appropriate attitudes and by setting a good example themselves. However, children are influenced by other figures in their lives, such as 'hero figures' in films and comics. The sight of Superman or famous sportsmen and women highlighting the lethal effects of cigarette smoking in the media has been used to deter children from taking up smoking, or to persuade them to stop. Similarly the media and parents have a significant role to play in educating children about appropriate sexual practices in order to limit the spread of such diseases as AIDS.

Direct experience

The third process by which attitudes are attained is direct experience of the object or person themselves. One way to obtain an attitude to pizzas is actually to try them. Many people are not happy to accept someone else's opinion of an object or a person and need to have direct experience of the item in question in order to form an opinion. Indeed, there is considerable evidence that attitudes acquired in this way are stronger and more vivid than attitudes acquired 'second hand' (Baron & Byrne 1991).

There are two main implications of the research on attitude formation for health professionals:

- It is much easier to influence a person's attitude whilst it is being formed than to try

to change it years later. Parents can have a very important influence on the development of their children's attitudes toward health.
- Social learning theory has illustrated the importance of exposing children to appropriate models. Thus, the media have a significant role to play in transmitting health education using characters that children respect and even idolise.

Attitude measurement

Sometimes it is possible to determine a person's attitude by observing her behaviour. It would not be too difficult to ascertain the attitude of a member of a group of CND demonstrators towards nuclear weapons, since they display their views for all to see. Sometimes simply asking people for their views on a particular topic will reveal their basic attitude. However, the majority of individuals do not put their attitudes on public display and formal techniques need to be designed to 'tease out' views on specific topics. One method used to measure attitudes is the attitude scale or questionnaire. Attitude scales consist of a series of statements about specific issues. Respondents are required to either agree or disagree with these statements.

The Likert attitude scale presents a choice between agreeing strongly with statements and disagreeing strongly with them. An example of statements on a Likert scale designed to investigate attitudes to smoking and health might be:

1. Smoking only 5 cigarettes a day will not cause any serious health problems.

   Agree strongly
   Agree somewhat
   Neither agree nor disagree
   Disagree somewhat
   Disagree strongly

2. Smoking should be banned in all public places.

   Agree strongly
   Agree somewhat
   Neither agree nor disagree
   Disagree somewhat
   Disagree strongly

The statements are equally balanced between those that are favourably disposed to smoking and those that are unfavourably disposed towards smoking. Respondents are required to ring the response that best corresponds to their view. In this way, the scale can be used to assess those individuals who endorse statements favourable to smoking and those that do not.

It is not difficult to construct an attitude scale, but it does not consist of dreaming up a number of statements and asking people whether they agree with them or not. Each attitude scale has to be valid and reliable. The procedures for ensuring validity and reliability of questionnaires are quite strict and do take some time to complete, yet they are not beyond the capability of individuals who are prepared to follow the procedures carefully.

Attitude change

Each day we are subjected to an onslaught of attempts to try to change our attitudes to all sorts of things. Advertisements try to get us to buy certain products, politicians want us to vote for them and the Health Education Authority attempts to persuade us to give up smoking and take more exercise. The 'battle' is conducted via TV, radio, magazines and newspapers, but not all attempts succeed, as some are much better than others. Producing an effective persuasive communication is important for advertising agencies as they need to satisfy their clients. But it is even more important for persuasive communications to be effective in changing attitudes to health. It is much more difficult to try to get people to stop doing something they like or start doing something they dislike than to suggest they continue to do what they want but with this particular product. It is an 'uphill battle' for health education, therefore the attempts to change individuals' attitudes need to be well produced. In order to produce effective persuasive communications it is necessary to consider those factors that have been found to influence the extent to which people change their attitudes. There are three main elements of persuasive messages;

characteristics of the communicator, characteristics of the communication and characteristics of the recipients.

Characteristics of the communicator

There are certain features of the person delivering the message that are likely to affect whether people will be persuaded or not.

The first is *credibility*. A communicator's credibility depends on his expertise and his intentions. People are much more likely to be persuaded by someone they perceive to be an expert in his field. Also, a communicator's intentions are taken into consideration; if people perceive that he is liable to gain by his message, they will be less likely to do as he says (Hennigan et al 1982). A number of advertisements for headache remedies show a scientist in a laboratory producing the 'best possible product' to relieve pain from headaches. The scientist is both an expert and presumably stands to gain little since she is engaged in scientific research.

Another feature of the communicator is *likeability*. Physical attractiveness and the possession of positive personality traits have been found to determine how persuasive the person will be (Snyder & Rothbart 1971). If the communicator is liked because he seems to be similar to his audience, then this will enhance his persuasiveness too.

Finally the speed of message delivery is important. 'Fast talkers' have always had a poor reputation, yet individuals who speak rapidly whilst delivering a message are often perceived as more persuasive than those who tend to speak more slowly (Miller et al 1976). This may be due to a feeling that those who speak at a fast rate know their subject very well and care a lot about it.

In order to persuade patients to change their attitudes health professionals must appear credible, that is, they must 'come over as both expert and unbiased. Secondly, appearance should be geared to maximise likeability. Thirdly, the message should be put in a clear, crisp fashion; speaking too fast will sometimes confuse the patient.

Characteristics of the communication

Is fear the key? Some clergymen have attempted to change the attitudes of their congregation by putting the 'fear of God' into them, but can the same technique be used to change people's attitudes towards health? The answer is 'yes', but only under certain circumstances. If emotional appeals are to work, then they must be emotional. Half-hearted attempts to invoke fearful emotions in people will have no effect whatsoever (Leventhal 1970). The first condition is that emotional appeals must be strong. Secondly, individuals must believe that they are at risk if they ignore the content of the message. Thirdly, individuals must believe that if they heed the advice contained in the message they will be in no danger. If these three criteria are satisfied, fear will help change attitudes.

Another feature of the communication is the type of argument to use. Are two-sided arguments always better than one-sided arguments? The answer depends on the predisposition of the audience. If people are generally friendly and well disposed to the speaker, then it is better to present only one side of the argument, since highlighting the opposite position will serve no purpose. However, if the audience is indifferent or antagonistic towards the speaker, then it is better to present the opposing view and attack it successfully.

Repeating the message over and over again can alter attitudes in a favourable direction. Continual exposure to a stimulus produces a kind of familiarity that consistently results in more favourable evaluations of that stimulus. This frequency of exposure effect might be one reason why commercials are repeated quite often on the television. Grush (1980) found that the frequency of exposure effect has been a significant factor in political elections. Under conditions where all the candidates were relatively unknown before the election, those that were more frequently exposed to the public during the campaign were the ones likely to win.

In the context of health care, it may be useful to adopt these research findings and promote familiarity with patients. Though familiarity should not be construed as involvement, it refers to frequent contact. Under certain circumstances familiarity breeds content.

Characteristics of the recipients

Early studies tended to concentrate on the personality characteristics of individuals that were likely to make them more or less susceptible to persuasive communications. Such traits as low self-esteem and a high need for social approval were thought to be related to ease of attitude change (Zellner 1970; Skolnick & Heslin 1971), that is, individuals who did not have a particularly high opinion of themselves and those that had a strong desire to be liked by others, were more susceptible to change. Also, Mackie & Worth (1989) have illustrated the importance of affect in attitude change. They found that people are more easily influenced when they are in a good mood. Recently, however, the emphasis has shifted away from feelings towards a cognitive explanation of attitude change.

If people are able to think of a number of counter-arguments to the message being proposed they are less likely to change their minds. It seems that those people who are good at accessing these items of information from their memories are more resistant to attitude change, particularly if they are given forewarning and time to rehearse counter-arguments (Wood 1982). Sometimes individuals will 'bend over backwards' to do the opposite of what is being proposed. This type of response to persuasive communications has been termed reactance (Worchel & Brehm 1971). It tends to occur when an individual feels that his freedom to think for himself is being limited in some way.

Most people like to think of themselves as able to make up their own minds and think in an autonomous fashion, but if there is a feeling that someone is trying to take away this freedom, then reactance will occur. Further, we also like to be perceived by others as autonomous thinkers and may speak out against a speaker in order to be seen by others as able to make up our own minds and think critically. Finally, previous exposure to attempts to change attitude will affect the degree of individuals' resistance to change.

An audience is about to be addressed by two individuals on the subject of fluoridation of water supplies. The first speaker knows that the second speaker is fervently against fluoridation. He himself is actually in favour of fluoridation. There are two options open to the first speaker: (1) he can present the best argument possible for fluoridation, utilising all the techniques of attitude change that have just been mentioned or (2) he can present an argument against fluoridation, but in a totally incompetent fashion. This latter procedure 'inoculates' the audience against the next speaker. By presenting an argument using bad ideas and adopting an unconvincing presentation style, the audience is stimulated into rehearsing counter-arguments which are still very much in mind when the next speaker starts his talk.

Cognitive dissonance

Dissonance theory attempts to determine relationships between attitude change and behaviour. An example of cognitive dissonance would be a person who smokes 60 cigarettes a day and believes smoking to seriously damage health. The behaviour of the person is at odds with his attitude towards smoking and health. It is an uncomfortable or dissonant situation and under these circumstances individuals try to reduce the discomfort or dissonance. This may be achieved in one of two ways: the person can stop smoking or he can change his attitude towards smoking and health. Festinger (1957), who proposed the theory, suggested that people tend to change their attitude rather than their behaviour. Thus the smoker would tend to rehearse arguments that reduced the health risks of smoking, such as, 'I knew a woman who lived to the age of 82 and she smoked 60 cigarettes a day,' or 'I admit I may be a bit short of breath but I've never felt really bad from smoking, and it helps me relax.'

Dissonance can also occur when a decision has been made between two equally attractive options. Most people have, at some stage in their lives, been faced with a difficult decision involving a choice between two courses of action. Having chosen one option there is a certain degree of dissonance because the alternative option has been lost. Take, for example, the case of the young person who cannot decide whether to take a degree in geography or psychology. She has to pick one or the other. Having selected psychology, she starts to think about whether she has made the correct choice, since all the advantages of a geography degree have now been sacrificed. This state of dissonance is reduced by emphasising the positive features of psychology degrees and the negative features of studying geography. After 3 years of studying the chosen option, the student may wonder why the decision seemed so difficult at the time. In order to justify her action the student has changed her attitudes in positive and negative ways to both geography and psychology.

Attitudes may be changed through contact with other people. If two people really like each other but have totally different political views, there is a state of dissonance in their relationship. Again, to resolve the discomfort, either the behaviour or the attitude tends to change. If the feelings for each other are strong, then neither one will want to change that behaviour, so what tends to happen is that their political views become less polarised. Through exposure to the ideas of each other and through mutual affection, the politics of both individuals move closer together.

So far there has been some element of individual choice, but what if a person is forced to do something that conflicts with her attitude? Under these circumstances the degree of attitude change will depend on the reward for engaging in the attitude-discrepant behaviour. Festinger & Carlsmith (1959) gave individuals very boring tasks to complete. The subjects were required to tell another person that the tasks were very interesting and were given either a large reward ($20) or a small reward ($1) for doing so. Afterwards, the subjects were asked about their own liking for the tasks. Those who had been given a small reward rated the dull tasks higher than those who had been given a large reward. Small rewards increase dissonance and thus induce greater degrees of attitude change. Further research has since refined the 'less leads to more effect'. Attitude change takes place when:

- individuals think they are free to engage in the attitude-discrepant behaviour
- they are publicly committed to the action
- they do not view the reward as a bribe (Schlenker et al 1980).

It is sometimes difficult for those who are involved in health education to understand why some people do not take any notice of professional advice despite being presented with overwhelming evidence that their lifestyle is endangering their health. The smoker may often refuse to stop smoking because he is aware of the risks of lung cancer, that is, he reduces cognitive dissonance by increasing his liking for smoking. He knows that the habit is killing him and thus says to himself, 'Well, I must really like it.' Dissonance may act against the health professional in this instance, but it can become an ally if used correctly. Since individuals are likely to move their attitudes towards those of someone they like and respect, health professionals can use this finding in their interaction with patients.

The research on attitude change can be applied to the prevention of diseases such as AIDS. Initially the characteristics of the target population need to be considered. Those individuals that are at high risk due to inappropriate sexual practices or use of drugs need to be assessed in terms of the reasons why they pursue these practices. Often it is more effective to 'modify' behaviour rather than attempt to change it completely. Rather than concentrating on attempting to stop people having many sexual partners, it is also necessary to recognise that many people will not be able to accommodate such changes in their behaviour and therefore one has to modify their sexual behaviour by promoting the use of condoms. In the case of drug abuse, the provision of 'clean needles' is a requisite in the prevention of the disease.

The characteristics of the persuasive communication itself need to be considered in the context of the determinants of compliance, that is, if messages use fear as a method of preventing the disease, this will only work if:

- people are afraid
- they think that they are at risk if they continue their present behaviour
- they believe that if they follow the advice they will be safe.

The latter condition seems to have been heeded; many people believe that having sex with one partner and using a condom will result in high levels of safety. It is the combination of the first two conditions that may not be working.

At the time of writing, many people who engage in multiple heterosexual relationships do not believe they are at risk from the disease. The 'messages' may have frightened them initially but cease to do so because they cannot see the evidence of AIDS around them. Unless individuals have had direct experience of patients who have contracted the disease and perceive the similarity between the affected patient and themselves, they will not think that they are particularly at risk. Thus the role of prevention is to convince people that they are at risk.

This also applies to other areas such as smoking and coronary heart disease—because people feel all right, they do not think that the horrible consequences that await them are real or likely to happen. Added to this, cognitive dissonance can operate to reduce the impact of the undesirable consequences of the 'at risk' behaviour. Prevention of such diseases as AIDS has to concentrate on illustrating to those who think they are unlikely to contract the disease that many of those affected thought the same. Highlighting the similarities between those affected and those who think they are not at risk is a necessary step.

ATTRIBUTION ERRORS

You have agreed to go on a 'blind date'. You knock on the door of the person you have arranged to meet and are invited in. It transpires that your 'date' is on the phone to the garage. The conversation starts amicably enough but gradually becomes more heated until he starts shouting down the phone. After a short while, your new acquaintance slams down the phone and storms out of the room saying that he will be back in a minute. You wonder whether it is a normal occurrence for your new date to lose his temper so easily.

Fundamental error

Meeting someone for the first time can be a hazardous business, especially if he starts slamming the phone down and storming off. To what should we attribute the cause of such behaviour? Is there something about the person's disposition that makes him short-tempered? Or would any person react in such a way if given similar treatment by a disreputable garage? At this stage we are unable to be sure whether dispositional or situational factors caused the angry behaviour. Under these circumstances, we are liable to opt for a dispositional attribution of causality, that is, when we lack information about the cause of a specific behaviour, we tend to think that it is due to some aspect of the person's personality rather than some external aspect of the situation. This 'error' is called the *fundamental attribution error*. The reason for the error is quite obvious. When meeting someone for the first time we tend to concentrate on the person's actions; the context in which they take place is less important. We are so taken up with assessing the person in front of us that we tend to ignore the background.

In the context of health care, the dispositional bias is particularly common. Maslach & Jackson (1982) call this bias 'blaming the patient'. They state:

Casting causal blame among patients becomes more frequent and probable when the operational paradigm is a medical model and when record keeping excludes contextual information but highlights personal problems.

They suggest that because health practitioners see patients on an individual basis, they are more likely to focus on what it is about that person that is causing the problem rather than looking for situational causes. Further, the way that medical records are structured contributes to the fundamental attribution error. There is little room in the records for situational variables and thus the patient's problems are conceptualised in terms of person-centred evaluations. Medical files tend to be made up of characterisations of patients rather than descriptive details of the circumstances underlying their problems.

Actor–observer bias

Exercise 2.1

Think of one of your best friends. Rate this friend on the following characteristics using the scale that follows.

Rating scale

−2	Definitely does not describe
−1	Usually does not describe
0	Sometimes describes, sometimes not
+1	Usually describes
+2	Definitely describes

Aggressive ....
Introverted ....
Thoughtful ....
Warm ....
Outgoing ....
Hard working ....
Ambitious ....
Friendly ....

Cover up your responses with a piece of paper, then think about yourself. Rate yourself on the following characteristics using the scale that follows.

Rating Scale

−2	Definitely does not describe
−1	Usually does not describe
0	Sometimes describes, sometimes not
+1	Usually describes
+2	Definitely describes

Aggressive ....
Introverted ....
Thoughtful ....
Warm ....
Outgoing ....
Hard working ....
Ambitious ....
Friendly ....

Add up the 8 scores for your friend's characteristics ignoring the − and + signs. Your friend should have a score between 0 and 16. Now add up your own scores, again ignoring the − and + signs. It, too, should be between 0 and 16.
Compare your best friend's score with your own. Is your friend's score greater than yours? If so, then you have succumbed to the actor–observer effect.

Imagine that you are walking down the street and observe another person on the other side of the road. Suddenly the person trips and falls over. With no other information at your disposal you might conclude that the person was clumsy, which would be consistent with the fundamental attribution error. However, let's say that while looking at the other person you then stumble. Do you think that you are clumsy? Chances are you do not and blame the council for not taking good enough care of the pavement. There is a tendency to attribute the cause of other people's behaviour to internal dispositional factors and the cause of our own behaviour to external situational factors. This phenomenon is termed the *actor–observer effect*.

Janis & Rodin (1979) suggest that the actor–observer effect poses problems for health professionals:

Thus, a patient not taking his or her medicine is viewed as recalcitrant and uncooperative. Patients, however, as actors would be inclined to attribute their reactions to environmental events. Thus, they would know that they had stopped the medication because it made them overwhelmingly sick, for example. Clearly, physician and patients may see the same event from two different perspectives as each attends to a different set of cues.

The effect can be minimised if individuals can be induced to empathise with patients. Role playing the needs and expectations of the patient can make one more aware of what it feels like to be a patient and, at the same time, reduce the risk of attributional bias.

Self-serving bias

Suppose you have just played a game of tennis doubles. Your opponents have a reputation for being difficult to beat, yet you and your partner have won the match convincingly. Quite rightly you are pleased with your performance and conclude that all the training and practice were worthwhile. The next week you and your partner are faced with opponents who have no reputation at all. In fact they are thought by some to be a 'pushover'. Disaster strikes and you lose the match. How do you explain what went wrong? Chances are you will tend to concentrate on such things as the tennis court being slippery, the light being awful and your partner not playing at her best. In other words, when you won, it was due to your skill and ability; when you lost, it was due to the weather, the state of the court, the performance of your partner etc. This tendency to attribute the cause of success to internal factors and attribute the cause of failure to external factors has been termed the *self-serving bias* (Miller & Ross 1975). The reasons why such attributions occur is due to a need to protect our self-image and a need to appear competent and present a positive public image.

The self-serving bias can lead to serious difficulties for health professionals, particularly when they are working as members of a team. Each member of the team may perceive success as stemming from her own contribution, but attribute the cause of failure to her partners. The difficulties may be made worse if a team is comprised of individuals from different disciplines. Instead of a person bearing the accusation of responsibility for failure, it is the discipline itself that is perceived to be at fault. Thus faulty attributions can be a source of prejudicial feelings and actions towards members of other groups.

The halo effect

Nisbett & Wilson (1977) showed students one of two films. One contained an instructor behaving in a warm friendly manner. The other contained the same instructor behaving in a cold and aloof fashion. The instructor spoke with a French accent. The students were asked to judge not only how much they liked the instructor, but how much they liked his French accent and his appearance. The students who were shown the 'warm' film liked the instructor's appearance and felt that the French accent contributed in a positive way to the lecture. Those students who were shown the 'cold' film disliked his appearance and felt that the accent hindered his performance. The students who liked the instructor said that this liking had not influenced their assessment of his specific attributes in anyway. The students who had been shown the 'warm' film developed an overall liking for the instructor. They then interpreted other aspects of his behaviour in a favourable light without realising that they had done so. This is called the *halo effect*.

A similar situation can arise at a job interview. If a person creates an overall good impression on the interview panel, they are likely to interpret his mannerisms in a positive way. For instance, a simple smile from the interviewee may be interpreted positively if the overall impression that has been created is a good one, but interpreted negatively if the impression has been a bad one. Also, people having made a first impression, tend to 'go beyond the information given', that is, a person who conveys a smart image might also be thought to be intelligent, highly motivated and punctual. Having formed a good overall impression of a person, interviewers tend to ask questions that support their initial hypothesis rather than asking questions that can disprove their initial impression. In so doing they receive the answers they expect rather than those which truly represent the characteristics of the interviewee.

Thus patients who have created a positive impression on health staff will have their traits and abilities evaluated in a favourable manner, whereas those who, unfortunately, have not made such a good impression may, as a result of unfavourable evaluations, receive less interest and attention.

Labelling

Even before we meet someone for the first time, we often have information about him or her. This information can affect the way in which we perceive the person when we meet. Because personality is difficult to define, people tend to resort to labels to simplify categorisation. 'Oh, you know the type, middle-class, reads *The Guardian*, member of the National Childbirth Trust, etc.' A midwife faced with such a description of a pregnant woman is bound to be influenced by the label. It is difficult enough making a good impression on people without having to cope with misleading labels. Sometimes we are unaware of the labels that have been assigned to us and may be surprised at people's first response to us. However, at other times, we are all too aware of our label and this may affect our behaviour.

Labelling leads not only to perceptual bias but to self-fulfilling prophecy as well. Rosenhan (1973) illustrated the powerful effect of labels in a famous study entitled 'On being sane in insane places'. Rosenhan arranged for 12 normal people to arrive at a psychiatric hospital complaining of 'hearing voices'. All were admitted and diagnosed as either schizophrenic or manic depressive. The amount of time spent in the institution ranged from 3–52 days even though the 'patients' acted completely normally once they were admitted.

When they were discharged, most were labelled 'schizophrenia-in-remission', which implied that they were still schizophrenic but were not showing any symptoms at the moment of their discharge. None of the staff in the hospital recognised that the people were perfectly normal. In part, this is accounted for by the medical model of physical illness, in which it is more harmful to fail to detect an illness than to detect one that is not there.

Rosenhan (1973) conducted a second experiment. This time the staff in the institutions knew about the first experiment. They were instructed that some time over the next 3 months 'pseudo-patients' would seek admission to the hospital. The task for the staff was to identify these individuals. They were required to rate all 193 patients admitted during the 3 months, on a 10 point scale according to whether they thought the individual to be a pseudopatient. 41 patients were rated as probably being pseudopatients by at least one member of staff; 23 were highly suspected by at least one psychiatrist. Actually, no pseudopatients were sent to the hospital.

Another labelling effect was produced by Rosenthal & Jacobson (1968). They went to a primary school and offered to test the children in one class on a number of intellectual ability scales. On the basis of their results, they isolated a number of children who performed particularly well. These children were labelled 'intellectual bloomers'. Their performance was monitored at regular intervals. After 1 year they were examined on a number of tests of intellectual ability and were found to score significantly higher than the other members of the class. This finding might not seem surprising if it were not for the fact that the intellectual bloomers were never given intellectual ability tests in the first place, they were picked out at random and given the label. Having been labelled as liable to succeed, after a period of only 1 year, they had. In this instance the labelling process worked to the advantage of the children, but consider those children that have been labelled as not likely to succeed—they face the challenge of reacting to a system designed to make success difficult to achieve and must at all costs refuse to believe that because they have been labelled 'an intellectual desert' it must become a self-fulfilling prophecy.

The evidence suggests that the use of labels causes problems for those that use them and more importantly for those they are applied to. It is difficult to have no preconceived ideas about people before meeting them, but it is important to try to maintain an open mind and be ready to accept information that does not fit into any set preconceptions.

Exercise 2.2 Cognitive set

Consider the following account:

A father and his son were driving along the highway when the father suddenly lost control of the car and crashed into the telephone pole. The father was killed instantly and his son was badly injured. The boy was rushed to the local hospital where it was found that he was suffering from serious internal injuries. A prominent surgeon was immediately summoned. When the surgeon arrived and went to the operating room to examine the boy, there was a gasp from the surgeon. 'I can't operate on this boy,' the surgeon said, 'He is my son.' How could the boy be the surgeon's son?

If you cannot resolve the apparent paradox, you are suffering from cognitive set and some would say you are prejudiced. A clue to the solution is that both men and women fail to solve the riddle.

The solution is that the surgeon is the boy's mother and the reason the majority of people fail to solve the riddle is that they have the idea that all surgeons are male. Thinking is confined to viewing behaviour along prescribed set lines according to certain common perceptions. Prejudice need not be conscious discrimination but may be a result of cognitive set or more simply 'blinkered thought'.

PREJUDICE
Formation

Prejudice describes a special type of attitude towards members of a social group. Prejudice leads to a negative evaluation of an individual stemming solely from his membership of a group. Prejudice may be defined in the same way as an attitude, that is, there are three main components: affective, cognitive and behavioural. The affective component of prejudice is much the same as the affective component of an attitude for it refers to negative feelings, but the cognitive and behavioural components have different names. Prejudicial thoughts that stem from an individual's membership of a specific group are called stereotypes. Not all stereotypes are unfavourable; the romantic French, the industrious Japanese and the dependable British are examples of stereotypes that do not cause much acrimony. It is the stereotypes that are both incorrect and demeaning that demand investigation.

The origins of stereotypes and other forms of prejudice will be dealt with later on in the chapter; for the moment, it is sufficient to pose questions regarding the truthfulness of stereotypes. There are two responses to individuals who say that 'there's no smoke without fire', or there is always some element of truth in a stereotype. The first is that one can always find examples of individuals' behaviour that supports the stereotype. Usually this behaviour is found at the expense of ignoring all other behaviours that do not support the stereotype. Examples supportive of stereotypical behaviour can always be found if one searches hard enough. Secondly, the stereotype itself may lead to a self-fulfilling prophecy in exactly the same way as labelling. A stereotype of people with red hair is that they are quick to anger. Thus if a person has red hair and is aware of the stereotype she may expect to be treated as having a fiery temper. After a period of time, she may come to behave in such a way because she is expected to do so.

Prejudicial actions or behaviours are called *discrimination*. These behaviours usually result in some form of harm to the subject. Discrimination may take the form of avoidance or it may result in more extreme actions such as exclusion from jobs or education and even assault. People who practise discrimination are not always open about their prejudice and often practise it in subtle ways so that they may remain undetected. An example of subtle discrimination is the use of 'token acts'. The use of small positive acts towards a disliked person or group deflects criticism of prejudice (Rosenfeld et al 1982). 'What do you mean I don't like coloured people? I was at lunch with one only the other week.' The term 'token black/woman' refers to the employment of one member of an unfavourable group so that this action may be used as an example of equal opportunity if accused of prejudice. Health professionals should not be convinced by tokenistic attempts to avoid genuine criticism of discrimination.

Measurement

It is easy to spot the bigots of this world for they reveal themselves by their words and actions. However, the majority of individual's prejudices are not so transparent and specific devices need to be constructed to assess degrees of prejudice. In developing measures of assessment, it is necessary to refer to the three components of attitudes and prejudice: cognitive, affective and behavioural.

- *Cognitive component.* Prejudiced beliefs and stereotypes may be measured by presenting individuals with a list of personality characteristics (traits) and asking them to indicate those traits that best describe some social group.
- *Affective component.* Emotional feelings may be measured using attitude scales designed to assess the strengths of individuals' feelings towards various social groups.
- *Behavioural component.* Discrimination is much more difficult to measure. The presence of discriminatory tendencies can be detected relatively easily, but assessing the strength of these tendencies is not quite so simple. One method is to use the *social distance scale*.

Exercise 2.3 Constructing a social distance scale

These scales are designed to measure the amount of distance or closeness people wish to place between themselves and members of specific social groups.

Step One: Choose the social group(s) to be examined. Start by choosing different racial groups, then consider using other groups, e.g. heterosexuals and homosexuals, mentally ill/handicapped and other professional groups in the caring professions.

Step Two: Construct a distance scale starting with a statement of the type of relationship you would find acceptable:

I would find it acceptable for (insert the group here) to:

1. Come to my country as visitor   Yes/No
2. Live in my country   Yes/No
3. Work in the same organisation as myself   Yes/No
4. Work at the same job as myself   Yes/No
5. Live in the same town/city   Yes/No
6. Live in the same street   Yes/No
7. Have lunch/a drink with me   Yes/No
8. Be neighbours   Yes/No
9. Be close friends with me   Yes/No
10. Marry or become involved with members of my family   Yes/No

The number of yes/no responses towards each group, and particularly the number of yes responses to statements 6–10, will give you an indication of the amount of social distance you would be willing to accept.

The social distance scale does give a useful indication of one's behavioural intentions to members of different social groups, but it does not give an indication of all aspects of discriminatory behaviour. It will not assess the degree to which organisations discriminate between members of different groups, nor will it work as an analysis of discriminatory tendencies between men and women; they may be perfectly willing to get married, yet still behave in a prejudiced way to each other.

The origins of prejudice

In order to reduce prejudice, it is necessary to examine its origins. There are a number of different theories that have been put forward to explain how prejudice is produced:

- intergroup competition
- us vs them
- authoritarian personality.

Intergroup competition

This theory states that prejudice arises out of competition between different groups. Thus prejudice would tend to occur in situations where there is competition and desired resources are at a premium. The role of competition and conflict in the development of prejudice was illustrated by Sherif and his colleagues (Sherif 1981). Young boys attending summer camp in the USA were divided into two groups. During the first week, the boys took part in numerous activities and developed a strong sense of identity with their groups. In the next week, the experimenters brought the two groups into direct competitive conflict with each other by way of a series of contests and sports events. Only one group could win and there was a substantial prize for the winner. After a short period of time, the two groups showed more and more animosity towards one another. The boys used positive adjectives to describe their own group and negative adjectives to describe their opponents. The two groups started calling each other names and fighting broke out. At the start of the summer camp there had been no bad feeling between the groups; towards the end they hated each other.

Sherif and his colleagues put this change in behaviour down to competitive conflict between the two groups. Their theory was given added support by the finding that the only way to reduce the negative feelings of hostility between the groups was to engage both of them in cooperative tasks. Both groups were required to work together to achieve a common goal. Thus, Sherif and his colleagues claim to have demonstrated the powerful effects of intergroup competition on the development of prejudice.

Us vs them

Tajfel (Tajfel 1982; Turner et al 1987) proposes that the process of social categorisation is the first stage in the development of prejudice, that is, people tend to categorise themselves into groups as this creates a sense of group affiliation or social identification. Membership of the group will enhance the self-esteem of the individual as long as the group compares favourably with other groups. Therefore there is a tendency for members of groups to perceive their group as superior to others as this maintains group self-esteem and by implication individual self-esteem. Further, Pettigrew (1981) has shown that attribution errors contribute to group polarisation. He states that when prejudiced people see what they regard as a negative act by someone from another group, they will tend to attribute the cause to personality factors, but when prejudiced people perceive what they regard as a positive act by someone from another group they will put the behaviour down to the 'exceptional case' or luck. These behaviours serve to widen the gap between groups emphasising the positive characteristics of one's own group at the expense of others.

Skevington (1981) has examined the applicability of Tajfel's theory in a nursing context. She gave 64 first- and second-year nursing students and pupils a questionnaire designed to measure status differences and desired social mobility. She found that there was some evidence for Tajfel's theory. The registered nurses had a higher status than enrolled nurses because they were attributed with more advantages. The registered nurses had more positive subjective characteristics and a high positive social identity. The lower status enrolled nurses were found to have 'a preponderance of attributed disadvantages' and a less positive social identity.

Not surprisingly, 50% of enrolled nurses wanted change. However, Tajfel (1959) and Doise & Sinclair (1973) claim that social comparisons between the two groups will enhance perceived differences. Contrary to these claims, Skevington (1981) found that the two groups of nurses tended to decrease the perceived differences between themselves. She suggests two explanations for her results:

- The nurses in the study worked closely with each other on the wards, which reduced stereotyped impressions obtained from groups in other studies.
- The enrolled nurses were trying to assimilate the role and become more similar to the registered nurse group as a means of achieving a similar social identity to the registered nurses.

These findings are important for the light they shed on ways to reduce prejudice. One step to take is to place groups together so that the close contact reduces the sort of stereotyping and misattribution mentioned by Tajfel and Pettigrew. As shall be seen later, however, this step is insufficient on its own.

The authoritarian personality

Adorno et al (1950) linked prejudice to a cluster of personality traits they termed the authoritarian personality. Individuals scoring highly on the 'F scale' (their measure of authoritarianism, F standing for fascism) are submissive and obedient to authority, reject groups other than their own and tend to view the world in 'black-and-white' terms. Thus the person with an authoritarian personality is filled with as much fear as hate and allies himself to an authority figure who promises to rid the world of his objects of fear and loathing. The authoritarian person develops these traits in part due to punitive child-rearing practices which create a pattern of submissive obedience to authority

and rejection of groups other than his own. There is evidence that certain strong, prejudiced reactions to 'other groups' are related to authoritarian personality characteristics (Cherry & Byrne 1976), but it would be wrong to conclude that all prejudice could be reduced to a simple analysis of personality dynamics.

Reducing prejudice

It is apparent from the diverse origins of prejudice that producing a strategy for reducing the problem will not be easy. Firstly, many individuals are unaware that they are prejudiced. Therefore an initial step in the reduction of prejudice is to make people aware of it in themselves. Most individuals are prejudiced in some way or another and realising this is a necessary stage in trying to change. Also, most individuals do not want to be prejudiced and would not wish to transmit their prejudices to their children. Thus, programmes designed to highlight how prejudice occurs and illustrate ways to manage inappropriate behaviour may prove fruitful.

There is one technique that has been used to reduce prejudice with some success—intergroup contact. It was noted earlier that one reason for the lack of prejudice between the nursing groups (Skevington 1981) was high levels of intergroup contact. It has been suggested that increased interaction between social groups reduces prejudice because:

- both groups start to realise that they are not quite so different and have a number of similarities
- repeated exposure often leads to liking as we have seen in the research on attitude change
- negative stereotypes may be destroyed through lack of evidence (Amir 1976).

Finchilescu (1988) conducted a study of nursing students in four different hospitals in South Africa. Two of the hospitals provided racially integrated training; two did not. The student nurses completed questionnaires that measured attitudes towards racial integration in the training of nurses and the work ability of nurses belonging to different racial groups. Nurses in the two hospitals with racially integrated training reported stronger support for such training than did the nurses in the segregated hospitals. However, the nurses in the the two integrated hospitals did not report more favourable views towards nurses of other races than those who worked in the hospitals without integrated training.

This evidence gives limited support toward a policy of desegregation. Indeed, school segregation in the USA was outlawed over 30 years ago. Did this act lead to a reduction in children's prejudice? The answer, unfortunately, is 'no'. Stephan (1978) reviewed the research and concluded that there was no single study that showed a significant increase in the self-esteem of minority children following desegregation; that in only 13% of school systems studied was there any reduction of prejudice; and that prejudice increased in as many cases as it decreased. Why should this be?

Aronson & Bridgeman (1981) say that such findings are in part due to the attitude of the education authorities, part due to lack of equal status contact, but more importantly due to the competitive nature of the typical classroom. Teachers are continually emphasising which child is first, which child is the best, which child can finish in the fastest time. Exams and tests are structured to reflect who is 'top' and who is 'bottom' of the class. Outside the classroom, sports and games reflect the same degree of competition. If one considers that one of the main origins of prejudice is competition (Sherif 1981), it is not surprising that desegregation on its own did not work. Aronson & Bridgeman (1981) point out that differences in ability between the children that existed before desegregation, were exaggerated by the competitive learning environment.

In order to investigate these assertions, Aronson et al (1978) devised a cooperative classroom structure. Pupils from different ethnic backgrounds were placed in groups of six. Each pupil was required to learn a segment of written material and convey it to the other members of the group. All six segments formed the answer to the problem. Each segment, like pieces of a jigsaw puzzle, had to be put together in order to

form the whole picture. Thus each child had equivalent importance and had to cooperate with other members of the group to determine the answer. The results of the teaching programme were found to be particularly encouraging.

- The pupils increased their liking for their workmates, irrespective of ethnic background.
- There was an increase in self-esteem.
- There was an improvement in academic performance.

It is not suggested that the whole of the educational and sport curriculum be turned into cooperative learning sessions, for these improvements were obtained in only three 45-minute sessions a week. However, it might be a good idea to introduce some element of cooperative learning into the school curriculum, particularly where there is a mix of ethnic groups.

The research on the origins and reduction of prejudice has a number of important implications for health professionals:

- Prejudice between different health groups may be reduced by constructing intergroup teams.
- Intergroup contact can be effective in the learning/training context.
- Groups must have common goals to work towards.
- There must be equal status between members of the group.

The last point may cause considerable problems due to the fact that many interdisciplinary and intradisciplinary teams or groups are made up of individuals who have considerable status differences, but if it can be made clear at the outset that each member of the group has a contribution of equal importance to make, the problem can be reduced.

Both society and the institutions of society are made up of many different groups of individuals. Differences between groups can lead to hate, fear and suspicion or, as Aronson has shown, these differences can be used to advantage and facilitate greater self-esteem, knowledge and respect for other people's points of view.

REFERENCES

Adorno T W, Frenkel-Brunswick E, Levinson D J, Sanford R N 1950 The authoritarian personality. Harper Row, New York

Amir Y 1976 The role of intergroup contact in change of prejudice and ethnic relations. In: Katz P A (ed) Towards the elimination of racism. Pergamon, Oxford

Aronson E, Bridgeman D 1981 Jigsaw groups in the desegregated classroom: in pursuit of common goals. In: Aronson E (ed) Readings about the social animal, 3rd edn. Freeman, San Francisco

Aronson E, Stephan C, Sikes J, Blayney N, Snapp M 1978 The jigsaw classroom. Sage, Beverley Hills

Baron R A, Byrne D 1991 Social psychology: understanding human interaction, 6th edn. Allyn & Bacon, Newton Mass.

Cherry F, Byrne D 1976 Authoritarianism. In: Blass T (ed) Personality variables in social behaviour. Erlbaum, Hillsdale NJ

Doise W, Sinclair A 1973 The categorisation process in intergroup relations. European Journal of Social Psychology 3: 145–157

Festinger L 1957 A theory of cognitive dissonance. Row Peterson, Evanston Ill

Festinger L, Carlsmith L M 1959 Cognitive consequences of forced compliance. Journal of Abnormal and Social Psychology 58: 203–210

Finchilescu G 1988 Interracial contact in South Africa within the nursing context. Journal of Applied Social Psychology 18: 1207–1221

Grush J E, 1980 The impact of candidate expenditure, regionality, and prior outcomes on the 1976 Democratic presidential primaries. Journal of Personality and Social Psychology 38: 337–347

Hennigan K M, Cook T D, Gruder C L 1982 Cognitive tuning, set, source credibility, and the temporal persistence of attitude change. Journal of Personality and Social Psychology 42: 412–425

Janis I L, Rodin J 1979 Attribution, control, and decision making: social psychology and health care. In: Stone G, Cohen F, Adler N E (eds) Health psychology. Jossey Bass, London

Leventhal H 1970 Findings and theory in the study of fear communications. In: Berkovitz L (ed) Advances in experimental social psychology. Academic Press, New York, vol 5

Mackie D M, Worth I D 1989 Processing deficits and the mediation of positive affect in persuasion. Journal of Personality and Social Psychology 57: 27–40

Maslach C, Jackson S E 1982 Burnout in the health professions: a social psychological analysis. In: Saunders G S, Suis J (eds) Social psychology of health and illness. Erlbaum, Hillsdale NJ

Miller D T, Ross M 1975 Self-serving biases in the attribution of causality: fact or fiction? Psychological Bulletin 82: 213–225

Miller N, Maruyama G, Beaber R J, Valone K 1976 Speed of speech and persuasion. Journal of Personality and Social Psychology 34: 615–624

Nisbett R E, Wilson T D 1977 Telling more than we can know: verbal reports on mental processes. Psychological Review 84: 231–259

Pettigrew T F 1981 The ultimate attribution error: extending Allport's cognitive analysis of prejudice. In: Aronson E (ed) Readings about the social animal, 3rd edn. Freeman, San Francisco

Rosenfeld D, Greenberg J, Folgar R, Borys R 1982 Effect of an encounter with a black panhandler on subsequent helping for blacks. Personality and Social Psychology Bulletin 8: 664–671

Rosenhan D 1973 On being sane in insane places. Science 179: 250–258

Rosenthal R, Jacobson L 1968 Pygmalion in the classroom: teacher expectation and pupil's intellectual development. Holt Rinehart Winston, New York

Schlenker B R, Forsyth D R, Leary M R, Miller R W 1980 A self-presentational analysis of the effects of incentives and attitude change following counter-attitudinal behaviour. Journal of Personality and Social Psychology 39: 553–557

Sherif M 1981 Experiments in group conflict. In: Aronson E (ed) Readings about the social animal, 3rd edn. Freeman, San Francisco

Skevington S M 1981 Intergroup relations and nursing. European Journal of Social Psychology 11: 43–59

Skolnick P, Heslin R 1971 Approved dependence and reactions to bad arguments and low credibility sources. Journal of Experimental Research in Personality 5: 199–207

Snyder M, Rothbart M 1971 Communicator attractiveness and opinion change. Canadian Journal of Behavioural Science 3: 377–387

Stephan W G 1978 School desegregation: an evaluation of predictions made in Brown versus Board of Education. Psychological Bulletin 85: 217–238

Tajfel H, 1959 Quantitative judgement in social perception. British Journal of Social Psychology 17: 115–120

Tajfel H 1982 Social identity and intergroup relations. Cambridge University Press, Cambridge

Turner J C, Hogg M A, Oakes P J, Reicher S D, Wetherell M S 1987 Rediscovering the social group: a self-categorisation theory. Blackwell, Oxford

Wood W 1982 Retrieval of attitude-relevant information from memory: effects on susceptibility to persuasive and intrinsic motivation. Journal of Personality and Social Psychology 42: 798–810

Worchel S, Brehm J W 1971 Direct and implied social restoration of freedom. Journal of Personality and Social Psychology 18: 294–304

Zellner M 1970 Self-esteem, reception and influenceability. Journal of Personality and Social Psychology 15: 87–93

RECOMMENDED READING

Abraham C, Shanley E 1992 Social psychology for nurses. Edward Arnold, London
A comprehensive analysis of social psychology as applied to nursing authored by individuals who have had considerable experience teaching health professionals.

Baron R A, Byrne D 1991 Social psychology: understanding human interaction, 6th edn. Allyn & Bacon, Newton Mass. There are a number of basic social psychology texts, most of which are fine. However, I think this one is good because it is easy to understand without sacrificing psychological sophistication.

Duck S 1992 Human relationships: an introduction to social psychology, 2nd edn. Sage, London
Duck is concerned with presenting social psychology in a context that is relevant to the reader as opposed to a more formal academic structure. He succeeds because he maintains academic rigour whilst discussing issues in a very readable fashion.

DiMatteo M R, Friedman H 1982 Social psychology and medicine. Oelgeschlager Gunn Hain, Cambridge Mass.

3

Communication process

The final chapter in this section examines the way in which the delivery of care is determined firstly by making decisions both individually and in groups, by communicating these decisions in ways that are more likely to increase compliance and by looking at other items such as conformity and obedience. Many people find difficulty in implementing the advice of health professionals and thus behaviour modification is discussed as a means of helping people to help themselves.

A woman has just had a miscarriage. If one out of every five pregnancies results in miscarriage, this means that she will have four successful pregnancies before experiencing another miscarriage. Do you agree?

A man comes up to you in the street and says, 'We are desperately short of blood. Could you give blood each month for a year?' You might think that such a request is asking too much. However, the man then says, 'OK, could you give blood just once?' The second request is more reasonable and you might well comply.

But, let us say that the same man had come up to you in the street and said, 'We are desperately short of blood. Could you put a blood donor sticker in your car window?' and then followed up this request by saying, 'OK, could you give blood just once?' You might not feel so inclined to comply with his second request. In both circumstances the second request is exactly the same, 'OK, could you give blood just once?', but putting a 'strong' request first is more likely to get you to give blood. Why?

A friend of yours has been told by her doctor that she must lose weight. She has come to you in tears because she has tried everything possible and just cannot manage to lose even a few pounds. She says that she is beside herself with worry and does not know what to do next. Could you help her?

Communication is not just talking effectively to people. It is a complicated process made up of a number of different elements. The three questions above illustrate some of the main elements of the process of communication. Firstly, decisions have to be made regarding the content of the communication. A decision regarding a specific course of action towards a person, or a group of people, is the initial stage in the communication process. Making the correct decision is by no means easy. Should decisions be based on statistical probabilities, or should they be based on the experience and knowledge of the clinician? An investigation of how individuals use inference and probability in decision-making can help to provide an answer.

Having decided on a course of action, it has to be communicated effectively to the patient. Research on social influence has shown that the communication process is affected by such items as conformity, compliance, obedience and modelling. In other words, individual behaviour is influenced by the actions of others in specific contexts. An analysis of the nature of this influence can inform ways to improve the communication process.

Finally, the decision has been made. It has been communicated effectively and the patient understands exactly what she should do, but for some reason she just cannot do it. In the example given above, the woman knows that she must lose weight and really wants to do so but is finding the task too difficult. Under these circumstances behavioural techniques can be employed to help the woman achieve her goal to lose weight. Programmes can be developed to help individuals change their behaviour and realise their aims.

DECISION-MAKING

When one thinks about decision-making and health care it is usually the health professional who is the focus of attention. However, one should not forget that many health decisions are made by 'patients'. For instance, deciding whether one feels ill; deciding to seek health care; deciding what to eat or drink, what exercise to take etc. are all decisions relating to health that are made nearly every day. This section is concerned with decisions made by health professionals (patient decision-making is discussed in Chapter 6). The two issues to be discussed are the psychological factors influencing the way individuals make decisions and how group decisions differ from those made by individuals.

Individual decisions

For many years there has been a debate about the relative effectiveness of the 'clinical decision' compared to the 'statistical decision'. The clinical decision would typically involve a health professional making some prediction about the effectiveness of a particular treatment based on the experience of the professional, the knowledge of the patient and sometimes intuition. Often, the clinician would be unable to identify how the decision was reached. The statistical decision is based on established quantitative methods. A prediction about the effectiveness of a particular treatment depends on statistical probabilities regarding the success of the treatment based on previous research studies. Proponents of the clinical approach emphasise the unique status of the human brain in being able to come up with insightful solutions beyond the capacity of statistical diagnosis, whilst those in favour of the actuarial approach highlight the often vague, subjective even unscientific attitude of health professionals to making decisions.

In actual fact, both the clinical and statistical positions are compatible with each other. If the health professional is willing to become informed of the typical mistakes that are made in the area of human inference and probability theory, then she will be able to combine her intuition with an increased statistical sophistication to arrive at decisions in a logical, yet human, fashion.

Let us examine some of the mistakes that are typically made in the areas of probabilities, inferences and decision-making. We are not always rational decision makers. If I said that every time I toss a coin and it comes up heads, I'll pay you £2 and every time it comes up tails, you pay me £0.50, would you accept the wager? Chances are you probably would. But if I now said that it will cost you £1 for each time the coin is tossed, would you accept? Let us see whether it would be worth your while.

Suppose you had two bets. With a fair coin, you would win £2 on the first toss and lose £0.50 on the second. Thus you would make £1.50. This represents a profit of £0.75 per toss and is known as the expected value. However, you had to pay £1 to play each game, therefore you stand to lose £0.25 each game you play. Thus you should not pay more than £0.75 per game, for this is the point of indifference and a rational decision maker would play any game whose cost to enter was lower than £0.75 since it guarantees a profit in the long run.

Let us increase the stakes. If a coin comes up heads I will pay you £2000 and if it comes up tails, you pay me £500. You pay £700 for each toss of the coin. Although a rational decision maker would have no hesitation in accepting the bet since the cost to play the game (£700) is lower than the point of indifference (£750), you might think twice. This is because there is a difference between the economic value of the bet and the psychological value of the bet. Unless you are used to dealing in such large sums of money, the psychological risk involved would deter you from accepting the bet. When stakes are high, rational decision-making is not so easy.

In many circumstances individuals do not even bother to work out the odds and are seduced by the opportunity to win. The only casino game that offers the player a reasonable chance with an expected value greater than zero is pontoon/blackjack/twenty-one; all the other games guarantee the casino will win (Bond 1974).

The reason for using the above example is not to help health professionals win at the casino (even assuming they could afford it), nor is it appropriate to compare decisions about betting with decisions about people's health. The example is meant to illustrate the importance of the subjective value or utility of a decision. Where the risk is high, people are less likely to follow rational, mathematical rules. Many decisions relating to the health of patients involve high degrees of risk and thus have a large subjective utility component and require careful consideration.

The ways questions are put to patients can influence their decision. Consider the following: a rare disease is expected to kill 600 people.

The exact scientific consequences of the disease are:

- If programme A is adopted, 200 people will be saved.
- If programme B is adopted, there is a 1/3 probability that 600 people will be saved and a 2/3 probabilty that no people will be saved.

Thus:

A = 200 saved
B = 1/3 chance 600 will be saved; 2/3 chance 0 will be saved.

Which of the two programmes would you choose?

The majority response is for programme A because of the risks involved in programme B. However, consider the same problem reformulated as follows:

- If programme C is adopted, 400 people will die.
- If programme D is adopted, there is a 1/3 chance that nobody will die and a 2/3 probability that 600 people will die.

Thus:

C = 400 will die
D = 1/3 chance 0 will die; 2/3 chance 600 will die.

Under these circumstances the majority choice is for the risk-seeking alternative D; the certain death of 400 people is less acceptable than the risky options.

The two versions of the problem describe identical outcomes, the only difference is that in the first situation the death of 600 people is the reference point and the outcomes are evaluated in terms of lives saved or gains. Whereas in the second situation the reference point is couched differently, thus the programmes are evaluated in terms of lives lost. Therefore the way the question is 'framed' influences the decision to act in terms of risk or safety. Kahneman & Tversky (1982) called this 'prospect theory'.

Decisions about specific courses of action in health care usually involve the evaluation of evidence. Decisions are seldom made without the presence of some form of inference or judgement relating to the evidence. In many cases inferences about probabilistic outcomes are incorrect.

Exercise 3.1

1. Which of the following is more likely:
   a. that an English word would begin with the letter 'r'?
   b. that the third letter of an English word would be 'r'?

2. A fair coin has been tossed five times with the result H H H H H. If you had to predict the outcome of the sixth toss, would you choose heads or tails?

3. In a particular city 80% of the taxis are owned by company A and are blue. The other 20% are owned by company B and are yellow. An accident occurred one night and a witness reported that the car involved was a taxi. Unfortunately it was much too dark for him to make out whether the taxi was coloured blue or yellow. What is the probability that the taxi belonged to company A?

4. If a fair coin is tossed six times, which of the following sequences of outcomes is most likely:
   a. H H H T T T?
   b. H H H H H H?
   c. H T T H T H?

5. Half of the white blood cells of healthy patients possess a particular characteristic, whilst 70% of the cells of patients suffering from a particular disorder possess this characteristic. 10 cells from Patient A are examined and 7 show the characteristic. 20 cells from Patient B are examined and 14 show the characteristic. Which of the following is true?
   a. Patient A is more likely to have the disorder than Patient B.
   b. Patient B is more likely to have the disorder than Patient A.
   c. They are equally likely to have the disorder.

6. In general, are people from your home town more successful than people from other parts of the country?

7. Which cause of death is more likely:
   a. lung cancer or stomach cancer?
   b. murder or suicide?
   c. diabetes or motor vehicle accidents?

Answers are on page 63.

Errors in human inference fall into a number of different categories (Kahneman & Tversky 1982). The first category refers to a tendency to view unrelated events as being related. Some gamblers expect a run of bad luck to be followed by a run of good luck, so that if presented with a coin that had just been tossed five times with the result H H H H H, they would be more likely to bet that the next toss would result in a tail than in a sixth head. This is known as the 'gambler's fallacy' and is incorrect. The result is equally likely to be a tail as a head, for each toss of the coin is independent from the next—they are unrelated. The coin cannot 'remember' the five previous heads and thus cannot be influenced by what occurred before. Thus in the example quoted at the beginning of the chapter one would have to disagree with the statement concerning the pregnancy—having had one miscarriage does not reduce the odds of it happening again.

A second category of errors is concerned with the availability of information relating to an event. Simply stated, events will be judged as likely or probable if examples of them come easily to mind. This explains why English words beginning with 'r' are judged more likely than English words whose third letter is 'r'. Objectively, the opposite is true, but it is much more difficult to produce examples of words whose third letter is 'r' than to produce words beginning with 'r'. Words beginning with 'r' are more available though in fact they occur less frequently in English than words whose third letter is 'r'.

Similarly, Lichtenstein et al (1978) found that individuals tended to overestimate the frequency of disorders that were well publicised, and underestimate the frequency of disorders that were under-publicised. Thus lung cancer is viewed as more frequent than stomach cancer, murder more frequent than suicide and diabetes more frequent than motor vehicle accidents. In fact, stomach cancer, suicide and motor vehicle accidents are more likely to occur than their counterparts. People from your local town might seem more successful than people from other towns because the information concerning these people is more readily available.

Another factor that tends to bias probabilistic judgement is representativeness. Kahneman & Tversky (1982) give the following information about a person. 'Intelligent but lacks creativity. Neat and tidy but rather a dull, mechanical person. Does not mix well with others but has a high need to achieve. He has a deep moral sense of purpose.' If this description of a person has been chosen at random from a group comprising 30 engineers and 70 social scientists, what is the probability that the person is an engineer? You might think that the probability is quite high, but Kahneman & Tversky (1982) say that this inference is misconceived. There are two sorts of information that are presented: a subjective, unreliable personality sketch and 'hard facts' concerning the ratio of engineers to social scientists. Rational decision makers would predict that there is a 7 in 10 chance that the person is a social scientist and ignore the relatively worthless personality sketch.

Similarly, in the taxi example, the fact that the accident occurs at night is neither here nor there but this information may mislead people into thinking that the chances of a blue taxi being involved in the accident are 50/50 instead of 80/20. Lack of representativeness occurs when irrelevant information clouds judgements based on reliable information.

These are just a few of the problems regarding inferences about probabilistic outcomes. (For a further discussion, see Bourne et al 1986.) How does this research relate to the clinician versus statistics debate? Probability theory does provide a concrete basis for decision-making, but to replace the clinician with a diagnostic computer would be met with horror by patients. The research does suggest that health professionals should be able to make use of a diagnostic computer with appropriate statistical packages and also be aware of the mistakes often made in the area of human inference. In this way the intuition and creativity of the health professional can be combined with the reliability of mathematical tools to produce decisions that are well informed and relevant to each patient's specific needs.

Group decisions

Decisions are not always taken by individuals on their own; often it is assumed that a more balanced decision can only be accomplished by a group of people. Whyte (1956) observed a large number of committees in the business sector and concluded that members of the group did not want to appear irresponsible through making extreme statements and thus tailored their contributions to meet with the group consensus. Decisions regarding health care are made in many cases by teams or groups of health professionals; therefore it is a good idea to gain an idea of the sorts of group dynamics that may affect the quality of the decisions produced.

Exercise 3.2

For this exercise a minimum of 12 people are needed. Five people will take part in a group discussion, the others will act as observers.

1. Ask for five volunteers to take part in a group discussion. Take them outside the room and brief them separately from the rest of the group. Explain to them that they will have to make a series of individual decisions on their own without consultation and then they will get together as a group and discuss the same dilemmas.

2. Each person has to imagine that he or she is advising a fictitious person who faces a choice between two alternative courses of action. One of the alternatives is more attractive than the other but involves a greater element of risk. Consider, for example, Dilemma 1 (below).

If the operation had a 9/10 chance of being successful, you might reasonably advise Mr R. to go ahead and have it. But what if the operation only had a 1/10 chance of success? This would be a very risky choice.

Each member of the discussion group has to choose the lowest probability of success that they would advise Mr R. to accept.

3. Each member of the discussion group works through the following five dilemmas on his or her own and decides on a probability that will reflect his/her cautious or risky advice to the fictitious person in the dilemma.

4. Write your individual decision (1/10, 3/10, 5/10, 7/10, 9/10 or 10/10) on a piece of paper. The dilemmas are:

Dilemma 1

Mr R. is 42 years old and has a serious heart condition. His life has become increasingly restricted due to his condition. He can no longer indulge in even slightly strenuous pastimes. Work, sport and sex are out of the question. His consultant has estimated that he has about 5 years to live. He has been told that he can have an operation which, if successful, will make him a 'new man'.

He should risk the operation if:

a. there is a 1/10 chance that it will succeed
b. there is a 3/10 chance that it will succeed
c. there is a 5/10 chance that it will succeed
d. there is a 7/10 chance that it will succeed
e. there is a 9/10 chance that it will succeed
f. he should not risk the operation under any circumstances 10/10.

Dilemma 2

Ms H. is a qualified nurse and has decided to further her career by enrolling for a Health Psychology course at a University. She has been offered a place at two Universities. The first has considerable status and a good reputation in the area of Health Psychology, but a large proportion of the students fail to pass the course. The second institution does not have such a good reputation but has a much higher pass rate. You have to imagine that you are advising Ms H. What is the lowest probability of her passing the difficult course that she should accept to go to the first University?

She should go to the first University if:

a. there is a 1/10 chance that she will succeed
b. there is a 3/10 chance that she will succeed
c. there is a 5/10 chance that she will succeed
d. there is a 7/10 chance that she will succeed
e. there is a 9/10 chance that she will succeed
f. she should not risk going to the first University under any circumstances 10/10.

Dilemma 3

Mr S. is a successful data processor in a computing firm. He is well liked by all his colleagues and his job is quite secure but he feels that it lacks excitement. Recently, he has had an offer from a new company that represents an exciting new challenge and an opportunity to diversify his talents. However, he cannot be sure that the new company will succeed. If he goes, he will not get his old job back. What is the lowest probability of the new company succeeding that you would advise him to accept?

He should join the new company if:

a. there is a 1/10 chance that it will succeed
b. there is a 3/10 chance that it will succeed
c. there is a 5/10 chance that it will succeed
d. there is a 7/10 chance that it will succeed
e. there is a 9/10 chance that it will succeed
f. he should not risk the move under any circumstances 10/10.

Dilemma 4

Mrs P. is married with two children aged 12 and 14. She is an infant teacher at a local school. Over the last few years, Mrs P. has felt in bit of a 'rut'. She regards her marriage as stable but largely unfulfilling. In order to make her life more interesting she has taken on a lot of work in the community and, as a result, met a man with whom she has fallen in love. This man is single and wants her to leave her unhappy marriage. She would leave but has doubts about whether the new relationship would succeed and be stable enough for herself and her children. What is the lowest probability that the new relationship should succeed in order for her to end her marriage?

She should enter into the new relationship if:

a. there is a 1/10 chance that it will succeed
b. there is a 3/10 chance that it will succeed
c. there is a 5/10 chance that it will succeed
d. there is a 7/10 chance that it will succeed
e. there is a 9/10 chance that it will succeed
f. she should not enter the new relationship under any circumstances 10/10.

Dilemma 5

Mr and Mrs A. have to send their son to one of two schools. The first has an excellent reputation for high educational attainment, but also has a reputation for emotional difficulties amongst its pupils. The second school does not have such a high academic reputation but neither does it have large numbers of emotional problems in its pupils. What is the lowest probability that the child will experience no emotional problems at the first school?

The child should go to the first school if:

a. there is a 1/10 chance of no problems
b. there is a 3/10 chance of no problems
c. there is a 5/10 chance of no problems
d. there is a 7/10 chance of no problems
e. there is a 9/10 chance of no problems
f. the child should not be sent to the first school under any circumstances 10/10.

5. Whilst the five discussion group members are making their individual decisions, return to the rest of the main group. The rest of the group should be split into two; one section with five members, the other will depend on the size of the whole group. Ideally, there should be four members, but it can be done with as few as two and as many as eight. The group of five is called the 'NVC' group and the group of two to eight, the 'Bales' group.

6. Bales (1958) developed a system for categorising group behaviour. He suggested that there were four main categories of communication: positive socio-emotional responses, attempted answers, questions and negative socio-emotional responses. All the verbal communication could be categorised into these four groups. Further two types of 'leader' tend to emerge. One is concerned with 'getting the job done' and is referred to as the 'task leader'. The other is concerned with the emotional tone of the group and is referred to as the

socio-emotional leader. The four categories can be represented as follows:

- *Socio-emotional area positive*. Shows tension release, jokes, laughs, shows solidarity, raises others' status, gives help, agrees, understands, concurs.
- *Tasks area attempted answers*. Gives suggestion, direction, gives opinion, evaluation, expresses feeling, wish, gives orientation, information, repeats, clarifies, confirms.
- *Task area question*. Asks for information, confirmation, repetition, asks for opinion, analysis, asks for suggestion, direction, possible ways of action.
- *Socio-emotional area negative*. Disagrees, shows passive rejection, withholds help, shows tension, asks for help, withdraws, shows antagonism, deflates others' status.

Each person is allocated to one of the four main categories. If there are more than four, they can be doubled up so that two people are in each category, if less combine 1 and 4; 2 and 3. They have to rate the members of the discussion group on their category of communication. Instruct each person to have in front of them five sheets of paper, one for each dilemma. Each sheet should be divided into five sections that refer to the five members of the discussion group. As the discussion proceeds, the frequency of a particular type of communication is noted along with who produced it. Thus the number of responses made by each participant in each category is observed.

7. As we have seen in Chapter 1, a great deal of communication is transmitted nonverbally. In order to gain information concerning the dynamics of a group, it is necessary to have some evaluation of the nonverbal signals that are being passed between members of that group. Each of the five members (ten can be used, two per person if necessary) of the NVC group are assigned to observe one of the five members of the discussion group. They should have five pieces of paper with the following categories of nonverbal behaviour on each:

- *Facial expressions*. Note the number of smiles, nods and frowns during each dilemma. Also note any other facial expressions that are used.
- *Posture/gesture*. Note the posture of the body; leaning forward, tense, relaxed. Note gestures such as clenched fist, palms up in the air, pointing. Note any fidgeting, movement of feet, legs etc.
- *Voice*. Note the changes in pitch/tone, the changes in volume. Note how fast/slow the person speaks and whether the voice is calm or excited.
- *Other*. Note any other features of nonverbal behaviour such as the overall time speaking, number of interruptions made and any other 'little idiosyncrasies'.

8. Arrange five chairs in the centre of the room, sufficiently far apart for the observers to get a good view of the group. Ask the observers to place themselves so that they are in a good enough position to make their observations. Finally, ask the observers if they are clear about the procedure and if there are any questions. Bring the discussion group back to the main room and collect their individual decisions. Inform them that they have to go through the five dilemmas again, this time discussing each one as a group. The people sitting around them will observe the discussion. Tell them to spend at least 5 minutes and no more than 10 minutes discussing each dilemma and they *must* come to a decision in the end. Before discussing each dilemma, ask one of them to read it out aloud so that the observers have some idea of the content of the discussion.

9. While the discussions are taking place, put the individual decisions on the board and calculate the means of the scores for each dilemma. The mean of the individual decisions can be compared with the group decision to see if it differs:

Dilemma	Individual					Mean	Group
	1	2	3	4	5		
1							
2							
3							
4							
5							

Points for discussion

Stoner (1961) carried out an experiment similar to the exercise that you have just completed. He used more people and more dilemmas, but the basic structure of the experiment was the same. He found that when the dilemmas were discussed in groups, the group decision tended to involve more risk than decisions made by the individuals on their own. This finding was contrary to the widely held opinion of that time, namely that group discussion would lead to a more carefully considered, cautious decision. The experiments were conducted using management students from Massachusetts Institute of Technology and the effect came to be known as the *risky shift*.

Group discussion leads to riskier decisions. One theory put forward to explain the effect was the diffusion of responsibility. Each member of the group feels less personal responsibility for the decision and is able to advocate more risk. Diffusion of responsibility does occur in group behaviour. One has only to observe the behaviour of groups of soccer hooligans to see how responsibility is diffused within the group and acts are committed in a group which would be unthinkable by people on their own. Did this occur in the exercise you have just completed? You might find that on some of the dilemmas there was indeed a shift to risk but on others there was in fact a shift to caution. This was the finding of Nordhoy (1962) who found that some items reliably shift in the cautious direction. Clearly the diffusion of responsibility theory cannot explain shifting to more cautious behaviour.

However, if you look at your results you will see that whether it is a change to risk or caution, a change of decision has taken place as a result of group discussion. Burnstein (1983) puts this 'polarisation effect' down to group discussion accentuating the views already held. Another explanation is based on the disproportionate influence of certain members of the group, that is, there may be some people who are exerting pressure on others to conform to their decision. The reason people change their views as a result of group discussion is because they are influenced by the 'leadership' qualities of certain individuals. In order to see whether this is the case, one needs to examine the dynamics of group behaviour.

The Bales analysis will provide an indication of the quantity and type of communication made by each of the participants. This information can be used to determine whether there is evidence of task leaders and socio-emotional leaders. This information can be combined with an analysis of the individual decisions of the leaders to examine whether there is a relationship between leadership and group decisions. Nonverbal communication can also provide evidence about who emerged as a leader. Such items as smiling and nodding, interrupting others' conversation and time 'holding the floor' are nonverbal indicators of leadership. Finally, ask how the participants felt during the exercise. Did the discussion group feel they were being swayed by one individual? How did they feel about being observed? Was there any diffusion of responsibility? Did the observers find it difficult to note the discussants' behaviour? Were there any significant events that occurred between individuals? Were any particular mannerisms used by the members of the discussion group?

If one compares the final group decision on each of the dilemmas to any one of the individual decisions, it is likely that no match will be found. This suggests that each person's decision was affected in some way by membership of a group. Many decisions about health care are carried out by groups or teams of health professionals. An analysis of the ways in which group dynamics can influence the decision-making process can produce more efficient, and importantly, more relevant decisions regarding specific options in the delivery of health care.

SOCIAL INFLUENCE

There are many tactics, strategies and procedures one can employ to exert influence over patients to adopt advice about health care. Indeed, a major feature of the communication process is the ability to present items of information in such a way as to guarantee action on the part of the recipient. Unfortunately, there is no magic formula for attaining such control as people have minds of their own and wish to appear able to use them. Yet there are ways of presenting information that are quite likely to achieve success.

Attempts to exert social influence take a number of different forms. *Conformity* occurs in situations where individuals yield to 'group pressure' without direct requests to do so. *Compliance* is a more direct form of social influence. It occurs in circumstances where people will alter their behaviour in response to a direct request to do so. *Obedience* involves commands, rather than requests and *modelling* takes place in situations where behaviour is changed through the observation of the actions of someone else.

Conformity

There are certain 'unwritten rules' in society that indicate ways in which people should behave. Forming a queue to wait for a bus; wearing a tie at a formal function and applauding a concert performance are examples of these rules and are called *social norms*. Some social norms serve a useful function, others do not. Forming a queue to wait for a bus prevents social chaos, but wearing a tie on certain occasions serves no

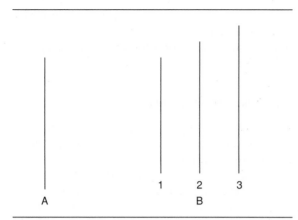

Figure 3.1 The Asch experiment.

obvious purpose. Useful or not, conformity is a pervasive aspect of human behaviour. A famous experiment conducted a number of years ago by Asch (1951) illustrated how individuals conform to group pressure. A group of eight subjects were asked to look at three lines of different length and one standard line (Fig. 3.1).

The members of the group had to estimate which of the three lines was the same length as the standard line. Seven out of the eight subjects were confederates of the experimenter, only one was a bona fide subject. On the first 12 trials, the confederates gave a truthful answer, but on the next 8 trials they were asked by the experimenter to give a false response. Thus, the experimenter would ask each of the members of the group in turn which of the three lines 1, 2 or 3 was the same length as the standard line. The first six members of the group all replied that number one was the same length as the standard line, when in fact it was obvious that the correct answer was number two. The seventh member of the group was the genuine subject. If a person was faced with the previous six members of a group reporting that number one was the correct answer and it was obvious that number two was correct, what would she do? Chances are that she would conform to group pressure and reply 'number one', going along with the rest of the group. In fact 75% of those tested by Asch in this situation, went along with the group's false answer on at least

one occasion. Clearly, many people prefer to go along with group decisions rather than disagree openly with the judgement of the group.

There are two explanations for conforming to group pressure. The first is called *normative social influence* and states that one reason why individuals conform is because they do not want to cause problems by openly disagreeing with everyone else. They do not want to 'rock the boat'. They can see the correct answer but feel it is not worth their while to go against group opinion.

Another explanation is called *informational social influence*. If all the people in front of you have answered in a way that disconfirms your opinion, you start to question your ability to make correct responses. In situations of uncertainty we look to others for information about how to deal with them. The subject in the Asch experiment may start to think that there is something wrong with her eyesight. Both explanations are appropriate and can often occur in conjunction with each other. Both normative and informational social influence play an important role in many social situations.

Conformity is a pervasive feature of group dynamics and thus requires some form of analysis to determine the nature of the factors that influence the effect. There are four main variables that can affect conformity:

- *Status.* Some groups elicit a greater degree of conformity than others. If a group is regarded as being 'of high status' then one is more likely to conform to group opinion than a group 'of low status'. The status of the group is determined by the individual.
- *Size.* The size of the group is important up to a point. Conformity increases as the size of the group increases from 3 to 5; however larger groups do not produce more conformity. Wilder (1977) says that it is not the number of people in the group that is important but the number of social entities. In some groups there may be 'cliques' or subgroups that are perceived as one social entity, making it inappropriate to treat them as separate and distinct individuals.

• *Sex differences*. Early experiments on conformity found that women conformed much more than men (Crutchfield 1955). More recent research has found no such differences and it is suggested that mistakes in the design of some of the early experiments were responsible for the incorrect findings (Bisanz & Rule 1989).

• *Having an ally*. The presence of someone else in the group who disagrees with group opinion significantly reduces conformity. In an experiment on visual judgements, Allen & Levine (1971) found that the reduction in conformity occurred even if the ally had 'inch thick' spectacles. Simply breaking the unanimity of the group is sufficient to reduce the effect. Further, it is better if the ally disagrees with the group right at the start rather than later on in the questioning procedure (Morris et al 1977). Therefore, it is suggested that to prevent conformity occurring in groups it is better to speak out right at the beginning of a group discussion rather than leave disagreements to later on in the proceedings.

Many health professionals find themselves in group meetings to discuss numerous issues. The format of the group may vary, but social influence does not. Sometimes the group may be made up of members from different professions, sometimes the health professional may find himself in the presence of what he regards as high status or influential individuals. In these circumstances conformity to group opinion needs to be avoided. Janis (1982) has proposed that 'group think' can occur when groups get together to discuss issues. As each member goes along with the group, there is a suppression of personal doubts and a shared illusion of unanimity, resulting in irrational decision-making. To protect against this effect occurring, each member of the group should be encouraged to express any doubts about a particular procedure as soon as possible.

Compliance

Health professionals are continually asking patients to alter some aspect of their behaviour.

This may seem quite straightforward, but psychologists have found that people tend to employ subtle and complex techniques to ensure compliance with their requests.

The 'foot-in-the-door' technique

This works on the principle that a small or trivial request followed by a much larger more important request is liable to ensure compliance. Freedman & Fraser (1966) conducted a number of experiments in this area. In one, a researcher posing as a volunteer worker knocked on people's doors and asked them if they would mind a sign being erected on their front lawns stating 'Drive carefully'. In order to get an idea of how the sign would look, they were shown a picture of a house with a poorly lettered sign on the front lawn that practically obscured the view of the house. Not surprisingly, only 17% agreed to the erection of the sign. However, in one instance a particular group of people gave a 76% favourable response. The reason for their compliance had occurred 2 weeks earlier. A different volunteer worker had come to their houses and asked them to display a very small sticker in their window saying 'Be a safe driver'. A reasonably trivial request that just about all the people agreed to, but the subsequent effects were considerable. Because these people had agreed to quite a trivial initial request, they were willing to put up with a huge inconvenience later on. Cialdini (1993) warns us to beware of agreeing to trivial propositions since they increase our compliance with much larger requests.

The 'door-in-the-face' technique

A large request followed by a small one also works. Cialdini et al (1975) stopped students in the street and asked them if they would agree to act as unpaid counsellors to juvenile delinquents for 2 hours a week over 2 years. Nobody agreed. The next request was to take a group of delinquents on a trip to the zoo and 50% of the students agreed. This compared to only 16.7% agreement when the second request was presented on its own. How can both techniques work when at first glance they seem to be advocating opposite approaches? The answer lies in an analysis of the underlying psychological processes responsible for exerting the social influence.

In order for the 'door-in-the-face' technique to succeed, the two requests have to be delivered by the same person. If the second request is delivered by another person it will not work. This is because the effect is based on mutual reciprocity. In most cases, we like to help people when they ask us to do something for them. Faced with a person willing to reduce her request we are usually willing to move from our initial unacceptance to meet her reduced request.

In contrast, the 'foot-in-the-door' technique will work even if another person makes the second request. This is because the individual has experienced a shift in perception. The initial request produced a commitment on the part of the person to the project. Having committed herself, it does not matter who subsequently requests cooperation because she has become involved. This latter fact enables the second request to be delivered days after the first and still be effective, whereas the 'door-in-the-face' procedure will only work if the interval between the requests is relatively short. Thus both techniques are effective because they are based on different underlying psychological processes.

'Low-balling'

If a psychologist were to ask a group of students if they could take part in one of her experiments which was an important feature of her research programme, wait for a response and only then tell the students that the experiment starts at 7.00 a.m. the following day, she would be much more likely to get her subjects than if she told them directly when the experiment was due to start. This has been called 'low-balling' from the term to 'throw a low ball'.

Cialdini et al (1978) asked graduate students to put a poster up in their rooms. In the low-ball condition, they agreed to display the poster and then were told that they had to collect it from the foyer downstairs, whereas in the control condition they were told that they would have to go downstairs to collect the poster before they made a decision whether to display it. The experimenters found that 60% of the students in the low-ball condition went downstairs to collect the poster, whereas only 20% of the control group did so. It pays to beware of things that sound too simple or too easy to be true and to be less hasty in making decisions.

Ingratiation

Increased liking can lead to compliance. If people like us, then they are more likely to yield to our requests. Getting people to like us can be achieved through flattery. Liden & Mitchell (1988) found that subtle forms of flattery were more effective in gaining compliance. A person who realises that she is being flattered with an ulterior motive in mind will react in a hostile manner. Less-direct techniques are more effective such as paying careful attention to everything the other person says and encouraging her to talk about herself. Personal similarity is another factor that can enhance a person's attractiveness to another. If people are convinced that others share their beliefs and opinions, they are more likely to be attracted toward them.

Guilt

Causing others to experience guilt is an effective way of gaining their cooperation. Children tend to be the most competent exponents of this technique. 'William's Mummy takes him to the swimming baths every Thursday afternoon, so please can we go too Mummy?' Freedman & Wallington (1967) stress that in almost all cases people induced to feel guilt show greater compliance than control groups not made to experience guilt. Many individuals engage in dramatic portrayals of their anguish to ensure the help and concern of others.

All of these techniques are used on members of the public every day to persuade them to change their behaviour along the lines directed by often unscrupulous individuals. An analysis of these techniques may make people less susceptible to them. An important question arises for health professionals relating to the use of such techniques in the provision of health care. The example given at the beginning of the chapter illustrating the use of the 'door-in-the-face' to get people to give blood serves as an example. Many people would say that getting more people to give blood is an admirable act, but what about other areas of health care? Should health professionals adopt these sorts of techniques to implement health care in general?

There are certain ethical restrictions that should be considered such as the patient's right to know exactly what is going on and how he is being manipulated. A second point relates to trust. If health professionals are to get patients to trust them, then the use of such techniques could seriously undermine the development of a trusting relationship. This does not mean that health professionals should abandon methods to improve compliance to therapeutic regimens; one does not have to ingratiate oneself to obtain people's affection and respect. Appearing to patients as a friendly and concerned person who 'practises what she preaches' can influence the extent to which they will comply with requests to change their behaviour in some way. There are a number of other factors that affect the important area of patient compliance and these will be discussed in more detail in Chapter 6.

Obedience

This procedure of social influence is concerned with telling or commanding people to do something rather than asking them to do it. That people obey the commands of authority figures is hardly surprising since failure to obey is often accompanied by some form of punishment. However, it is the influence of powerless authorities to command obedience and the extent of people's willingness to go along with the commands of the person 'in the white coat' that has interested many psychologists.

Milgram (1963, 1974) devised a dramatic experiment to illustrate the extent of people's obedience to authority. He advertised for members of the public to come to Harvard University to take part in a psychology experiment on learning. When they arrived they met another person who was to take part in the same experiment. They were asked to toss a coin to determine who would be the 'experimenter' and who would be the 'subject' in the experiment. It was a two-headed coin and the person they met was a confederate of Milgram. The situation was fixed so that the unknowing person was the experimenter and Milgram's confederate the subject.

The experiment was described to both individuals as that of delivering electric shocks to the subject to facilitate learning. The shocks were to be administered by means of a control panel in front of the 'experimenter'. They were graded according to strength:

1. Slight
2. Moderate
3. Strong
4. Very strong
5. Intense
6. Extreme intensity
7. Danger: severe shock
8. XXX 450 volts.

The 'experimenters' were told to deliver an electric shock every time the subject made a mistake and to increase the shock the more mistakes were made. Actually, the confederate never received any shock. But a mild pulse of 45 volts was used on the 'experimenter' to convince him that the shocks were real. The experiment began and after a while the confederate started to make mistakes. Gradually the shocks were increased by the experimenter till they reached a worrying level. Meanwhile Milgram gave encouragement to proceed:

> 'Please go on.'
> 'It is absolutely essential that you carry on.'
> 'You have no choice, you must go on.'

The dilemma facing the 'experimenter' was whether to continue up the shock scale or to defy Milgram. All the people that enrolled for the experiment were volunteers and could have terminated the situation at any moment, but

Milgram found that fully 65% of the subjects showed total obedience and proceeded right up the scale delivering what might be construed as lethal doses of electric shock to the other person.

In this, and other experiments, Milgram (1974) found that subjects (62.5%) would administer large electric shocks to the confederate perceiving him to suffer from a heart condition and hearing him pounding on the wall for relief. Further, 30% continued to obey even when this required that they grasp the victim's hand and force it upon the shock plate.

Many people protested and certainly not everyone obeyed the instructions of Milgram. Two factors seem to be important in resisting and countering obedience to authority:

• *Responsibility for one's actions.* In the experiments, some subjects were told that they would not be responsible for anything that happened to the 'victim'. It has been found that when people are given responsibility for their actions, they are far less obedient to authority (Kilham & Mann 1974).

• *Disobedient models.* After exposure to people who categorically refused to obey commands to administer shock, many subjects (90%) refused to give the highest level of shock available to the confederate. Thus exposure to people who disobey authority figures and giving people more responsibility for their actions reduces social influence and facilitates a more autonomous behaviour pattern.

Modelling

Sometimes social influence may be exerted unintentionally. Suppose a person is in the park and she is extremely thirsty. She finds a drinking fountain only to discover that there is a sign saying 'Water unsuitable for consumption'. She is just about to go away and find another source of refreshment when another person comes along and starts to drink from the drinking fountain. Under these circumstances, it is probable that the thirsty woman would disregard the warning and drink the water. Her behaviour has been influenced by someone else and in this instance the 'model' is unaware of the effect he has had. This is an example of what might be termed response disinhibition, since initially, the woman had inhibitions about drinking the water which were subsequently extinguished by the presence of another person's actions.

Modelling can also lead to inhibition of action. Suppose you are waiting in a queue of traffic and are late for an appointment. You are considering overtaking but realise that such action is not allowed. However, you decide that you have to get to your destination and are about to overtake. Suddenly, one car pulls out, starts to overtake and immediately falls back in line. Having seen someone act in the way you proposed and return to the queue, you may decide that overtaking is not worth your while. In this situation, the model has inhibited your proposed action.

In both these instances the models are unaware of the influence they are exerting over others' behaviour. Therefore, it is important that health professionals are aware that their behaviour is being observed by patients, even though they are unaware of this attention. Modelling is a powerful form of social influence, whether it is intentional or not, and can be used to improve the provision of health care. But, telling patients to give up smoking and then smoking a cigarette is a totally counterproductive modelling procedure.

Craig & Prkachin (1978) have shown how pain can be reduced by social models. Volunteers were exposed to a series of electric shocks of five different intensities. Subjects were asked to rate the painfulness of the shocks. Physiological measures of skin conductance and heart rate were taken. The shocks were administered to the subjects in the presence of a confederate of the experimenter. In one condition the confederate always rated the shock after the subject and on each occasion her ratings were 25% lower. (The confederate never received any shock.) In the control condition the subject was unaware of the confederate's perception of the shock. The results of the study indicated that subjects exposed to the 'tolerant model' experienced less discomfort than the subjects in the control condition. Further, the physiological data indicated that heart rate and skin conductance were significantly lower for the subjects exposed to the pain-tolerant model. The experimenters suggest that exposure to someone who seems to be experiencing less pain actually reduces the experience of pain itself.

BEHAVIOUR MODIFICATION

The last stage in the process of communication is concerned with trying to ensure that the patient is able to act on the information that has been provided. Many individuals lack the ability, or skill, to operationalise instructions. Behaviour modification refers to a group of techniques that can be used to help people change their behaviour in a desired fashion. No unequivocal definition of behaviour modification exists, but, in the context of the communication process, it may be defined as 'the application of a broadly defined set of procedures, based on the principles of conditioning, to facilitate desired changes in behaviour'. Before examining these procedures, it is necessary briefly to describe the principles of conditioning on which the procedure is based.

Conditioning

Both classical and operant conditioning have been mentioned in Chapter 2. To recapitulate briefly, classical conditioning involves the process of association. If a baby is touched on the cheek, she will turn toward the touch and begin to suck. The touch on the cheek is the *unconditioned stimulus* and the turning and sucking is the *unconditioned response*. The baby has not learned this behaviour; it is automatic. Suppose the sound of the mother's footsteps and the feeling of being picked up always precede the touch on the cheek. The sound and the feelings eventually become associated with the touch on the cheek and start to 'trigger' the responses of turning and sucking. The footsteps and the picking up have become *conditioned stimuli*.

Operant or instrumental conditioning involves the use of rewards and punishments to change behaviour. Any behaviour that is reinforced will be more likely to occur again in the same or

similar situation. There are two types of reinforcement: positive and negative. Positive reinforcement provides the subject with a reward such as a smile or food. Negative reinforcement is not punishment—it occurs when something unpleasant is stopped and increases the likelihood of an operant. For instance, if it is raining and a person is getting wet, she might put up an umbrella to stop the rain reaching her. This is an example of negative reinforcement which is likely to increase the use of an umbrella. Both positive and negative reinforcement strengthen behaviour. Punishment, on the other hand, weakens some undesired behaviour.

Behaviour does not have to be rewarded at every instance; if a mother smiles at her child every fourth or fifth time she brings her a toy, she will keep on bringing it. *Partial reinforcement* leads to or results in a very strong form of conditioning and will take longer to extinguish than giving a reward every time the behaviour occurs. The subjects can be rewarded according to the number of times they exhibit a particular behaviour or they may obtain a reward contingent upon a time period. Even random, unpredictable partial reinforcers can exert considerable influence to maintain response levels (fruit machines/one-armed bandits).

Before considering different behavioural techniques, a fundamental necessity of behaviour modification is the establishment of 'baseline responding', that is, an in-depth analysis of current reinforcers needs to take place before attempting to change them. For example, the teacher who always sends the disruptive child outside the room as punishment for his behaviour may believe that this action is a punishment; yet it may well be the case that some children actually want to stand outside the classroom, and see the teacher's punishment as an actual reward. Clearly, under these circumstances actions will sometimes lead to the opposite of the desired outcome. The teacher has failed to make a detailed analysis of what constitutes a reward and punishment for each child.

There is a clear necessity to be absolutely certain that conditioning procedures are underpinned by exact analysis of appropriate rewards and punishments. Using the threat of prison confinement as punishment ignores the exact schedules of punishment and reinforcement. It is assumed that punishing offenders by sending them to prison will deter them from offending again, but if the exact schedules are considered this is not the case. The thief steals the goods (reward) and is caught and goes to prison (punishment). The thief is punished for getting caught not for stealing the goods. Under these schedules the thief is much more likely to avoid getting caught than to stop stealing.

Techniques

The basic principles of conditioning have been applied in a number of different ways. This has led to the development of behaviour modification techniques designed to help individuals change their behaviour.

Positive reinforcement

Providing appropriate rewards for appropriate behaviour is a central feature of behaviour modification. A psychiatric hospital had a problem with one of its patients. David tended to vomit over everyone and everything at meal times. This behaviour needed attention due to the effect it was having on his physical condition and also because he did not have too many friends. After ascertaining that there was no physiological cause for the condition, it was decided to implement a behaviour modification programme to try to extinguish the vomiting behaviour. The first step was to determine the rewards that were associated with his vomiting. It was found that two rewards featured prominently in his behaviour: having a bath after vomiting and the attention of staff. Therefore it was decided to extinguish these responses. In their place socially acceptable behaviours were substituted and reinforced. David was rewarded every time he did not vomit, and he was encouraged to gain attention from other patients through social interaction rather than with staff. After a number of months extinguishing undesirable behaviours and reinforcing positive

ones, David stopped vomiting at meal times and was able to gain the attention he desired from everyday interaction with other patients.

Punishment

If it is necessary under certain conditions to use punishment, then it should always be used in conjunction with positive reinforcement. Punishing a behaviour will, if successful, extinguish it and leave a 'vacuum'. This vacuum may be filled by some other behaviour worse than the first. Therefore one needs to substitute an appropriate behaviour and reinforce it to maintain control over the variables.

Another feature of punishment is the need for it to be administered as soon as possible after the event. If this does not happen, then punishment can have an opposite effect. Consider parents who spank their children a considerable time after the misdemeanour. If the child fails to make the connection between the punishment and the behaviour to be extinguished then there is no reason to suppose that the child will cease to perform that behaviour. Worse, the child may come to believe that it is perfectly acceptable to hit others without cause, since that is exactly what his parents do.

Bee (1989) thinks that whatever short-term benefits may accrue from spanking, there are three long-term effects to consider: (a) the child observes the adult using force to solve problems and may model her behaviour accordingly. Telling a child that it is all right for adults to do this but not for children will have little effect since children will do what adults do, not what they say; (b) by repeatedly pairing the parent's presence with unpleasant events, the positive value of the parent is undermined. After a while, this may result in the beneficial effects of positive reinforcement being reduced; so (c) anger is frequently associated with spanking. Young children can read facial expressions quite clearly, thus an atmosphere of rejection is created instead of warmth and caring. There are other forms of punishment besides physical punishment and it is suggested that other forms of control should be used (Patterson 1975).

Time-out

This is a procedure designed to isolate the person from an environment that is creating disruptive behaviour. Nordquist (1971) described how the time-out technique was used to control the tantrum behaviour of a 5-year-old boy. The boy refused to do what his parents said and was particularly disruptive just before bedtime. He used to kick, scream, throw objects, hit his parents and his younger sister as well. He also frequently wet his bed. An analysis of the parent–child interaction was performed. This revealed that when the boy was quiet, the parents took this opportunity to talk to each other or read a book. When the boy started to be disruptive they very quickly responded to this behaviour. The time-out programme started by asking the parents to stop maintaining his disruptive behaviour by discontinuing to bargain with the child and threaten him. They were told to place the child in a corner of his bedroom for 10 minutes whenever he refused to obey his parents' instructions. All bed wetting was ignored. After a while the boy's disruptive behaviour ceased and so too did his bed wetting. Douglas (1992) describes the use of this technique in greater detail with 'problem children'.

Systematic desensitisation

This is a technique designed by Wolpe (1958) which is particularly effective in dealing with phobias. It is based on the principle that a response that is antagonistic to anxiety in the presence of anxiety-provoking stimuli will weaken the bond between the anxious response and the stimuli that elicit it. The technique has three stages: (a) muscle relaxation; (b) development of a hierarchy of anxieties; (c) countering the conditioning. The following case history reported by Rardin (1969) illustrates the technique in action.

An 18-year-old first-year student nurse was very nervous about seeing blood and had felt anxious about it for a number of years. However, it had not been a serious concern until she entered nursing. She reacted to the sight of blood with discomfort, dizziness and nausea. When faced with films depicting various medical conditions, on many occasions she had to leave the room for she felt that she would faint or vomit if she continued to look at the film. Not surprisingly, this phobia interfered considerably with her performance as a nurse.

Before starting the systematic desensitisation programme a fear hierarchy was constructed, including items that included blood resulting from surgery, injury and childbirth. Then the programme would start with asking the subject to visualise an instance of the anxiety-provoking stimulus and getting her to rate her anxiety on a scale from 1 to 10. The therapist, during this period, would provide continual reinforcement relating to her ability to cope with the stimulus.

Slowly the subject would work through ever more anxiety-provoking situations with the therapist asking the subject to quantify her anxiety and then providing positive reinforcement, until the subject was able to maintain control over her anxiety. It should be noted that the technique does not remove the anxiety engendered by the stimulus, but enables the person to manage her anxiety to such an extent that she is able to cope with situations that previously would have been unthinkable. After 1 year, the nurse in question was able to cope with the most anxiety-provoking situation in her hierarchy.

More recent research has suggested that the basic technique proposed by Wolpe has some flaws. Miller & Morley (1986) suggest that graded hierarchies are not necessary and the development of a deliberately induced counter-response is not necessary either. Further, a close relationship between therapist and patient is not important. Nevertheless, the technique has proved successful in many cases of anxiety and phobia.

Applications

Two programmes of behaviour modification will be considered as they illustrate not only the wide variation in the application of the technique, but also an indication of how programmes are operationalised. The first concentrates on the reduction of obesity. Many millions of people are overweight and some wish to do something about it. Often, peoples' attempts to lose weight prove unsuccessful; Jeffrey (1976) provides an example of one technique that may help individuals to obtain the weight loss they desire. Secondly, behaviour modification has been applied to marriage guidance. If it can help promote marital harmony, as Hops (1976) suggests, then it is worth careful consideration.

Obesity

The first point to make is that punishment and avoidance procedures have proved consistently ineffective in the reduction of obesity. Rather than focusing on just weight loss, it is more important to influence eating and exercise habits. Jeffrey (1976) describes an obesity reduction programme consisting of three stages: assessment, treatment and maintenance.

Assessment. This stage consists of three 1-hour interviews with the client/patient. The first interview is concerned with establishing a 'baseline'. The therapist introduces the programme to the client and discusses the components. The client is asked to complete an inventory to determine onset of obesity, previous attempts to lose weight, eating habits, exercise patterns, reasons for wanting to lose weight and whether any of the person's social networks will help or hinder the programme. The therapist stresses the importance of keeping a daily record of the person's weight, food consumed and all physical activity.

The second interview evaluates the client's self-monitored weight, eating and exercise habits. Such items as snacking, 'binges' and particular situations that elict eating are analysed. The advantages of staying obese or doing something about it are discussed. Then a behavioural contract is prepared which specifies the required guidelines and the consequences of not fulfilling them. If a contingency contract is used, then a certain amount of money, or equivalent, is deposited with the therapist only to be returned on completion of the relevant stages in the programme.

The third interview reviews the programme and the contract. If the client desires, she can opt out of the programme. The terms of the contract are agreed and both the therapist and the client sign a contract document.

Treatment. This, too, is divided into three phases. Phase one is concerned with food and exercise management. The client is given guidance on the sorts of foods to eat and a food-exchange plan is constructed. The individual is allowed to eat within his food preferences, but these have to lead to a weekly weight loss of between 1 and 4 pounds.

Food buying habits need to be altered. The client is told to buy only those foods that meet the agreed list of food-exchange diet requirements. The individual is instructed to prepare a list before shopping and to buy items only from the list. Also, he is told never to shop when hungry and to avoid buying extra quantities of food.

Food that is out of sight is often out of mind. It is essential to store food so that it cannot be easily reached or seen. Placing food in cupboards and in opaque containers can help. Menus are constructed that include some of the client's favourite foods as well as the food-exchange items. Smaller portions on smaller plates are also encouraged.

Sometimes people eat so fast that they are unaware of when they are full up. Eating is meant to be an enjoyable experience, therefore patients are encouraged to eat slowly and savour each bite. Putting smaller amounts of food on the fork, pausing between mouthfuls and stopping eating when the stomach feels slightly full, help to regulate food consumption.

As soon as the meal is over, leave the table. Often overweight people will remain at the table and finish off any leftovers. A solution is to buy and prepare smaller portions of food, but when this is impractical, it is perfectly all right to encourage people to leave food they do not want on the plate.

Snacking is a primary cause of overeating. Sometimes it is necessary to develop a specific plan to counteract snacking, for example, substituting low-calorie foods for the usual snacks will result in a smaller calorific intake. Skipping meals to indulge in snacks is often a problem. If individuals are encouraged to eat at regular intervals, snacking can be reduced.

Family and friends must be encouraged to help and not hinder the individual in his attempt to lose weight. They should be asked not to criticise obesity but reward progress in the programme; to buy and prepare low-calorie meals; to talk about other things than food and engage in non-food activities.

Stress and anxiety are often managed by eating more. Clients should be taught new ways of handling stressful circumstances other than eating more food. Exercise and hobbies can be substituted as alternative ways of managing stressful circumstances.

The final feature of this phase is the development of an exercise plan. It is often helpful to engage the help of a friend to exercise with the individual. Arranging a daily activity that fits in with the client's regular schedule facilitates activity. It might be considered useful if the client enrols in a health club or physical fitness class.

The second phase in the treatment programme examines the problems that the client may be experiencing with the programme. The client is encouraged to provide his own rewards when he meets his weight-management goals.

The third phase in this section focuses on stabilising new eating and exercise habits. The client is encouraged to continue rewarding himself as he continues to lose weight. As the desired goals are achieved, a proportion of the initial monetary deposit is refunded.

Maintenance. The emphasis of this stage is the maintenance of eating and exercise habits to preserve the weight loss. The meetings with the therapist become shorter but if problems are encountered, then access to guidance should be easy. Some contact should be maintained for a year, at which point the rest of the client's money is returned, if he has maintained his desired weight loss.This programme will only work if the person genuinely desires to lose weight and is motivated to do so; little can be done for the individual who refuses treatment.

This type of technique can be applied to other problems such as drug abuse, smoking and sexual problems (Craighead et al 1976). However, one other example of behaviour modification will be described that deals with personal relationships, a context not always thought to be affected by behavioural outcomes.

Marriage guidance

The behavioural approach to relationships is based on mutual reward. Relationships are maintained as long as both members continue to supply each other with positive reinforcement. If both partners cease to provide appropriate rewards, the relationship breaks down and the couple drifts apart. Unfortunately, married individuals have signed a contract to stay with each other for life and there are legal, social and religious sanctions to prohibit them from divorcing. Many couples stay together in the most disharmonious circumstances rather than go through a divorce. Although approximately one marriage in three ends in divorce, it is quite surprising that the numbers are not greater. A couple may have to face illnesses, financial difficulties, changes in homes and jobs, the needs of children, the attractiveness of others etc. If one considers the lack of practice in learning how to live together in difficult circumstances, the divorce rate might not seem so surprising at all.

An example of an unsatisfactory relationship in behavioural terms is provided by Hops (1976) who cites the case of the husband who comes home from work and, as the marriage is in its infancy, is eager to discuss his day at work with his wife. However, as the marriage progresses the frequency of this behaviour decreases. The husband, who is talking and interacting with people all day is satiated but his wife is anxious to talk and starts to ask a lot of questions. Unfortunately, the husband is exhausted and just wants to put his feet up in front of the television and maybe read the newspaper. A likely result of this behaviour is the continual nagging of the wife to try and get some response from her husband. Hops (1976) says that this is one of the most frequently noted scenarios reported by marital therapists. A sequel to this behaviour pattern is the establishment of mutual punishment rather than reinforcement. In order to get some reaction from her husband, the wife may punish him in some way. He in turn responds with some verbal jibe and mutual punishment ensues. The result is often long silences at meal times and boring, lifeless evenings.

A behavioural programme designed to help married couples is described by Hops (1976). There are four stages:

- pinpointing
- communication skills training
- problem solving and negotiation
- contingency contracting.

Pinpointing

Before any change in behaviour can take place, it is necessary to pinpoint those behaviours that need changing. Many couples are unable to discriminate between positive and negative behaviour and use broad undefined statements to describe each other. 'He always treats me like dirt' and 'She doesn't love me any more' are statements that fail to define precisely the problem. Statements like 'He never kisses or hugs me' are much more precise and pinpoint the problem in behavioural terms. Couples are taught to specify behaviours precisely and are then given the task of recording behaviours that produce pleasure or displeasure in their spouse. In this way, a list is produced of the exact behaviours that need to be changed by the couple.

Communication skills training

One result of pinpointing may be an increase in communication between the partners, but in the majority of circumstances, some training in communication skills is required. Sometimes people are so intent on getting over their own point of view that they fail to listen to what their partners are saying. The first communication skill to learn is the ability to listen to what the other person is saying. In certain situations it is necessary to teach a person to paraphrase his or her partner's last few sentences in order to ensure active listening.

Sharing the time spent speaking to each other is another important communication skill. Many interactions are dominated by one person so that the partner cannot 'get a word in edgeways'. Training can take the form of both partners speaking for a set period of time, say 2 minutes, with active listening to the content of the conversation.

Some people have nonverbal responses that are 'put-down' behaviour. Often individuals who behave in this way are unaware of the effect that they have on their spouses. Therefore, it is necessary to give them feedback about what they look like when behaving in this way. Couples are taught to reduce their aversive verbal behaviours. They are asked to think of something positive the spouse has done during the week and state it. If a verbal or nonverbal put-down occurs as a response, it is pointed out to the client.

Problem solving and negotiation training

The goal of this stage is to provide couples with the skills necessary to solve problems together. A wife complained to her partner that he never hung up his clothes in the bedroom. He replied that he would hang them up if the wardrobe was not full up with all her clothes that she never used. The argument continued until the wife compromised by saying that she would make space in the wardrobe if he would agree to hang his clothes up more often. He agreed. The solution was facilitated by the wife's ability to compromise and seek a mutual solution to the problem.

Contingency contracting

If the previous three stages have failed to help the couple reconcile their problems, contingency contracting can be used. This represents the final stage in the behavioural approach to marriage guidance. Contracts are set up between the two individuals concerning their behaviour toward each other. The couple get together and discuss those features of each other's behaviour that they find rewarding and those they find unrewarding. They then discuss the types of rewards that they would like if they behave in the desired fashion.

The contract is not permanent and can be renegotiated. Notice that there is no mention of love and affection in this approach. Psycho-logists who adopt the behavioural perspective are only concerned with the modification of observed behaviours; they do not study the thoughts and emotions of people and have been criticised for neglecting to do so. Nevertheless, in some circumstances, behaviour modification can help individuals implement behaviour changes that otherwise would have remained incomplete.

REFERENCES

Allen V L, Levine J M 1971 Social support and conformity: the role of the independent assessment of reality. Journal of Experimental Social Psychology 4: 48–58

Asch S E 1951 Effects of group pressure on the modification and distortion of judgement. In: Guetzkow H (ed) Groups, leadership, and men. Carnegie, Pittsburgh

Bales R F 1958 Task roles and social roles in problem-solving groups. In: Maccoby E E, Newcombe M, Hartley E L (eds) Readings in social psychology, 3rd edn. Holt Rinehart Winston, New York

Bee H 1989 The developing child, 5th edn. Harper Row, New York

Bisanz G I, Rule B G 1989 Gender and the persuasion schema. Personality and Social Psychology Bulletin 15: 4–18

Bond N A 1974 Basic strategy and expectation in casino blackjack. Organisational Behaviour and Human Performance 12: 413–428

Bourne L E, Dominowski R L, Loftus E F, Healy A F 1986 Cognitive processes, 2nd edn. Prentice Hall, Englewood Cliffs NJ

Burnstein E 1983 Persuasion as argument processing. In: Brandstatter M, Davis J, Stocker-Kreichgauer G (eds) Group decision processes. Academic Press, London

Cialdini R B 1993 Influence: science and practice, 3rd edn. Harper Collins, New York

Cialdini R B, Vincent J E, Lewis S K, Catalan J, Wheeler D, Darby B L 1975 Reciprocal concessions procedure for producing compliance: the door-in-the-face technique. Journal of Personality and Social Psychology 31: 206–215

Cialdini R B, Cocioppo J T, Bass H R, Miller J A 1978 Low-ball procedure for producing compliance: commitment then cost. Journal of Personality and Social Psychology 36: 463–476

Craig K D, Prkachin K M 1978 Social modelling influences on sensory decision theory and psychophysiological indexes of pain. Journal of Personality and Social Psychology. 36: 805–815

Craighead W E, Kazdin A E, Mahoney M S 1976 (eds) Behaviour modification: principles, issues, and applications. Houghton Mifflin, Boston

Crutchfield R A 1955 Conformity and character. American Psychologist 10: 191–198

Douglas J 1992 Behaviour problems in young children. Routledge, London

Freedman J L, Fraser S C 1966 Compliance without pressure: the foot-in-the-door technique. Journal of Personality and Social Psychology 4: 195–202

Freedman J L, Wallington S A 1967 Compliance without pressure: the effect of guilt. Journal of Personality and Social Psychology 7: 117–124

Hops H 1976 Behavioural treatment of marital problems. In: Craighead W E, Kazdin A E, Mahoney M S (eds) Behaviour modification. Houghton Mifflin, Boston

Janis I L 1982 Groupthink, 2nd edn. Houghton Mifflin, Boston

Jeffrey D B 1976 Behavioural management of obesity. In: Craighead W E, Kazdin A E, Mahoney M S (eds) Behaviour modification. Houghton Mifflin, Boston

Kahneman D, Tversky A 1979 Prospect theory: an analysis of decision under risk. Econometrica 47: 263–291

Kahneman D, Tversky A 1982 On the study of statistical intuitions. Cognition 11: 123–142

Kilham W, Mann L 1974 Level of destructive obedience as a function of transmitter and executant roles in the Milgram obedience paradigm. Journal of Personality and Social Psychology 29: 696–702

Lichtenstein S, Slovic P, Fischoff B, Layman M, Coombs B 1978 Judged frequency of lethal events. Journal of Experimental Psychology: Human Learning and Memory 4: 551–578

Liden R C, Mitchell T R 1988 Ingratiatory behaviors in organizational settings. Academy of Management Review 13: 572–587

McCauley C 1989 The nature of social influence in groupthink. Journal of Personality and Social Psychology 57: 250–260

Milgram S 1963 Behavioural study of obedience. Journal of Abnormal and Social Psychology 67: 371–378

Milgram S 1974 Obedience to authority. Harper Row, New York

Miller E, Morley S 1986 Investigating abnormal behavior. Erlbaum, Chichester

Morris W N, Miller R S, Spangenberg S 1977 The effects of dissenter position and task difficulty on conformity and response to conflict. Journal of Personality 45: 251–266

Nordhoy F 1962 Group interaction and decision making under risk. Unpublished Masters thesis. School of Industrial Management, MIT, Mass.

Nordquist V M 1971 The modification of a child's enuresis: some response–response relationships. Journal of Applied Behavioural Analysis 4: 241–247

Patterson G R 1975 Families: applications of social learning to family life. Research Press, Champaign Ill

Rardin M 1969 Treatment of a phobia by partial self-desensitization. Journal of Consulting and Clinical Psychology 33: 125–126

Stoner J A F 1961 A comparison of individual and group decisions involving risk. In: Brown R (ed) Social psychology. Free Press, New York

Whyte W H 1956 The organization man. Simon & Schuster, New York

Wilder D A 1977 Perception of groups, size of opposition, and social influence. Journal of Experimental Social Psychology 13: 253–268

Wolpe J 1958 Psychotherapy by reciprocal inhibition. Stanford University Press, Stanford

RECOMMENDED READING

Cialdini R A 1993 Influence: science and practice, 3rd edn. Harper Collins, New York
This is an excellent book not only for the 'easy to read' style, but also because it provides an invaluable insight into the ways we are influenced by other people. It is backed up by the author's prodigous research.

Craighead W E, Kazdin A E, Mahoney M S 1982 (eds) Behavior modification: principles, issues, and applications, 2nd edn. Houghton Mifflin, Boston
This book contains a practical review of the use of behaviour modification in a wide range of settings including a number of chapters on the application of behaviour modification to health care settings.

Janis I L 1982 Groupthink, 2nd edn. Houghton Mifflin, Boston

A very readable account of the processes involved in groupthink. Illustrated by a number of examples where groupthink has led to disastrous decisions being made by eminent people.

Kahneman D, Tversky A 1982 On the study of statistical intuitions. Cognition 11: 123–142
Contains a wealth of information on the psychological factors that influence decision making. Sometimes a good deal of concentration is required to follow the logic of the arguments but such effort is well worth the while.

Milgram S 1974 Obedience to authority. Harper Row, New York

Wright G N 1984 Behavioural decision theory. Penguin, Harmondsworth

Answers to the decision-making questions

1. (b)
2. Neither
3. An 8 in 10 chance
4. All three
5. Patient B
6. No
7. The second item in each pair.

Content

4

Psychobiological perspective: pain and stress

This chapter deals with two of the most important features of psychobiological behaviour: pain and stress. The emphasis is upon how pain and stress may be managed and how the maladaptive consequences can be reduced. Pain is defined and examined in terms of the factors that influence pain and the techniques for reducing it. Similarly stress is defined in terms of cognitive appraisal with a view to discussing the effectiveness of stress management techniques.

The term 'psychobiology' has been applied to the scientific study of the relation between biological processes and behaviour (Taylor et al 1982). However, in the context of health psychology, the term has been used to distinguish the psychological approach to health and disease from the biochemical approach. Accordingly, some authors have included topics that had little to do with biology (patient compliance, illness behaviour and behaviour modification). This chapter uses the term to refer to areas in health psychology that have a connection with biology or physiology. Two important psychobiological areas of health psychology are undoubtedly pain and stress. Both have physiological components but, it is argued, are psychologically determined. The experience of pain and stress takes different forms (acute, chronic), yet an examination of these forms is particularly difficult since one is unable to experience the stress and pain of someone else. Most would agree on the need to reduce both pain and stress, but how to do it is another matter. This chapter investigates the nature of the concepts themselves, looks at the factors that influence the experience of pain and stress, but, more importantly, tries to establish ways in which individuals can learn to manage pain and stress and reduce the negative consequences to tolerable levels.

THE NATURE OF PAIN

Melzack (1973) reports the case of the young Canadian student who was highly intelligent and seemed perfectly normal apart from having never felt pain at any time during her life. When she was a child she had bitten off the tip of her tongue while chewing food and had burnt herself after kneeling on a hot radiator to look out of a window. She apparently felt no pain in response to electric shock, scalding water and an ice-bath. 'Equally astonishing was the fact that she showed no changes in blood pressure, heart rate or respiration when these stimuli were presented' (Melzack 1973).

This example of congenital insensitivity to pain, whilst rare, illustrates that pain is much more than a simple sensory experience. It might seem desirable never to feel pain but in fact it is a serious disorder placing the individual in a very dangerous position. The girl mentioned above died at the age of 29. As pain is such a complex phenomenon, it is proposed to answer three questions. What is pain? What factors influence pain? What can be done to reduce pain?

WHAT IS PAIN?

The first distinction to make is between *sensory pain* and *reaction to pain.* Sensory pain refers to the pain threshold. At some point stimulation becomes painful, at another point it becomes unbearable. These points differ from individual to individual, that is some individuals will feel pain when others do not; some people will be able to withstand more pain than others. Reaction to pain is the observable component. We can only assess the degree of pain by observing individuals' reactions to pain, for we cannot feel another person's pain. Again there are large individual and cultural differences in the ways

in which reactions to pain manifest themselves. This distinction presumes that we can actually discriminate between sensory pain and reaction to pain.

Unfortunately this is not quite so simple since objective methods designed to quantify pain rely almost exclusively on measuring people's reactions to pain in some way or another. Wall (1984) states that an alternative way of viewing pain is that it is a *need state,* just like hunger and thirst. In other words, the purpose of hunger is to remind the body that it needs food. The purpose of thirst is to remind the body that it needs water. The purpose of pain is to signal to the body impending injury or that it needs to rest. This description might be applicable to acute pain but is not necessarily applicable to chronic pain, which is the second distinction.

People show a differential response to acute and chronic pain. Sternbach (1968, 1984) said that the physiological, subjective and psychological responses to acute pain were different to those of chronic pain. Acute pain involved often short-lived and reversible discomfort. Further, the relationship of injury to pain is extremely variable after acute injury. There are periods of time when the person may be pain free; when the body is capable of producing its own analgesic in certain sites of the body, thus enabling the person to function independently of the injury. Chronic pain often has no identifiable cause, is not transient and involves intense psychological adjustment. Some of the signs associated with chronic pain are sleep disturbance, verbal attacks on others, decreased activity, depression, lowered pain tolerance, exhaustion and fatigue. The majority of research has been concerned with the examination of acute pain under 'laboratory' conditions, but this does not represent the majority of pain as many people suffer from chronic pain. The distinction between acute and chronic pain is particularly important when considering methods to control pain later in this chapter.

There are three major theories of pain. The first two rely heavily on purely physiological components, and the third includes psychological factors.

Specificity theory

The idea that there are specific pathways responsible for transmitting pain messages to a centre in the brain originated with the French philosopher, René Descartes. In 1894, however, von Frey presented a model proposing that the quality of skin sensation (touch, cold, warm, pain) depends, initially, on the type of sensory nerve endings stimulated. The difference in structure of these nerve endings makes them highly sensitive to one kind of stimulus and unresponsive to others. Pain is associated with stimulation of the *free nerve endings*. This model proved oversimplistic, as it was found that stimulation of free nerve endings was also capable of eliciting other sensations. When the outer part of the ear is stimulated, the individual experiences warmth, cold, touch, itch and pain. This is strange, since there are only free nerve endings in this part of the ear.

Lyn (1984) has pointed to a number of structures within the nervous system that contribute to pain. Two groups of nerve fibres have been implicated: the myelinated A-delta fibres; and the unmyelinated C fibres. Some investigators believe that the A-delta fibres mediate immediate or sharp pain, whereas C fibres mediate dull or aching pain. Thoracic and abdominal organs differ from skin in many respects. They are relatively protected from injury, and have a different type of nerve supply. Most thoracic and visceral tissues can be the source of severe pain, though the damage usually has to be quite extensive before it becomes painful. However, the passage of renal stones (minimal tissue damage) may cause severe pain. Further, the localisation of pain from these areas is not good; gall bladder pathology can give rise to pains in the shoulder. There is no evidence for the pain centre in the brain as postulated by von Frey. Specificity theory does help to explain why injury is perceived as pain. Pain is felt when pain pathways are stimulated. The theory does not explain essentially psychological features of pain such as phantom limb pain, congenital insensitivity to pain and environmental factors that distract the individual to the extent that no pain at all is perceived.

Pattern theory

Pattern theories relate pain perception to particular patterns of impulses in the nervous system. Pain may occur with any kind of stimulation as long as the stimulation is excessive. Anything very hot, very cold, or pressing very hard on the skin causes pain. The differences in quantity, rather than quality, of peripheral nerve fibre discharge produce differences in quality of sensation. Small stimulation of the cornea causes a feeling of touch, whereas strong stimulation causes pain. The same kind of nerve fibres are discharging, but the difference in sensation is due to an increased discharge and spatial summation of the effect.

Livingstone (1943) put forward a theory suggesting that reverberating circuits sent volleys of impulses to the brain which were interpreted as pain. These reverberating circuits have been put forward to explain the presence of pain even when there are nerve lesions and the nervous system is no longer intact. Minimal stimulation can set them off. Thus the pattern theory is able to account for minimal and maximal tactile stimuli.

Gate control theory

The central idea of gate control theory is the presence of neural mechanisms in the spinal cord which can somehow 'close a gate', and so prevent pain messages from travelling to the brain. There are certain neurons (interneurons) located in the spinal cord which receive input from two sources:

- nerve fibres carrying pain messages
- nerve fibres carrying information from the skin senses such as temperature and pressure.

When the interneurons are stimulated mainly by fibres from the skin senses, the 'gate' is closed, and pain messages arriving at the spinal cord are blocked. In contrast, when the interneurons are stimulated mainly by fibres carrying pain messages, they are inhibited, the gate remains open and pain messages reaching the spinal cord are transmitted onward to the brain. The whole process bears some relation to the old adage 'rubbing it makes it better'. There still remains the question of accounting for such phenomena as phantom limb pain. Melzack & Wall (1965) propose that information descending from the brain can also open and close the gate. Thus psychological factors such as past experience, emotional state and the meaning of the situation can affect the perception of pain.

The validity of gate control theory has been debated over the past 15 years. The majority of discussions have centred on the exact nature of the specific anatomical and neurophysiological mechanisms that can account for triggering the perceived pain. Melzack & Wall (1965) assumed that the substantia gelatinosa was the primary vehicle for the gating process, but there were questions regarding the exact function of the substantia gelatinosa in the gate model. These questions led to a revision of the theory (Melzack & Wall 1988).

This revision attempted to state the multiple functions of the substantia gelatinosa; to propose a descending inhibitory input to the gate and to provide evidence for neuropeptide involvement. As yet there is still doubt regarding the exact location and function of elements of the gate control theory, nevertheless, it represents a useful conceptual tool in the area of pain research. It is the best we have got.

The experience of pain is comprised of three components:

- sensory/perceptual
- emotional
- cognitive.

The sensory/perceptual system transmits basic sensory information, such as the location of pain in the body and whether it is a burning, aching or piercing pain. Essentially it provides information about where we hurt and what it feels like. The emotional component influences the degree to which we desire to escape from pain, by either removing the pain source or removing ourselves. It also includes our emotional response to pain. The cognitive aspect of pain determines the meaning of the sensory experience. Pain after a serious car accident may signal rest and relaxation, whereas the pain of terminal cancer may signal frustration, anger and guilt. This latter appraisal may make the pain more difficult to tolerate.

FACTORS INFLUENCING PAIN

The majority of the research investigating the factors influencing pain has been concerned with pain tolerance as opposed to pain threshold. There has also been a disproportionate emphasis on laboratory pain stimulation as opposed to research on clinical pain. Some of the factors that have been thought to influence mainly pain tolerance are: degree of injury, culture, anxiety and personality.

Degree of injury

Beecher (1959) compared US soldiers injured on the battlefield with civilians hospitalised for major surgery. He found that 4 out of 5 hospitalised patients requested morphine, as compared with approximately 1 in 3 of the soldiers. As this was not a function of shock or trauma-induced analgesia, Beecher suggested that the meaning of the situation was affecting the pain being felt. The soldiers' pain was offset by the fact that they had escaped death on the battlefield, whereas the civilians' pain had singularly negative connotations. Thus the degree of injury is not necessarily proportional to the amount of pain experienced.

Culture

Melzack (1973) presents evidence of the way in which culture can affect the experience of pain. In some remote Indian villages, an annual hook swinging ceremony takes place. Two steel hooks are placed into the lower back of a youth who is to experience the ceremony. He is then hoisted on to a pole and transported from village to village. During the whole of this process the youth displays no pain whatsoever, despite what must appear to be excruciating pain. Of course, we are unable to measure the degree of pain experienced and can only infer from the youth's reaction that little pain was present. However, there are observable cultural differences in response to pain.

Zborowski (1969) reports that behavioural expressions of pain differ among ethnic groups of patients in medical settings. The differences were thought to be due to the attitudes and values of the ethnic groups. Third-generation Americans tended to respond to the pain in a matter of fact way, and acted as if they should be 'good, uncomplaining patients'. The Irish were similar in their pain expressions, but their suffering was communicated to observers. On the other hand, more overt responses to the pain were forthcoming from Italian and Jewish subcultures. The Italians felt that pain had to be avoided at all costs, and their expressions were aimed at the elimination of the pain. The Jewish group were more concerned with the memory of pain and its implications.

The idea that culture in its broadest terms affects the expression of pain and the view that health professionals should be aware of these differences is laudable, but care must be taken to avoid falling into the trap of stereotyping patients' pain responses on the basis of their cultural origin. Davitz & Davitz (1985) said that if nurses are asked directly about the question of cultural stereotypes and pain, they resent any implication that they operate on the basis of cultural stereotypes. To find out whether nurses are influenced by stereotypes they presented American nurses with a brief vignette describing an adult patient (see Box 4.1).

The experimenters first of all varied the cultural background of the person, so that each patient had the same physical condition, age and sex but a different ethnic background. The

six ethnic background variables were: Oriental, Mediterranean, Black, Spanish, Anglo-Saxon/Germanic and Jewish. They also investigated varying the severity of the illness (mild, moderate and severe). The mean ratings of physical pain and psychological distress for each group of patients and for each level of severity of illness were measured.

For both physical pain and psychological distress, nurses believed that Jewish and Spanish patients suffered most, while Oriental and Anglo-Saxon/Germanic patients suffered the least. Jewish patients were perceived as suffering relatively greater pain and psychological distress in cases of psychiatric and cardiovascular illnesses.

Davitz & Davitz (1985) say:

> The results of this research clearly indicate that one aspect of American nurses' belief systems about suffering involves the ethnic or religious backgrounds of their patients. In discussing our research with nurses, we have found that some nurses react defensively to our findings. They strenuously insist that they never generalise, that they treat all patients as individuals. That may indeed be the case for particular nurses, but our data do indicate that in general, American nurses in fact tend to share certain generalised beliefs about patients.

To summarise, whilst one cannot objectively measure the experience of pain, the fact that people in excruciating circumstances do not seem to be in pain due to the social nature of the event suggests that culture may indeed affect the pain experience. Secondly, there does seem to be consistent evidence that people from different cultures and subcultures respond to pain in overtly different ways. Thirdly, stereotypical views of pain are held by health professionals.

Box 4.1 Sample vignette

Name of patient: Michael O'Hara
Age: 37
Background: Irish

Michael O'Hara, struck by an automobile, was admitted to the hospital with a fractured femur and facial injuries. Currently in traction, he is to remain hospitalised for an indefinite period.

Anxiety and personality

Anxiety can have a considerable effect on both the quality and intensity of the pain experiences. Patients who are anxious are more sensitive to pain and, as might be predicted from this, neurotic patients (who generally have high levels of anxiety) complain of pain more than others (Rachman & Philips 1975). Pain threshold is reduced in the presence of elevated anxiety and anxiety contributes to the aversiveness of the pain experience. The fear of pain or anticipation of high pain levels will increase anxiety, which in turn will lead to a self-fulfilling prophecy, because an increase in anxiety will lead to an increase in pain sensitivity (Melzack 1973).

Walding (1991) found that there was a relationship between pain, anxiety and perceived powerlessness. She suggested that each of the three factors affected each other and that a decreasing perception of powerlessness lessened the postoperative pain experience. Bond (1971) studied 52 women with cancer of the cervix to see how their personality traits and attitudes to disease related to the pain they felt and to their complaints. He found that pain-free patients were less emotional and more sociable, while patients experiencing pain but not complaining of it were emotional but not sociable. The patients who were both sociable and emotional experienced and complained of considerable pain and received most attention. Further research by Bond et al (1976) has indicated that introverts are more sensitive to pain stimuli, but extroverts complain more at lower levels of pain.

Finally, Connolly et al (1978) investigated the relationship between personality, anxiety and pain during the labour of childbirth. The sample of 80 women were given the Minnesota Multiphasic Personality Inventory and their pain/anxiety levels were monitored during the labour. Not surprisingly, pain and anxiety levels rose during the course of the labour. Pain and anxiety were similar for normal and 'hysterical' MMPI groups but the 'anxious–depressive' MMPI groups displayed higher levels of pain and anxiety. Sternbach (1968) reviewed several studies that had investigated the relationship between anxiety and pain. He concluded that increasing anxiety enhanced pain responses, and decreasing anxiety reduced such responses.

Memory for pain

Lander et al (1992) examined 138 children aged between 5–17 years who were attending an outpatient lab for venipuncture. The children reported their anxiety and expected pain: before venipuncture, immediately after and 2 months after their visit. Four patterns of responses were identified when prediction recall and accuracy were examined. The largest group (n = 74) was labelled 'realistic' since experienced and recalled pain scores were comparable. Many children in this group also had expected pain that was equivalent to experienced and recalled pain. A second group was identified for whom the experience seemed irrelevant (n = 23). Recalled and expected pain were the same no matter whether the experienced pain was high or low. A third group was designated overreactors because more pain was recalled than had been experienced or expected (n = 23). Finally, the last group was labelled the denial group as they recalled having very little pain despite expecting and experiencing mid- to high levels of pain. The findings indicate that memory for pain is not always accurate and that children possess different types of coping strategy to deal with painful experiences.

PAIN REDUCTION AND MODIFICATION

The most common method for reducing pain is the pharmacological approach and the use of drugs, but there are a number of psychological approaches that have been put forward to modify tolerance and thresholds of pain.

Acupuncture

The ancient Chinese believed that all life energy flowed through meridians, or pathways, radiating throughout the body under the skin. Too much life energy passing through these meridians caused pain and could be reduced by the insertion of needles at certain points in the body. Whilst there is no evidence to support the existence of the meridians, it has been claimed that the insertion and manipulation of a needle in certain sites in the body can relieve pain. Some Chinese physicians believe in the importance of inserting the needle in the correct site, while others think that the site is irrelevant (Kepes et al 1976). Although the acupuncture process may be ostensibly physiological, some observers have pointed out that the technique may achieve its effects largely through psychological factors. Firstly, only approximately 20% of the population are likely to benefit from acupuncture. Secondly, acupuncture anaesthesia is only practised on selected individuals who have shown themselves to be open to suggestion and easily hypnotised (Taub 1976). The processes involved in acupuncture and hypnotism are not thought to be the same.

Mayer et al (1976) induced pain in subjects by the electric stimulation of a tooth. One group of subjects were given acupuncture and another group of subjects were hypnotised. Acupuncture was found to increase the pain thresholds by about 27%, whereas hypnosis increased the pain threshold by as much as 85%. Following naloxone injections (a pharmacological antagonist), the acupuncture group's pain thresholds dropped drastically. Naloxone was found to have little effect on the hypnosis group. The authors propose that the two processes of acupuncture and hypnosis are quite distinct, the former achieving its effect by stimulating the secretion of morphine-like substances from the central grey matter; the latter achieving its analgesic qualities through higher order cortical mechanisms.

Acupuncture can moderate pain for some people, in some situations, for short periods of time. It has not proved particularly effective in the treatment of chronic pain (Murphy 1976), nor can it be used for the majority of the population. A better bet for psychological research into techniques of pain relief, therefore, would seem to be an analysis of hypnotism.

Hypnotism

Since the days of Dr Cloquet's remarkable claims about the analgesic effects of Mesmerism in over 300 operations, there has been a great deal of interest in the mechanics of Mesmerism, or, as it is now called, hypnotism. A widely held view of hypnosis pictures the hypnotist seated in front of the patient swinging a watch on a chain before the patient's eyes. The actions are accompanied by the hypnotist saying such things as, 'You are going to sleep, you are going to sleep.' The hypnotic procedure is in fact a variable process, and it can involve altering the patient's negative perceptions of pain, enhancing positive self-statements, improving health-related attitudes and developing deep feelings of relaxation that are incompatible with pain.

Barber (1982) reviewed the literature on the use of hypnotism in the treatment of clinical pain. The conclusions were:

- Subjects often show as much pain relief when given suggestions for reduced pain as under hypnosis.
- Many types of suggestion have proved effective in pain relief.
- Those people who are generally highly suggestive respond well to suggestions for reducing pain.
- When subjects are provided with pain relief suggestions, they often use distraction as a technique to relieve the pain.

Barber (1982) has been one of the main protagonists of the position that hypnosis does not involve a unique state of mind or consciousness. He rejected the idea that the state of hypnosis is similar to sleepwalking and proposed a more appropriate analogy of becoming engrossed in a good book. Temporarily, one is unaware of what is going on around and about, becoming totally involved in the world of the book. Thus Barber (1982) suggests that it is just as ridiculous to say that the hypnotised person is in a trance as it is to say that a person engrossed in a novel is in a trance. The idea that concentrating hard on a particular task blocks out pain sensations is quite commonplace.

Pennebaker (1984) relates this to the cognitive components of the sensations emanating from the body, that is, one is apt to feel more pain when the external environment is boring than when it is able to absorb the individual. Similarly one is less conscious of pain if the external environment is particularly stimulating.

Hilgard & Hilgard (1975) believe that suggestions may reduce pain by modifying the emotional response to pain (teaching the person to relax in the presence of pain), whereas hypnosis actually blocks a major portion of the pain response from awareness. They cite as evidence the *hidden observer* phenomenon. A hypnotised subject is required to immerse one arm in a bucket of ice-cold water while under the suggestion to feel no pain in that arm. The subject is asked to rate how much pain she is experiencing in her arm on a scale of 1 to 10. The typical report is 0. The subject had also been instructed to record the degree of pain on the same numerical scale, using the arm that had not been hypnotised. Whilst the subject was overtly reporting 0 pain, the hand out of awareness was writing 2, 5, 7, and 9. The hidden observer was reporting essentially normal pain while the hypnotised part of the subject was experiencing no pain at all. The experimenters suggest that the mind is capable of blocking and monitoring pain at the same time. Olness (1989) has commented that more than 80% of children over the age of 2 years can benefit from hypnosis used in action and emergency settings, even though the children have had no experience of hypnosis.

Cognitive restructuring

The occurrence of pain may sometimes be anticipated before the event. Particular attention has been paid to psychological preparation with an emphasis on enhancing 'cognitive control'. There are two forms of cognitive control: informational control and strategic control.

Informational control

This involves the provision of information which enables the individual to predict accurately what is about to happen to him. Johnson (1975) exposed male subjects to pain in the laboratory. One group was given information regarding the physical sensations they might expect as a result of the procedure. Another group was given information about the procedure, but no information about the sorts of sensation to expect. It was found that the information about the sorts of physical sensation to expect significantly reduced the distress, whereas merely providing information about the procedure itself was no different from a control group who had no instructions. The intensity of the sensations experienced was the same for both groups. More accurate expectations were associated with less distress.

Similar findings have been reported in the context of preparation for surgery by Hayward (1975), but, wherever preparation involves a number of additional components, such as reassurance, emotional support and coping techniques, it has been found that information about sensations alone is not enough in itself to significantly reduce distress, but needs to operate in conjunction with the other components to prove effective (Johnson et al 1978).

Strategic control

This is demonstrated by the work of Turk et al (1983). Subjects are encouraged to increase their resistance to stress and pain by firstly being given general instruction about the nature of pain. Secondly, subjects are trained to relax, and are provided with a selection of strategies such as redirecting attention or reinterpreting the whole experience, with which to confront the pain. Thirdly, the subjects are asked to imagine the painful situation and their reaction to it, and subsequently play the role of a teacher instructing someone else in this procedure.

Turk et al (1983) provide evidence of the effectiveness of this procedure in reducing pain. It could be argued that this sort of structural control training requires considerable time and effort on the part of the trainer and the patient and it is not always practical. Of course, in many situations, it is not practicable to go through the whole procedure, but in the context of chronic pain and in other situations where there is sufficient time to prepare the patient, it represents an important step forward in the reduction of distress due to pain.

McCaul & Malott (1984) have reviewed the role of cognitive approaches to pain control and have concluded that distraction is an effective strategy for coping with mild levels of pain.

Sensation redefinition, however, is more effective for higher levels of pain. Thus, an injection, dental drilling and early stages of childbirth would benefit from distraction techniques, whereas sensation focusing and redefinition are more effective in the reduction of higher levels of pain associated with later stages of childbirth, noxious medical procedures and perhaps chronic pain.

Pain behaviour

Since pain can only be a subjective phenomenon, we rely on observations of people's response to pain. As such it has been argued that an approach which concentrates on the observable features of behaviour would have great significance for an analysis of pain. The three learning mechanisms that characterise the learning theory approach are:

- operant conditioning
- classical conditioning
- observational learning.

Reward and punishment are the key concepts in the operant approach to pain. Chronic pain often has little to do with nociceptive activity, and is more often associated with pain in the absence of nociception or with affective and environmental factors. Indeed, Loeser & Fordyce (1983) state that chronic pain and acute pain have nothing in common save for the four letter word pain.

Pain behaviour is frequently related to some form of reward (something desirable happens if the patient manifests pain behaviour, such as attention from one's spouse or financial compensation). Sometimes pain behaviour involves avoidance of something undesirable (such as getting out of a stressful job or avoiding contact with a threatening individual or situation). It might seem that an appropriate response to someone who is in pain is to appear supportive and provide attention and reassurance. According to the operant approach this will only serve to reward the 'pain behaviour' because it rewards the person by giving her attention every time she reports feeling pain. If the individual is rewarded for appearing to be in pain she will do

it more and perhaps subjectively feel more pain as well.

Block et al (1980) obtained information from a sample of patients about how their spouses usually responded to their pain behaviour. The patients were divided into two groups according to whether their spouses were essentially supportive or nonsupportive. The patients were interviewed in a room with a one-way mirror. For half of the interview they were informed that their wife was observing them from behind the mirror; for the other half of the interview they were told that a health professional was watching them and sequence effects were controlled. During each half of the interview, patients were asked how much pain they were experiencing. When the spouse observed the interview, more pain was reported from those individuals who had a supportive spouse than those whose spouse was thought to be nonsupportive. When a 'neutral' health professional observed the interview there was no difference between the two groups with reference to pain. The spouses' presence had, for the supportive spouse subgroup, become a conditioned stimulus, which had evoked increases in pain behaviour. Conversely, where the spouse had come to be discriminated as nonsupportive, a decrease in suffering was reported.

Conditioning can also explain how initially unconnected features of the environment can take on significance for the chronic pain patient. Suppose a person experienced back pain whenever they walked about a 100 feet. Over the course of time, the distance of 100 feet would become associated with the development of the back pain. Thus the person would have become conditioned to responding to the distance of 100 feet rather than the amount of walking and when the critical distance was imminent, increased anxiety about the pain would develop.

Another example of the conditioning process is the case in which a patient with chronic lumbar pain reports consistent aggravation of the pain with muscle spasm in the evening, particularly around the time when he is going off to sleep. He begins to associate the muscle spasm with sleep, experiencing considerable anxiety before going to bed for the evening. This anxiety exacerbates the pain and pain behaviour. The phenomena may occur in relation to movement in certain patients, when such movement produces excruciating increases in pain. Simply the thought of moving can then lead to increased anxiety about the pain, thus increasing the pain and pain behaviour.

The role of modelling behaviour in determining the experience of pain has been illustrated by the work of Craig & Prkachin (1978) in Chapter 3.

Children's pain

It might seem reasonable to suppose that health professionals are particularly sensitive to children suffering from pain. Eland (1985) suggests that this is not the case. She states that 66% of children between the ages of 4 and 10 years hospitalised for any reason in private, public, primary, secondary and tertiary settings across the US received no analgesics for the relief of their pain. Eland (1985) compared 18 adults and 18 children who had the same diagnosis of their condition. The children received a total of 24 doses of analgesics (13 non-narcotics, 11 narcotics) whilst they were in the hospital. The adults received 372 doses of narcotic and 299 non-narcotic analgesics. Eland (1985) states that there are a number of 'Old Health Professionals' Tales' pertaining to paediatric pain.

- *Active children are not in pain.* Children are apt to be up and about after surgery much quicker than adults. This activity is often taken to mean that the child is not feeling any pain. However, children do not always realise that staying still may limit the pain and thus are inclined to re-establish their normal activity levels as quickly as possible. There is also an inclination to get up and avoid the room or bed that is so often associated with discomfort in the form of injections or being 'messed about'.
- *Children tell the truth about pain.* The fact is, according to Eland (1985), that children do not always tell the truth about pain and the nurses' predisposition to believe the child stems in part from their reluctance to engage in unpleasant activities, like giving injections, with children.

- *Children and adults have a similar view of injections.* Adults realise that the momentary pain associated with an injection is only transitory and will result in the subsequent benefit of pain relief. Children do not necessarily associate pain relief with the injection and see the pain of the injection as unnecessary. Eland (1985) says: 'If a nurse's response to an adult's admission of pain were striking the patient with a baseball bat, the patient would deny all pain from that moment. To a young child, the shot is the baseball bat.' Because children often report that the events that hurt the most during their hospital stay were the injections, Eland proposes that the intravenous administration of analgesics should be used instead of intramuscular injections, and where this is impracticable to use the ventrogluteal site as this is less painful than the vastus lateralis and the rectus femoris sites.
- *Parents have insight into their child's pain.* Parents may have little or no insight into their child's pain because (a) they may never have seen their child in a similar situation, (b) they may be so stressed themselves that they cannot concentrate on their child's pain, or (c) they may trust the health care team to take care of the pain because it has taken care of many children with similar problems and knows what to do. This does not mean that parents have no function for the hospitalised child, they can serve as excellent distracters and reduce significant amounts of anxiety. Sometimes in cases of severe pain the child requires pharmacological intervention.
- *Young children do not feel as much pain as adults.* Even very young children experience pain. Williamson & Williamson (1983) found that newborns who were given a dorsal penile nerve block with lignocaine hydrochloride responded differently to circumcision than those who were not given a nerve block.
- *Children will become addicted to the drugs used.* The incidence of addiction to narcotics during acute illness episodes is extremely low and undertreatment of pain with narcotic analgesics may increase the chances of addiction because inadequate pain relief may cause the patient to concentrate on the pain

and the drug (McCaffrey & Hart 1976). Narcotics do depress respiration but again the incidence is low. Miller & Jick (1978) evaluated the evidence for depression due to narcotics and found only 3 hospitalised patients out of 3263 developed clinically significant respiratory depression which were all due to meperidine.

• *Children cannot tell you where they are in pain.* There are difficulties in communicating information about pain when the vocabulary to do so is limited. The Eland Colour Tool uses different coloured crayons to represent 'no hurt, middle hurt, worst hurt'. Children use these crayons to indicate on a body outline where the pain is occurring. Eland (1985) suggests that the use of this technique greatly facilitates the communication of pain information between children and health professionals.

Nearly ten years have elapsed since the Eland (1985) paper. Do these myths about children's pain still exist? Collier et al (1993) sent questionnaires on pain myths to 47 doctors and 33 nurses in the Nottingham area. There were twelve statements (see Box 4.2).

The participants were asked to indicate whether they thought the statements were true or false. They could also indicate whether they were unsure or did not know the answer. There were similar response patterns for both doctors and nurses. One statement was thought to be true by nearly 60% of the sample: 'It is often being restrained during procedures, rather than any pain involved, that children find distressing'. The other results were as follows:

• Approximately 1 in 4 doctors and nurses responded 'true' to the following statements:
— Children forget pain quicker than adults.
— Children cannot tell you accurately where it hurts.
— Generally there is a 'usual' amount of pain associated with any given procedure.
• Approximately 1 in 10 doctors and nurses responded true to the following statements:
— Narcotics always depress respiration in children.

> **Box 4.2** Statements in the Collier (1993) questionnaire
>
> • Active children cannot be in pain.
> • Children will always tell you when they are in pain.
> • Children feel pain less than adults.
> • Children forget pain quicker than adults.
> • It is unsafe to administer narcotics to children because they become addicted.
> • Narcotics always depress respiration in children.
> • Children cannot accurately tell you where it hurts.
> • The best way to administer analgesia is by injection.
> • Parents know the best way to manage their children's pain.
> • Generally there is a 'usual' amount of pain associated with any given procedure.
> • The less analgesia administered to children the better it is for them.
> • It is often being restrained during procedures, rather than any pain involved, that children find distressing.

— Parents know the best way to manage their children's pain.
— The less analgesia administered to children the better it is for them.
• There was no support for the remaining five statements.

It is encouraging to note that some of the myths received little support; however, the fact that some doctors and nurses appear to go along with seven of the myths signals that there is still some work to be done.

Finally the problems associated with prescribing pain relief for children with terminal cancer are highlighted by an extract from the case notes of the last days of a 7-year-old boy (Case History 4.1).

The problem of children's pain is a complex one for everyone. To be young and dying of a malignancy is a terrible thing but to be young and dying in totally uncontrolled pain is horrible. It is important for health professionals and the health system itself to be sensitive to problems associated with the provision of adequate pain control. This particular case study is not indicative of general practice, however the fact that it occurred at all is a cause for concern.

Sofaer (1985, 1992) proposes that one of the major problems in caring for patients in pain is

CASE HISTORY 4.1 GARY

Gary is 7 years old and has a Burkitt's lymphoma. He sits all the time in one position (about 45 degree angle) and moves only under severe protest. He has developed pneumonia and sepsis. His eye contact is almost nonexistent. Whenever he can, he just stares at the TV and occasionally drifts off to sleep. It's known pathologically that he has compression of the bowel, stretching of his abdominal tissues and now compression of the ureter. Now it's got to the point that he can't concentrate on TV or tapes any more and the nursing staff has realised that all of this is severe pain and is lobbying anyone from the first year resident, to the surgical team, to the oncology team to order narcotic analgesics to alleviate his pain. So far all have refused and the reasons have ranged from 'We don't want to stop his bowel function,' even though it's a known fact that he is totally obstructed and receiving total parenteral nutrition, to 'It might interfere with his breathing and he already has pneumonia,' and 'He may not be terminal yet and we don't want to start him on anything that strong too soon.'

The intravenous cortisone has been stopped. One of the nurses took the first year resident who actually was writing the orders and directly in charge of Gary's care into the room and told him to stay there for at least an hour and then tell her why he wouldn't change his analgesic orders. He came out after 5 minutes and said, 'I can't take that,' but wouldn't change his orders and would not give the reason(s) why. The experienced medical staff should have helped the young man with his feelings and should have told him what to order to alleviate Gary's pain.

Nursing redoubled their efforts with comfort measures, touch, allowing Gary's pet ferret to be brought to the room etc. and in general broke every rule in the book to make him feel better but nothing alters the pain for more than a minute or two. So nursing has to watch Gary's agony 24 hours a day until he dies.

The only thing nursing and medicine could have done for Gary in his last month was provide pain relief. Nursing tried every pain relief option at their disposal to make Gary comfortable. Medicine failed miserably by not prescribing strong analgesics and, as a result, Gary died in agony. On one day shortly before his death, he told me 'I want to die and go to be with Jesus. It's just too awful here.'

Gary finally died and a post-mortem was performed. The final pathology report included the following pathologies:

- entire GI tract ulcerated from mouth to anus
- compression of right ureter and invasion of right kidney by 13 × 15 cm mass
- complete bowel obstruction by the same 13 × 15 cm mass
- 90% of the bone marrow involved
- systemic candida.

poor communication between patients, nurses and doctors. There is a need for in-service-training courses as well as basic training courses for all health professionals in the area of pain relief. There is a great deal of ignorance concerning the nature of pain relief which is exacerbated by lack of communication skills. Health professionals must be able to work together and show sensitivity not just to the needs of patients, but also to the different conceptions of pain that abound. It is necessary to respond to each situation with tact and awareness in order to promote cooperation and not confrontation between individuals. Sofaer (1985) provides the following anecdote to illustrate some of these points:

A patient experienced severe postoperative pain following major gynaecological surgery. The staff nurse administered the prescribed postoperative analgesia and assessed its effect with the patient at hourly intervals. After 2 hours the effect wore off. The nurse telephoned the doctor, 'We have assessed the pain with Mrs Brown postoperatively and together we feel that the analgesia is providing relief only for 2 hours. Could you suggest a way of making her more comfortable and pain-free?' The doctor represcribed the analgesia on a more frequent basis. On other occasions, I have known nurses to telephone a doctor and say, 'Mrs. Jones is complaining of pain. Can you write up some more analgesia?' This different approach has not endeared the doctor to either the patient (complaining and disagreeing with his prescription) or to the nurse, effectively telling him his job.

STRESS

Baum et al (1984) state that 'Stress has become a popular concept for explaining a wide variety of outcomes, mostly negative, that otherwise seem to defy explanation.' They suggest that stress has been used as a label for the psychological symptoms preceding an illness, anxiety reactions, discomfort and many other conditions. An analysis of the use of the term reveals a fairly broad definition, yet the processes involved are quite specific. The purpose of this section is to outline the major models of stress, to discuss the role of cognitive appraisal in coping with stress and to investigate the different techniques that may be used to manage stress.

MODELS OF STRESS

Cox (1978) divides models of stress into those that conceptualise the phenomena as stimulus-based, those that conceptualise it as response-based and those that suggest that it is an interaction between the two. Stress can be regarded as a stimulus to which an individual responds in some way. However, there are those that think the opposite, that stress is more a response to some noxious stimulus. Who is correct? Cox suggests that both groups are right and illustrates his thinking by asking us to consider the case of fatigue. Is it a stressful stimulus or a stressful response? It can be both. Sometimes people become so tired that they worry about whether they can do their job properly, and sometimes having a particularly demanding task to accomplish can induce in some people sensations of fatigue. Neither stimulus models nor response models are entirely adequate on their own. This has led some psychologists to put forward models of stress that emphasise an interaction, or tran-saction, between an individual and her environment. The first explanations, however, tended to concentrate on the physiological features of the phenomenon.

A physiological explanation

In 1935, Hans Selye was studying the effects of injecting hormones into rats. He found that the rats suffered ulcers, enlarged adrenal glands and shrunken thymus and lymph nodes. The effects were the same regardless of the concentration of the injections. Selye (1956) called this the 'stress syndrome' and suggested that it occurred in response to all forms of stressful stimulus. The body's response to any stressful stimulus occurs in three stages which Selye called the *general adaptation syndrome* (GAS).

Stage 1: The alarm reaction. This includes the effects of autonomic nervous system activation and is characterised by a drop in bodily resistance to stress. The adrenal medulla in turn secretes adrenaline and noradrenaline. Adreno-corticotrophic hormone (ACTH) is produced by the pituitary gland, which stimulates the adrenal cortex to release glucocorticoids. If the initial stress is too severe, the organism may die in this stage.

Stage 2: The resistance stage. The pituitary continues to secrete ACTH, which goes on stimulating the adrenal cortex to secrete gluco-corticoids, important to the resistance to stress because the glucocorticoids stimulate the con-version of fats and proteins to sugars providing energy to deal with the stressor. During this stage, resistance to the specific stress increases, and accordingly, the generalised response dis-appears. Many stress-related diseases develop in the resistance stage. Some may relate to the effects of the glucocorticoid hormones which inhibit the formation of antibodies, and decrease the formation of white blood cells. Another part of the resistance stage of the GAS is the suppression of many of the bodily functions related to sexual behaviour and reproduction. In males, sperm production drops, as does secretion of male sex hormones; in females, the menstrual cycle is disrupted or suppressed.

Stage 3: The exhaustion stage. If the specific stress continues, the body's ability to contain it and to resist other stresses ultimately collapses.

Under prolonged stress, body mechanisms are geared to defend the body, but the cost is mani-fest in the weakening of resistance to disease and infection. This physiological response pattern occurs regardless of the source of the stress, for example, extreme cold, illness and emotional conflict. Over a prolonged period of time, the ability to react to stress in this manner takes its toll of the body, that is, the individual's system gradually becomes 'worn out', resulting in increased susceptibility to illness and a reduced resistance to stress itself. There is evidence that this pattern of responses is dangerous over long periods of time (Innes 1981).

The fundamental flaw in the physiological approach to stress, though, is that the model does not incorporate individual differences in the perception of the stressful event. What is a stressful experience to one person is not to another. Evidence that the perception of the event, or cognitive appraisal, is a critical factor in the experience of stress comes from a number of sources.

Lazarus (1991) cites evidence of unconsciousness and anaesthesia eliminating the adrenal effects of psychological stress. Patients who were dying showed normal adrenal cortical conditions as long as they remained unconscious during the period of the fatal condition. They were unable to perceive the situation as dangerous and thus GAS could not occur. Bakal (1979) states:

A historical paradox of stress research is that 20 years ago, physiologists, in their studies of the physiological effects of heat, shock, and trauma, maintained that psychological variables were not important. Now the shoe is on the other foot, for the investigator of physical stressors must be very careful to rule out the possibility that any observed changes might have been due to the animal's psychological reaction to the situation.

The psychological perspective

The psychological perspective emphasises the role of interpretation of stressors on the stress response. A series of studies by Lazarus and his associates (Speisman et al 1964; Lazarus et al 1965) produced support for a psychological interpretation of stress.

In one study, Lazarus et al (1965) showed subjects an industrial accident film 'It Didn't Have To Happen'. This was a 13-minute black and white film devised as an educational tool to promote industrial safety. The film depicted three accidents. The first showed a man running the tips of his fingers through a ripsaw; the second, a man losing a finger; the third accident involved a worker being impaled by a plank of wood that had flown out of a machine.

One group of subjects (control) were given no explanation of the events other than to pay close attention to the film. Another group of subjects (intellectualisation) were told to analyse the film from the point of view of the interpersonal dynamics of the situation, to try to assess the

effectiveness of the techniques used by the foreman to influence the men's safety procedures. They were encouraged to view the film in a detached, analytical fashion. The third group of subjects (denial) were told that the events had all been staged by actors and nobody really got hurt. The accidents had been developed using special effects. The experimenters found that both the intellectualisation and the denial instructions were effective in reducing the emotional response to the film because they allowed the subjects to appraise the stressful stimuli in a less threatening fashion.

Cognitive appraisal and coping

The outcome of Lazarus's research into the psychology of stress was a cognitive model that emphasised individual differences in the way stress is perceived. Lazarus (1966) proposed a model that was made up of two sections. The first section was concerned with appraisal of stress and the second with coping mechanisms to deal with it. The first stage in the perception of stress is the primary appraisal of threat. If a lion suddenly burst into the room primary appraisal would be: 'How much am I in danger from this situation?' This would be followed by secondary appraisal: 'What am I going to do about it and what are the likely consequences of such action?' In this instance an individual's social and cultural background and his previous experience of similar situations is likely to influence his perception of threat.

Coping mechanisms are also classified into two categories: direct action and palliative action. Direct action involves an 'attack' on the stressful stimulus itself. The individual tries to remove or reduce the threat. An example of direct action coping with the stress of an imminent exam would be either to revise harder or to not bother to take the exam. Both actions directly seek to either reduce or eliminate the source of the stress. In contrast, palliative action modifies the individual's internal response to the stimulus. The threat is still present but the individual is better able to cope with it.

In many situations direct action coping may

be too costly for people and the only alternative is to alter their internal response to the threat. An exam cannot always be avoided and more revision may seem unnecessary, but the threat of the exam may be reduced by 'having a few drinks' or indulging in relaxation training. Both coping mechanisms may operate in conjunction with each other, indeed in managing stress it is important to consider techniques that consider using them together. This early model has been refined and revised (Lazarus & Launier 1978; Cohen & Lazarus 1979; Lazarus & Folkman 1984) but provides a useful focus for the analysis of recent research on cognitive appraisal and coping.

A major issue in stress research is the role of denial and intellectualisation. Bakal (1979) suggests that the reason why health professionals are good at 'hiding their emotions' is that they are in fact not feeling any emotion. They have defused the threatening aspects of the situation by cognitive reappraisal. Denial and detachment are capable of changing the emotion itself. Continual exposure to stressful situations may result in a 'distancing' of the health professional from the source of stress. If the object of the distancing is the patient, then this may affect the interpersonal skills of the health professional. A high score on the personality scale in Chapter 1 could indicate a level of depersonalisation, a coping style that has resulted from continuous exposure to stress.

A recent experiment by Steptoe & Vogële (1986) investigated the use of intellectualisation in dealing with emotional stimuli. They presented the industrial accident film used by Lazarus et al (1965) to 36 London medical students. The students were allocated at random to one of three conditions. In the first condition (control), subjects were given instructions similar to the control group studied by Lazarus et al (1965); a synopsis of the film content. In the second condition (intellectualisation), subjects were given instructions modelled on the procedure described by Lazarus et al (1965). They were designed to encourage a detached, analytic attitude towards the film. The third condition was called sensation focusing. Subjects were asked to concentrate on their emotional feelings and their experience of physical sensations while watching the film. During the film, heart rate and skin conductance were measured to indicate physiological levels of stress. Subjective emotional responses to the film were recorded using a symptom–emotion checklist based on the one used by Pennebaker (1982). Subjects used the checklist to report the sensations they were currently experiencing 15 seconds after each accident in the film.

The results indicated that there were no significant differences between the intellectualisation condition and the control on measures of heart rate and skin conductance. In this experiment, intellectualisation did not reduce physiological measures of stress. However, the sensation-focusing instructions did produce significantly lower levels of physiological stress than the other two. There were no significant differences between any of the conditions on the subjective measures of stress.

These results pose some difficulties for proponents of intellectualisation as a means to reduce the emotional response to stress. This experiment did not mirror the findings of Lazarus et al (1965). This does not mean that detachment, distancing and intellectualisation of stressful stimuli are irrelevant. It may be that they develop as coping mechanisms over a longer period of time. However, in this instance, intellectualisation did not prove as effective as sensation focusing in the reduction of physiological stress.

Why did sensation focusing work? Steptoe & Vogële (1986) put forward two explanations. The first suggests that internal and external stimuli compete for the attention of the subject: 'Physiological reactions may have been reduced because subjects spent so much time attending to bodily sensations that they were distracted from the film.' The authors maintain that this technique may well be unsuccessful for modest or minimal threats, but appropriate under the present experimental circumstances. The second explanation is derived from the work of Leventhal et al (1979). Concentrating on one's emotions may serve to 'objectify' the experience.

Sensation focusing enables the subject to interpret the sensory inputs in a nonemotional manner.

Both explanations are equally applicable, but further research is needed to determine the exact nature of the response. It is interesting to note that the subjective emotional reactions to the accidents did not differ between conditions. This finding indicates a discrepancy between physiological and subjective responses to threat. In terms of cognitive appraisal, the main finding of this experiment is that telling people to pay attention to their bodily feelings during stress can lead to substantial reductions in physiological response to threat. The categories of coping responses proposed by Lazarus (1966, 1991) have been extended by Billings & Moos (1981). They asked 360 families to indicate a recent personal 'crisis' or stressful life event. They gave the families a list of 'coping responses' and asked them to indicate which ones they used to handle the situation. The experimenters grouped the items in terms of whether they were problem-based or emotion-based (Box 4.3).

On the basis of this, and other research, Moos (1986) has elaborated a model for understanding, coping and adapting to stress. The first

---

Box 4.3 Coping response categories (Billings & Moos 1981)

Active cognitive—emotion-focused
1. Tried to see the positive side
2. Tried to step back from the situation
3. Prayed for guidance

Active cognitive coping—problem-focused
1. Considered several alternatives for handling the problem
2. Took things one step at a time
3. Drew on past experiences

Active behavioural coping—problem-focused
1. Tried to find out more about the situation
2. Talked with a professional person
3. Took some positive action
4. Talked with spouse or other relative about the situation

Avoidance—emotion-focused
1. Prepared for the worst
2. Sometimes took it out on other people
3. Tried to reduce tension by eating more
4. Kept my feelings to myself

---

stage consists of three elements that relate to the individual, type of event and his environment: (a) background of the individual and personal factors, (b) the type and context of the event, and (c) the physical and social environment. The second stage starts with cognitive appraisal or the perceived meaning of the event, which leads into adaptive tasks and coping mechanisms. The third stage is the outcome of the event itself. This model is discussed in further detail in the next chapter in the context of people's responses to life stress/transition.

STRESS MANAGEMENT
Relaxation and meditation

Relaxation training can be considered the 'aspirin' of the clinical health psychologist.

Feuerstein et al (1986)

Relaxation may be thought by some to be lying back in a comfortable armchair or 'curling up' with a good book. However, many individuals find it difficult to relax in such ways and find it necessary to have some form of instruction in how to relax. One technique is called progressive muscular relaxation (Jacobson 1978). Every time a muscle contracts it creates a series of neural impulses that are sent to the brain. This creates tension, especially if many muscles are activated. Progressive muscular relaxation tries to teach people to recognise when excessive contraction of the skeletal muscles occurs and how to relax these muscles to reduce tension.

Progressive muscular relaxation involves the successive tensing and relaxing of various muscle groups. Throughout training, the patient typically sits or reclines in a comfortable chair in a quiet, dimly lit room with closed eyes. In order to enhance the relaxation effect, the therapist speaks in a slow and quiet tone of voice and usually has the patient successively tense and relax the following muscle groups: hands and forearms, upper arms (biceps), wrists, forehead, eyes, mouth, neck, shoulders, chest, stomach, buttocks, thighs, calves, and feet. The patient repeats the procedure twice for each muscle group. The therapist may explain to the patient that it is not necessary to obtain the maximum muscle tension possible. Also, it is up to the therapist to determine the rate at which the patient should relieve muscle tension, that is suddenly 'letting go' versus gradually relaxing the muscle.

Feuerstein et al (1986)

The evidence for the effectiveness of the technique in the reduction of stress is equivocal. Borkovec & Sides (1979) list studies that have found little or no difference between relaxation groups and control groups. A problem of such studies is the lack of systematic biochemical measures of the stress response, thus the differing results may be due to the different measures involved in each study.

Another type of relaxation technique is akin to meditation. Benson (1975) has described a procedure designed to help individuals who are faced with stressful situations called the relaxation response. The technique requires four basic elements:

- *A quiet environment*—the individual is usually asked to close his or her eyes.
- *A mental device*—this is usually a syllable that is repeated over and over again silently or in low tones to oneself. Benson suggests the syllable 'one' because of its simplicity and neutrality. The purpose is to reduce distractability.
- *A passive attitude*—distracting thoughts will occur during the relaxation period. It is important to disregard them and concentrate on the technique. However, one should not think about how well one is performing the technique.
- *Decreased muscle tone*—the individual should sit in a comfortable position.

Having satisfied these criteria the technique can begin.

The person sits in a comfortable quiet environment with his eyes closed. All muscles are relaxed starting with the toes and progressing to the face. This state of deep relaxation is maintained. The person is asked to breathe through his nose, and concentrate only on this breathing. As he breathes out, instruct him to say the word 'one' silently to himself. He breathes in. If a thought starts to enter his mind, he must ignore it. This practice should be continued for 20 minutes, with a gentle reminder when the time is up. Keep the individual seated for a few minutes with eyes closed. When finished, do not dwell on whether the procedure was a success or not. Try to repeat the procedure at some other time during the day.

Benson (1975) claimed that the relaxation response helped to reduce blood pressure, to produce changes in oxygen consumption by 5% and to affect the frequency of alpha waves. In a review of the literature on the effects of relaxation response techniques on the control of arousal in threatening situations, Holmes (1984) concluded that there was no evidence to show that the relaxation response is more effective in reducing somatic arousal than is simple rest. Younger et al (1975) claimed that electroencephalograph patterns of experienced meditators, rather than resembling an altered state of consciousness, are closer in appearance to somebody asleep. Benson's claim was that those who engaged in the relaxation response were better able to reduce their intake of alcohol and cigarette smoking; however, this might also be the result of a change of lifestyle of the meditators. It seems, therefore, that further controlled studies need to be conducted to establish whether relaxation is an effective method of stress management.

Biofeedback

Biofeedback involves procedures in which minute changes occurring within the body or brain are detected and amplified by complex electronic devices. These changes are then represented to people in a visual or auditory manner. Budzynski (1973) described biofeedback training as having three main goals:

- to develop an increased awareness of internal physiological states
- to establish control over these physiological states
- the transfer of control from the clinic or laboratory to areas of everyday life.

Hypertension is a considerable problem for many people in the community and has been shown to occur in 5–10% of the general population. Wolkind & Zajicek (1981) found that 47% of their sample of pregnant East End women suffered from hypertension at some time during their pregnancy. The success of the biofeedback technique in reducing hypertension unfortunately is limited. Miller (1978) found that a few patients were able to reduce their blood pressure to some extent using biofeedback training, but after returning to their natural environment the changes in the patients' metabolism were not always maintained. More success has been obtained with patients suffering from muscle contraction and migraine headaches.

Budzynski (1973) assigned patients to one of three treatment conditions. One group received biofeedback training; another group were told to practise relaxation; and a third group were asked to monitor their headache activity. After 8 weeks of 'treatment', the patients who had received the biofeedback showed the greatest reduction in frequency of headaches. However, exactly what the patients were learning in this experiment is not clear and it is unlikely that direct control over the appropriate physiological variable is acquired. Although the effectiveness of biofeedback as a direct agent of control may be questioned, as an indirect technique for accomplishing modification of physiological functioning it might have more success.

Bakal (1979) reports the case of one of his patients who was an outstanding success in his treatment programme. After 12 sessions of biofeedback training she reported a 'near-total disappearance of headache'. The physiological data indicated that she had gained 'little or no control over the muscle activity of her forehead'. The patient had adopted a new strategy toward herself and her work. The biofeedback technique enabled her cognitively to distance herself from a previously upsetting situation.

The effects of the process are similar to those described by the sensation-focusing technique of Steptoe & Vogële (1986). Concentrating on the internal physiological state distracts the individual from the external sources of stress and tension. Concentration is able to be maintained due to the need to alter or modify physiological functioning. Stroebel & Glueck (1973) describe biofeedback as the ultimate placebo because it 'provides the patient with an effective means of preventing illness and/or potentially curing himself by helping him regulate the pace of his daily lifestyle, of his thought patterns, of his body processes, his habits, and his perceptual style, hopefully reducing susceptibility to pathological levels of hyperactivation when faced with stressful life events.'

Carroll (1984) has reviewed the research on the effectiveness of biofeedback and concludes that:

Expectations ran high in the early days; much was promised. Has that promise been fulfilled? A cold, hard look fifteen years on would indicate that it has not. In most of the areas of application, biofeedback is poorly indicated. Either its effects are variable and/or short-lived, or they are no greater than those produced by simpler, less expensive alternatives, or they can be attributed to the agency of expectancy and placebo.

Stress inoculation

Meichenbaum (1977) and Meichenbaum & Cameron (1983) have proposed that a central feature of the experience of stress is maladaptive responses to faulty cognitions. A patient may not be aware that irrational beliefs are the source of stress. The stress inoculation technique begins with a phase designed to educate the individual with a conceptual framework for understanding her problem (Box 4.4).

The programme begins with an educational phase that provides the patient with a conceptual framework for understanding the nature of the problem. The purpose of this initial phase is to try to get the patient to talk to himself differently about the problem. Instead of reacting emotionally to the situation, the patient is encouraged to analyse the problem in an objective fashion. Thus a patient who experiences severe anxiety attacks would first be encouraged to discover the situations that produce the anxiety. A diary is kept whereby the patient records the thoughts that occur during the attack. It is

Box 4.4 Stress inoculation training (Meichenbaum & Cameron 1983)

Conceptualisation
1. *Data collection*
   - Identify the causes of the problem using an interview, image-based reconstruction, self-monitoring and observing behaviour.
   - Distinguish between making a mistake and a skill deficit.
   - Formulate a treatment plan.

2. *Assessment*
   - Train individuals to analyse problems independently.
   - Conduct an analysis of the 'true' situation.
   - Ask individuals to seek evidence that disconfirms their misperceptions.

Skills acquisition and rehearsal
1. *Skills training*
   - Training coping skills such as: communication, assertion and problem solving.
   - Training palliative coping skills such as: distraction, taking a different perspective, using social support, adapting emotional responses and relaxation.
   - Develop an extensive repertoire of coping responses to aid flexible responding.

2. *Skills rehearsal*
   - Promote utilisation of coping responses using imagery and role play.
   - Develop self-instructional training.

Application and follow-through
1. *Application skills*
   - Use cues of early stress as signals to cope.
   - Role play anticipated stressful situations.
   - Role play the patient coaching someone with a similar problem.
   - Expose the patient gradually to stressful situations.

2. *Maintenance and generalisation*
   - Identify 'high risk' situations and develop coping self-efficacy.
   - Develop strategies for dealing with failure.
   - Arrange follow-up sessions.

General guidelines for training
1. Consider training patients' friends and family to conduct treatment.
2. Be approachable.
3. Establish realistic goals and expectations.
4. Have plenty of rewards in the course of the treatment.

illustrated to the patient that thoughts can affect emotions. The work of Valins has shown that cognitive factors are the most important determinants of emotional responses. It is the individual's beliefs about his physiological state, rather than the actual state itself, that determine emotional behaviour.

Valins & Ray (1967) showed snake-phobic subjects a series of slides. The slides were made up of pictures of snakes and other anxiety-arousing pictures. One group of subjects was told that their heart rate was going to be monitored and they would be able to hear it via the monitoring equipment. The experimenters manipulated the heart-rate feedback so that the subjects believed that their heart rates were unaffected by slides of snakes but increased to the other anxiety-arousing slides. The other group heard the same sounds but believed them to be meaningless. Both groups were subsequently exposed to real snakes. Valins & Ray (1967) found that giving snake-phobic subjects false feedback of their heart rate enabled them to approach the real snakes more closely than the control group. The way in which emotions are conceptualised determines the nature of the emotional experience.

Meichenbaum (1977) uses this information to tell patients that anxiety involves physiological responses such as sweaty palms, increased heart rate, muscular tension etc. and the interpretation of the meaning of the responses. If the patient can be taught to use the physiological signs of anxiety as cues to utilise coping techniques, the experience of anxiety can be significantly reduced. Different cognitions about the situation lead to different emotions. The coping thoughts 'usually take the form of instructions to do several things, including instructions to engage in strategies to reduce physiological arousal such as relaxation techniques and regulated breathing. The client will also be told to focus his attention on the task in hand and not on his feelings of fear and this can involve specific advice as to what to do. For example, the socially anxious client may be asked to maintain eye contact and not avoid the gaze of the other person. How to manage the feelings of being overwhelmed by the emotion will also be dealt with' (Miller & Morley 1986). Instructions about intensity and time-span of the emotion are given and an evaluation of the patient's coping strategy is provided at the end. The therapist usually demonstrates coping techniques and requires the patient to undergo a series of graded exercises to practise his skills, gradually exposing the patient to more 'real' examples of the stressor. At the end of the training programme the patient will have replaced all his maladaptive thoughts with positive coping responses.

Novaco (1975) has used stress inoculation to help people control their anger. The first stage requires the individual to conceptualise her anger reactions as a series of cognitions and arousal states. Next, relaxation exercises and adaptive self-statements are taught for the four stages of anger management:

- *Preparing for provocation:* 'This could be a rough situation, but I know how to handle it.'
- *Impact and confrontation:* 'As long as I keep my cool, I'm in control of the situation.'
- *Coping with arousal:* 'Muscles are getting tight. Relax, time for problem solving. He wants me to get angry, but I'm not going to.'
- *Reflection:* 'I actually got through that without getting angry.'

The final part of the process asks patients to imagine provoking situations and grade them from mild to strong. They then have to work through the situations starting with the least provoking and ending with the most provoking. Stress inoculation has been used in wide-ranging areas, from pain (Turk 1978; Turk et al 1983) to mucous colitis (Youell & McCullough 1975), but has achieved most success in the area of stress and anxiety management. The use of inoculation techniques in the treatment of men at risk for coronary heart disease is described in Chapter 6.

Perceived control

People who feel that they have no control over what is happening to them have been found to experience high levels of stress (Cohen 1980). Glass & Singer (1972) suggest that people prefer activities where they think they have control over their environment. Two experiments by

Weiss and Seligman illustrate the power of control in reducing stress. Weiss (1972) emphasised the importance of predictability in reducing stress. Three rats were given a combination of electric shock and tones. Two of the rats received electric shocks to their tails, the third did not. The first rat heard a tone 10 seconds before the shock. The second rat heard random tones and therefore could not predict when the shock would come. The third rat heard the tones but did not receive any shock. Autopsies were performed and the degree of ulceration was measured. The third rat that received no shock, not surprisingly, had little ulceration. The second rat, however, was found to have extensive ulceration. The first rat, that was able to predict the electric shock, had a level of ulceration similar to the rat that had received no shock at all. The interesting point is that both the first and the second rats got exactly the same physical stimulus, it was the psychological variable of predictability that determined the degree of severe gastric ulceration.

The experiments of Weiss (1972) were conducted on animals and therefore their applicability to human behaviour is limited. However, many other studies have found similar effects using human subjects (Gatchel & Proctor 1976; Staub et al 1971). Being able to predict when stressful events are about to occur significantly reduces the emotional experience of the event. When children are told what a dentist is doing and what to expect, they report less anxiety and physical discomfort (Siegel & Peterson 1980). Perceived control is a significant factor in what Seligman (1975) termed learned helplessness. Seligman & Maier (1967) divided dogs into three groups. The first group were strapped into a hammock and were given electric shocks. They could switch the electricity off by pressing a pad with their nose. The second group of dogs were yoked to the first group and thus experienced the same amount of shock, but were unable to do anything about it. The third group were strapped into hammocks but experienced no shock.

In the next stage of the experiment, the dogs underwent training in a two-way shuttle box.

The shuttle box was divided into two sections separated by a barrier. The dogs were placed on one side of the box and a light was flashed 10 seconds prior to them experiencing a shock to their feet.

Under normal conditions the dogs soon learn to avoid the shock by jumping over the barrier when the light goes on. This is exactly what happened for the dogs from groups one and three. Those dogs who were able to terminate the shock by pressing a pad in the initial session, and those dogs who experienced no shock at all in the training session managed the escape–avoidance task with little difficulty. The dogs from the second group who were unable to control the shock in the initial training session did not perform so well. Approximately 75% of the yoked group completely failed to escape shock in the shuttle box. Like the other dogs, they would rush around the box to start off with, but then, instead of jumping over the barrier, they would typically lie down and become very passive as if they were 'depressed'.

Seligman (1975) claimed that the dogs in this group had learned to become helpless. During the initial training period they had been exposed to a situation where they had no control. Over a period of time this experience of lack of control developed in them a feeling that no matter what happened they would not be able to do anything about their circumstances. So when actually faced with an escape route in the second condition, they did nothing about it.

There is evidence that the learned helplessness phenomenon occurs in people too (Peterson & Seligman 1984). Seligman (1975) in fact argues that learned helplessness can result from any situation where people think that they have no control over events. It does not matter whether there is a solution to their predicament or not, as long as they perceive the situation as hopeless then they will cease to find a way out. Individuals who think that they have no control over events will learn to become helpless. Perceived control is relevant in a wide range of stressful conditions: from childbirth to crowding. It has even been suggested by some psychologists that whole communities can become helpless if they

perceive events to be beyond their control and one of the roles of the community health professional is to prevent this happening by producing a 'competent community' (Sue & Zane 1977).

In the hospital environment perceived control influences stress factors. Volicer et al (1977) devised the Hospital Stress Rating Scale to assess the degree of stress associated with various hospital practices. Medical and surgical patients were asked to rate hospital practices in terms of perceived stressfulness. The events rated as most stressful were, not surprisingly, thinking they might have cancer, losing their sight and knowing they had a serious illness. However, other events that were rated highly included not being told the nature of the diagnosis, not knowing the results of or reasons for treatment and having questions ignored. The latter group of events represents the stress caused by 'not knowing what is happening' and can be easily reduced by communicating more effectively with the patient.

The importance of perceived control in the reduction of stress cannot be overstated. In almost all circumstances where people are facing stress of one kind or another, giving them the idea that they have some control over events will reduce the levels of stress experienced. Health professionals should try to create in people the notion that they have a certain degree of control over their circumstances. The psychological and physical benefits of gaining a sense of control over events are to be found in the dentist's surgery as well as people's fight for the mastery of cancer (Taylor 1991). People need to feel that they have some control over the events that occur in their lives. When the perception of control is lost, stress and anxiety often follow, therefore health professionals should look to enhancing people's predictability and perceived control when constructing any stress management programme.

Social support

Most health psychologists would agree that social support can be a crucial factor in stress management, but there is considerably less agreement about what constitutes social support. Cobb & Jones (1984) suggest that social support can be measured by looking at three elements:

- the actual supportive behaviour of friends and kin
- the nature of the social network (whether it is a closely knit group of individuals or more widely spread out)
- the way that an individual feels about the support provided by her friends and kin.

This represents a good attempt to isolate the practical constituents of social support. It suggests that there are two important perspectives:

- *The individual perspective.* This represents the view of the individual about the people in the social network. A person may feel secure in the knowledge that she has a fully functioning social support network of friends and kin who are ready to help if the need arises. She also feels perfectly able to contact them and discuss with them her personal concerns.
- *The social network perspective.* This represents the actual behaviour of the people who constitute the network toward the individual.

This distinction is echoed by Gottlieb (1981, 1985) who says that coping depends on both the manifestation of support and on the belief that others would provide help if asked. But he also says that it is necessary to find out about what people do when they support each other.

Coyne & Lazarus (1980) use the terms *social network* and *perceived social support* to distinguish between quantity and quality of support. The social network is the number of people involved and the nature of the friendship. The perceived social support involves the individual's feelings and thoughts about how helpful the relationships are to him. Schaefer et al (1981) compared social network variables with perceived social support in relation to the physical health status, stressful life events, depression and morale of 100 people aged between 45 and 65 years. They found that social network had a weaker overall relationship to outcomes than perceived social support. However, it is necessary to determine what constitutes perceived social support.

Wills & Langner (1980) propose that possible determinants might be:

- copying or modelling influential friends or kin who have successfully coped with stressful life events
- assistance in solving problems
- guidance
- predictability
- giving information
- security and boosting self-esteem.

Social networks are not the only means of social support. Levitt et al (1986) investigated social network relationships as sources of maternal support and well-being. They examined the social networks of 43 mothers of 13-month-old infants to determine the degree to which the networks provided social support. They found that the mothers had an average of 13 persons in their network but support was provided primarily by the husband. The authors conclude that 'maternal well-being is a function of the difficulty of the infant, the quality of the mother's relationship with her spouse, and the amount of support provided through the marital relationship'. It was only when the marital relationship broke down that the support network assumed significance.

Finally, Cohen & McKay (1984) present a model of the conditions under which one's support network would reduce or prevent stress. It is based on the principle that the social network provides a 'buffering effect' to stressful events. There are three types of support mechanism:

Tangible support. Although virtually anyone with the required resources could provide those in need with money or care, tangible support is most effective when it is viewed by the recipient as appropriate. Offers of tangible support that result in feelings of inadequacy and indebtedness, will simply add to the stress of the individual.

Appraisal support. The support group may affect an individual's perception of the threat. Social support buffers people against stress by helping them to redefine the situation as less threatening. One turns to similar people who have experienced similar situations for advice and help. However, social support will only help if the stressor is socially acceptable; cancer patients generally do not want to discuss their illness because of the stigma attached to the condition and fail to seek out the help of other cancer patients in order to avoid publicly stating that they have cancer (Wortman & Dunkel-Schetter 1987).

A support group that acts as a comparison group may serve to reduce threat by allowing individuals to compare themselves to others who are perceived as being worse off. Social support can also help enhance a person's coping strategies by suggesting alternative strategies based on previous experience and by getting people to focus on more positive aspects of the situation.

Emotional support. If stress lessens one's feelings of belonging or being loved, emotional support can replace or strengthen these feelings. Uncontrollable stress can result in a loss of self-esteem. If this happens, then the support network can play a significant role in elevating low self-opinion. Events that result in depriving somebody of the feeling of belonging may be ameliorated by a form of support that develops relatively intimate personal relationships.

Thus social support can only be effective when a person's interpersonal relationships provide the resources that fulfil the coping requirements of a particular stressful event. Hobfoll (1988) argues that stress is facilitated by the loss, or threatened loss, of resources, whether personal, physical or psychological. People feel stress when resources seem likely to be expended. Thus stress and social support are strongly related to personal and social network factors. In summary, many people gain information about how to deal with stressful situations from their friends and relatives; often they would much rather have information and support from their social network rather than health professionals; health professionals have to negotiate ways of influencing members of an individual's network to provide information, care and support in the most appropriate manner.

REFERENCES

Bakal D A 1979 Psychology and medicine. Tavistock, London

Barber T X 1982 Hypnosuggestive procedures in the treatment of clinical pain. In: Millon T, Green C, Meagler R (eds) Handbook of clinical health psychology. Plenum, New York

Baum A, Singer J E, Baum C S 1984 Stress and the environment. In: Evans G W (ed) Environmental stress. Cambridge University Press, Cambridge

Beecher H K 1959 Measurement of subjective responses: quantitative effects of drugs. Oxford University Press, Oxford

Benson H 1975 The relaxation response. William Morrow, New York

Billings A G, Moos R H 1981 The role of coping responses and social resources in attenuating the stress of life events. Journal of Behavioural Medicine 4: 139–157

Block A R, Kremer E F, Gaylor M 1980 Behavioural treatment of chronic pain: the spouse as a discriminatory cue for pain behaviour. Pain 9: 243–252

Bond M R 1971 The relation of pain to the Eysenck Personality Inventory, Cornell Medical Index and the Whitely Index of Hypochondriasis. British Journal of Psychiatry 119: 671–678

Bond M R, Glynn J P, Thomas D G 1976 The relation between pain and personality in patients receiving pentazocine (Fortral) after surgery. Journal of Psychonomic Research 10: 369–381

Borkovec T D, Sides J 1979 Critical procedural variables related to the physiological effects of progressive muscular relaxation: a review. Behaviour Research and Therapy 17: 119–125

Budzynski T 1973 Biofeedback procedures in the clinic. In: Birk L (ed) Biofeedback: behavioural medicine. Grune Stratton, New York

Carroll D 1984 Biofeedback in practice. Longman, London

Cobb S, Jones J M 1984 Social support, support groups and marital relationships. In: Duck S W (ed) Personal relationships 5. Academic Press, London

Cohen F, Lazarus R S 1979 Coping with the stresses of illness. In: Stone G C, Cohen F, Adler N (eds) Health psychology. Jossey Bass, San Francisco

Cohen S 1980 After effects of stress on human performance and social behaviour: a review of research and theory. Psychological Bulletin 87: 578–604

Cohen S, McKay G 1984 Social support, stress, and the buffering hypothesis: a theoretical analysis. In: Baum A, Taylor S E, Singer J E (eds) Handbook of psychology and health. Erlbaum, Hillsdale NJ

Collier J, Pattison H M, MacKinlay D R E, Watson A R 1993 Pain in children: myths and attitudes of health care professionals. Paper presented to the Special Group in Health Psychology Conference, Nottingham

Connolly A M, Pancheri P, Lucchetti L et al 1978 Clinical psychoneuroendocrinology in reproduction. In: Carenza L, Pancheri P, Zichella L (eds) Clinical psychoneuro-endocrinology in reproduction. Academic Press, New York

Cox T 1978 Stress. Macmillan, London

Coyne J C, Lazarus R S 1980 Cognitive style, stress perspective, and coping. In: Kutash I L, Schlesinger L B (eds) Handbook on stress and anxiety. Jossey Bass, San Francisco

Davitz L L, Davitz J R 1985 Culture and nurses' inferences of suffering. In: Copp L A (ed) Perspectives on pain. Churchill Livingstone, Edinburgh

Eland J M 1985 The role of the nurse in children's pain. In: Copp L A (ed) Perspectives on pain. Churchill Livingstone, Edinburgh

Feuerstein M, Labbé E E, Kuczmierczyk A R 1986 Health psychology: a psychobiological perspective. Plenum, New York

Gatchel R S, Proctor J D 1976 Physiological correlates of learned helplessness in man. Journal of Abnormal Psychology 85: 27–34

Glass D C, Singer J E 1972 Urban stress. Academic Press, New York

Gottlieb B H 1981 Social networks and social support. Sage, Beverley Hills

Gottlieb B H 1985 Social support and the study of personal relationships. Journal of Social and Personal Relationships 2: 351–375

Hayward I 1975 Information: a prescription against pain. Royal College of Nursing, London

Hilgard E R, Hilgard J R 1975 Hypnosis in the relief of pain. Kaufmann, Los Altos

Hobfoll S E 1988 The ecology of stress. Hemisphere, New York

Holmes D S 1984 Meditation and somatic arousal reduction: a review of the experimental evidence. American Psychologist 39: 1–10

Innes J M 1981 Social psychological approaches to the study of the induction and alleviation of stress: influences of health and illness. In: Stephenson G, Davis J (eds) Progress in applied social psychology. Wiley, Chichester

Jacobson E 1978 You must relax. McGraw-Hill, New York

Johnson J E 1975 Stress reduction through sensation information. In: Sarason G, Spielberger C D (eds) Stress and anxiety. Wiley, New York, vol 2

Johnson J E, Rice V H, Fuller S S, Endress M P 1978 Sensory information, instruction in a coping strategy, and recovery from surgery. Research in Nursing and Health 1: 4–17

Kepes E R, Chen M, Schapira M 1976 A critical evaluation of acupuncture in the treatment of chronic pain. In: Bonica J J, Albe-Fessard D (eds) Advances in pain research and therapy. Raven Press, New York, vol 1

Lander J, Hodgins M, Fowler-Kerry S 1992 Children's pain predictions and memories. Behaviour Research Therapy 30: 117–124

Lazarus R L 1966 Psychological stress and the coping process. McGraw-Hill, New York

Lazarus R S 1975 The self-regulation of emotion. In: Levi L (ed) Emotions: their parameters and measurement. Raven Press, New York

Lazarus R S 1991 Emotion and adaptation. Oxford University Press, Oxford

Lazarus R S, Launier R 1978 Stress-related transactions between person and environment. In: Pervin L A, Lewis M (eds) Perspectives in interactional psychology. Plenum, New York

Lazarus R S, Folkman S 1984 Stress, appraisal and coping. Springer, New York

Lazarus R S, Opton E M, Nomikos M S, Rankin N O 1965 The principle of short-circuiting of threat: further evidence. Journal of Personality 33: 622–635

Leventhal H, Brown D, Schacham S et al 1979 Effects of preparatory information about sensation, threat of pain, and attention on cold pressor distress. Journal of Personality and Social Psychology 37: 688–714

Levitt M J, Weber R A, Clark M C 1986 Social network relationships as sources of maternal support and well-being. Developmental Psychology 22: 310–316

Livingstone W K 1943 Pain mechanisms. Macmillan, London

Loeser J D, Fordyce W E 1983 Chronic pain. In: Carr J E, Dengerink H A (eds) Behavioural science in the practice of medicine. Elsevier Biomedical, New York

Lyn B 1984 The detection of injury and tissue damage. In: Wall P D, Melzack R (eds) A textbook of pain. Churchill Livingstone, Edinburgh

McCaffrey M, Hart L L 1976 Undertreatment of acute pain with narcotics. American Journal of Nursing 76: 586–591

McCaul K D, Malott J M 1984 Distraction and coping with pain. Psychological Bulletin 95: 516–533

Mayer D J, Price D D, Barber J et al 1976 Acupuncture analgesia: evidence for activation of a pain inhibitous system as a mechanism of action. In: Bonica J J, Albe-Fessard D (eds) Advances in pain research and therapy. Raven Press, New York, vol 1

Meichenbaum D 1977 Cognitive-behaviour modification: an integrative approach. Plenum, New York

Meichenbaum D, Cameron R 1983 Stress-inoculation training: toward a general paradigm for training coping skills. In: Meichenbaum D, Jaremko M E (eds) Stress reduction and prevention. Plenum, New York

Melzack R 1973 The puzzle of pain. Penguin, Harmondsworth

Melzack R, Wall P D 1965 Pain mechanisms: a new theory. Science 150: 971–979

Melzack R, Wall P D 1988 The challenge of pain, 2nd edn. Basic Books, New York

Miller N E 1978 Biofeedback and visceral learning. Annual Review of Psychology 29: 373–404

Miller E, Morley S 1986 Investigating abnormal behaviour. Erlbaum, East Sussex

Miller R R, Jick H 1978 Clinical effects of meperidene in hospitalised medical patients. Journal of Clinical Pharmacology 18: 180–189

Moos R H 1986 Coping with life crises. Plenum, New York

Murphy T M 1976 Subjective and objective follow-up assessment of acupuncture therapy without suggestion in 100 chronic pain patients. In: Bonica J J, Albe-Fessard (eds) Advances in pain research and therapy. Raven Press, New York, vol 1

Novaco R W 1975 Anger control: the development and evaluation of an experimental treatment. Heath Lexington, Lexington MA

Olness K 1989 Hypnotherapy: a cyberphysiologic strategy in pain management. Pediatric Clinics of North America 36: 873–884

Pennebaker J W 1982 The psychology of physical symptoms. Springer, New York

Pennebaker J W 1984 Accuracy of symptom perception. In: Baum A, Taylor S E, Singer J E (eds) Handbook of psychology and health. Erlbaum, Hillsdale NJ

Peterson C, Seligman M E P 1984 Causal explanations as a risk factor for depression: theory and evidence. Psychological Review 91: 347–374

Rachman S J, Philips C 1975 Psychology and medicine. Temple Smith, London

Schaefer C, Coyne J C, Lazarus R S 1981 Social support, social networks and psychological functioning. Journal of Behavioural Medicine 4: 381–406

Seligman M E P 1975 Helplessness. W H Freeman, San Francisco

Seligman M E P, Maier S F 1967 Failure to escape traumatic shock. Journal of Experimental Psychology 74: 1–9

Selye H 1956 The stress of life. McGraw-Hill, New York

Siegel L J, Peterson L 1980 Stress reduction in young dental patients through coping skills and sensory information. Journal of Consulting and Clinical Psychology 48: 785–787

Sofaer B 1985 Pain management through nurse education. In: Copp L A (ed) Perspectives on pain. Churchill Livingstone, Edinburgh

Sofaer B 1992 Pain: a handbook for nurses, 2nd edn. Chapman & Hall, London

Speisman J C, Lazarus R S, Mordkoff A M et al 1964 Experimental reduction of stress based on ego-defense theory. Journal of Abnormal and Social Psychology 68: 367–380

Staub E, Tursky B, Schwartz G 1971 Self-control and predictability: their effects on reactions to aversive stimulation. Journal of Personality and Social Psychology 18: 157–162

Steptoe A, Vögele C 1986 Are stress responses influenced by cognitive appraisal? An experimental comparison of coping strategies. British Journal of Psychology 77: 243–255

Sternbach R A 1968 Pain: a psychophysiological analysis. Academic Press, London

Sternbach R A 1984 Acute versus chronic pain. In: Wall P D, Melzack R (eds) A textbook of pain. Churchill Livingstone, Edinburgh

Stroebel C F, Glueck B C 1973 Biofeedback treatment in medicine and psychiatry: the ultimate placebo? In: Birk L (ed) Biofeedback: behavioural medicine. Grune Stratton, New York

Sue S, Zane N 1977 Learned helplessness: theory and community psychology. In: Gibbs M, Lachenmeyer J R, Sigal J (eds) Community psychology. Gardner Press, New York

Taub A 1976 Acupuncture 'anasthesia': a critical view. In: Bonica J J, Able-Fessard D (eds) Advances in pain research and therapy. Raven Press, New York, vol 1

Taylor A, Sluckin W, Davies D R et al 1982 Introducing psychology, 2nd edn. Penguin, Harmondsworth

Taylor S E 1991 Health psychology, 2nd edn. McGraw Hill, New York

Taylor S E, Singer J E (eds) Handbook of psychology and health. Erlbaum, Hillsdale NJ

Turk D C 1978 Cognitive behavioural techniques in the management of pain. In: Foryt J P, Rathjen D P (eds) Cognitive behaviour therapy: research and application. Plenum, New York

Turk D C, Meichenbaum D, Genest M 1983 Pain and behavioural medicine: a cognitive behavioural perspective. Guildford Press, New York

Valins S, Ray A 1967 Effects of cognitive desensitisation on avoidance behaviour. Journal of Personality and Social Psychology 7: 345–350

Volicer B J, Isenberg B J, Burns M W 1977 Medical–surgical differences in hospital stress factors. Journal of Human Stress 3: 3–13

Walding M F 1991 Pain, anxiety and powerlessness. Journal of Advanced Nursing 16: 388–397

Wall P D 1984 Introduction. In: Wall P D, Melzack R (eds) A textbook of pain. Churchill Livingstone, Edinburgh

Weiss J M 1972 Influence of psychological variables on stress-induced pathology. In: Porter R, Knight J (eds) Physiology, emotion and psychosomatic illness. American Elsevier, New York

Williamson P S, Williamson M L 1983 Physiologic stress reduction by a local anasthetic during newborn circumcision. Pediatrics 71: 36–40

Wills T A, Langner T S 1980 Socioeconomic status and stress. In: Kutash I L, Schlesinger C B et al (eds) Handbook of stress and anxiety. Jossey Bass, San Francisco

Wolkind S, Zajicek E (eds) 1981 Pregnancy: a psychological and social study. Academic Press, London

Wortman C B, Dunkel-Schetter C D 1987 Conceptual and methodological issues in the study of social support. In: Baum A, Singer J E (eds) Handbook of psychology and health. Erlbaum, Hillsdale NJ, vol 5

Youell K J, McCullough J P 1975 Behavioural treatment of mucous colitis. Journal of Consulting and Clinical Psychology 43: 740–745

Younger J, Adriance W, Berger R J 1975 Sleep during transcendental meditation. Perceptual and Motor Skills 40: 953–954

Zborowski M 1969 People in pain. Jossey Bass, San Francisco

RECOMMENDED READING

Carroll D 1992 Health psychology, stress, behaviour and disease. Falmer Press, London
The emphasis of this book is on the relationship between stress and behaviour. It discusses the psychophysiology of stress and relates the findings to coronary heart disease. It also looks at stress in the broader context of health psychology as a whole.

Fontana D 1989 Managing stress. British Psychological Society/Routledge, Leicester
This is one of the 'problems in practice' series and thus concentrates on the practical features of stress

management. It incorporates many of the items discussed in this chapter into a functional programme.

McCaffery M, Beebe A 1989 Pain, clinical manual for nursing practice. Mosby, St Louis
It is important to view pain not just from a psychological perspective but from other standpoints too. This book takes a multidisciplinary perspective and illustrates how the studies on pain from different areas can be incorporated into practice.

Sofaer B 1992 Pain: a handbook for nurses, 2nd edn. Chapman & Hall, London

The advantage of this book is that it seems to cover most of the relevant points about pain in just 99 pages. This must be a boon for all time-pressed health professionals.

Sutherland V J, Cooper C L 1990 Understanding stress, a psychological perspective for health professionals. Chapman & Hall, London

This book examines the psychological aspects of stress in a health psychology context. Thus the examples and illustrations used are particularly relevant for health professionals as they mirror everyday concerns.

Bakal D A, 1979 Psychology and medicine. Tavistock, London

Copp L A (ed) 1986 Perspectives on pain. Churchill Livingstone, Edinburgh

Cox T 1978 Stress. Macmillan, London

Lazarus R S, Folkman S 1984 Stress, appraisal and coping. Springer, New York

Melzack R, Wall P D 1982 The challenge of pain. Penguin, Harmondsworth

5

Life transitions and crises

During the life span, people experience a series of transitions and crises. This chapter seeks to map out these events and discusses two conceptual frameworks that have been put forward to explain the experiences of people undergoing crisis and transition. The effectiveness of the two models is examined with respect to parenthood and bereavement.

> Like the lobster or the soft-shelled crab, humans seem sometimes to outgrow their 'shells' and become somewhat more vulnerable as they move from one phase of life to another.
>
> Kimmel (1980)

Developmental life-cycle approaches attempt to map out the course of human development throughout the life span. During the life span there are certain stages, or periods, in people's lives where they face a transition from one state to another. Some psychologists have referred to these periods in life as 'crises', in that they have to be resolved before the individual is able to proceed to the next stage. All individuals proceed through each of the stages of development, but it is the way in which they resolve the crises in each particular stage that shapes their personality.

Another approach accepts that there are certain stages in human development that have crucial significance for individuals, but states that there are other events during the life span that can also shape development. These events may be experienced by some individuals but not by others. The aim is to determine the sorts of life event that have psychological significance and to study how individuals adapt and cope with them. This approach has been called the 'marker' approach because it views life events as significant points in human development and seeks to mark them out.

Others view crises and transitions as processes and attempt to illustrate the common features of these processes and how individuals utilise specific coping mechanisms to deal with them. Two models are reviewed that have attempted to give an indication of the sorts of problems people experience during life crises. Most individuals experience the prospect of parenthood in some way or another. Similarly, at some stage, most of us will experience bereavement and will cope with it in different ways. Therefore it was decided to investigate these two particular crises/transitions in greater detail with a view to assessing the relevance and applicability of the two models of coping and adaptation.

DEVELOPMENTAL PERSPECTIVES

The two names most commonly associated with developmental psychology are Piaget and Freud. When life-span human development is being discussed, however, it is the work of Erik Erikson that immediately springs to mind. There are other theories of development that take a life-span perspective such as Buhler & Massarik (1968), Havighurst (1972) and Levinson et al (1978), but Erikson's is the best-known theory.

Although Erikson began his career as a student of Freud, his theory of personality development differs from Freud's in some important ways. Firstly, he emphasises the psychosocial nature of development. He believes that any theory of psychological development must take into consideration social, political and geographical influences on individuals and the significant effects of individuals on society. Development is defined partly by maturation and partly by the society in which the person grows. Secondly his theory does not view personality development ending at adolescence, but continuing to develop throughout the life span.

Erikson's theory

Erikson (1980) proposes eight stages of development. He calls these *developmental crises*, but crisis should be viewed more as a dilemma or period of difficulty rather than a catastrophe.

They are times when individuals face a transition or turning point in their lives, often accompanied by a degree of stress associated with having to resolve the dilemma. Each stage is phrased in terms of an opposition between two characteristics and the individual is required to successfully negotiate the stage or task in order to move on to the next one.

Stage 1: Basic trust vs mistrust (birth to 1 year)

The first crisis or dilemma occurs during the first year of life. The issue is whether the infant will be able to develop a sense of trust in the predictability of the world, or whether he will become mistrusting of the people and events that occur around him. The central role in this stage is played by the mother or caregiver. The children who emerge from the first year with a sense of trust are those with parents who are loving and respond predictably and reliably to the child. Not only is trust in the mother or caregiver a key element in an early secure attachment, but a child who has developed a sense of trust will go on to other relationships carrying this sense with him.

Stage 2: Autonomy vs shame and doubt (1 to 3 years)

The crisis is between developing a sense of confidence and independence versus shame and doubt. Parents again play a crucial role in determining the successful resolution of this conflict. If the child is able to experience new situations with confidence and a belief in himself, then he will go on to develop self-control and self-worth in later life. If, however, his efforts are met with continuous failure and ridicule, then shame and self-doubt will emerge. Since toilet training usually occurs during this stage, it is important for parents to exercise care in how they deal with the child's mistakes.

Stage 3: Initiative vs guilt (3 to 6 years)

A central problem of this stage is where the child 'goes too far'. He begins to pursue activities on his own, playing games with other children and offering help around the house. Sometimes his initiative will result in overdoing things as his knowledge of 'the rules' is incomplete. The risk is that when the child oversteps the mark, parents might respond with restrictions and punishment; both resulting in the development of guilt. Some guilt is normal, but too much guilt will inhibit initiative.

Stage 4: Industry vs inferiority (7 to 11 years)

At this time in the child's development the influence of the peer group gains ascendancy in the child's list of priorities. Schooling provides the vehicle for the development of new skills and the child is continually striving to achieve levels of competence comparable to his peers. Difficulties occur when the child is unable to develop expected skills and may instead develop a sense of inferiority. Pressure from parents to succeed at all costs can be extremely counterproductive; instead of the child growing up able to master his environment, he will grow up to feel inferior and shrink from trying out new things.

Stage 5: Identity vs role confusion (12 to 18 years)

It is not surprising that the adolescent boy or girl may experience a certain degree of role confusion during this stage. At the age of 16 the adolescent can, with the consent of parents, get married and start a family. This is one of the most responsible and important decisions an individual has to make during his or her life. In our society the 16-year-old is adjudged to be 'adult' enough to make that decision, yet not mature enough to drive a car, drink alcohol in a bar or view an 18-rated film. This is a time when the individual is continually seeking a sense of identity; a sexual identity, an occupational identity and an ethnic identity. The crisis is resolved when an integrated sense of self emerges, that is, the adolescent now knows what he or she wants to do and be.

Stage 6: Intimacy vs isolation (young adulthood)

Only if a well-integrated identity emerges from stage 5 can psychological intimacy with other people be possible. Erikson sees intimacy as the sharing of oneself with another and argues that there will be nothing to share if a sense of identity has not developed. Although young people usually form relationships with the opposite sex at this time, their friendships with the same sex and even their access to their own intimate feelings also mark this stage. People whose sense of identity is fragile see danger in letting others glimpse their dilemma and avoid all close contacts, choosing isolation instead of intimacy.

Stage 7: Generativity vs stagnation (middle adulthood)

Erikson defines generativity as 'the interest in guiding and establishing the next generation'. This is usually accomplished through child rearing and 'productive endeavours'. However it is not simply about bringing up children, but has to do with a faith in the future; a belief in the species. Instead of having children, one may work to create a better world for others. A lack of generativity may be expressed in stagnation, self-indulgence, boredom and lack of psychological growth.

Stage 8: Integrity vs despair (late adulthood)

If one has successfully managed to negotiate the previous six stages, then a sense of integrity will have developed. It refers to the acceptance of the limitations of life, a sense of being part of a larger whole that includes previous generations. It enables one to approach death without fear. Despair occurs if one looks back on one's life and wonders what it was all about; seeing it as unsatisfactory, yet realising that there is no time to start again. A feeling of 'was that it?' prevails.

The main strength of Erikson's theory is that he offers one of the few frameworks for describing change in childhood and adulthood. His theory has been criticised however for being overtly 'fuzzy' (Bee 1992) in that it represents a set of assumptions rather than precise descriptions of causes and relationships. Further Buss (1979) points out that Erikson considers psychological growth and health to be possible only if the behaviour of the individual is consistent with the society in which it develops. This benign view of society denies the fact that the social reality of the individual may be extremely repressive. Under such conditions, the healthy response would be one of shame and doubt rather than autonomy, or identity diffusion rather than identity. 'His view of society as a cosy, beneficial social institution promulgates a conformist theory which is excessively supportive of the status quo' (Roazen 1976).

The theory also suffers from the criticisms that have been directed towards psychoanalysis in general, that is, lack of empirical evidence to substantiate claims, retrospective analysis of data, etc.

The main advantages of the theory are that it provides markers to those events in people's lives that are likely to prove more difficult than others. It illustrates that these 'crises' are in fact transitions from one stage to another and individuals may need help to negotiate these transitions. Finally the theory emphasises that our personalities are not formed at birth but go on developing throughout the life span (Stevens 1983). Thus health professionals can use the approach of Erikson to highlight the sorts of problems that are likely to affect people at specific stages in their lives. As such it provides a marker to the time of the problem, but does little to provide guidelines on how to help people through their crisis or transition.

A competency model

Danish & D'Augelli (1980) have chosen a life-span human development perspective for their personal competency model. Unlike Erikson, they are concerned with developing techniques to help individuals negotiate life transitions with as little disruption as possible. Indeed, the authors propose that critical events during a person's life are not destructive episodes but in fact serve to intensify a restructuring process that can 'marshal resources toward further growth'.

The model has the following attributes: '(1) a central focus on life events; (2) a developmental as opposed to a disease conception; and (3) a belief that past life events help one prepare for future life events.' The authors suggest that if events are only viewed as markers the importance of the context of events is underestimated. Further, viewing events as markers also ignores the importance of the individual's experience of the event. The developmental intervention model they propose is centred on the enhancement of personal competence. 'The development of personal competency, a goal of the intervention, is defined as the ability to be self-reliant and to do life planning.' The more resources at the disposal of individuals, the better able they are to deal with life events and benefit from the experience. Resources are interpersonal skills (relating effectively to others), intrapersonal skills (competence in such things as setting goals, acquiring knowledge, making decisions, taking risks, developing self-control and understanding oneself) and social support networks (family and friends).

Danish & D'Augelli (1982) consider there to be consistent similarities between life events, hence individuals should be encouraged to reflect on past events, whether successful or unsuccessful, in order to utilise those skills that were successful in the past or reflect on the sorts of skills that they might have used to make the encounter more successful.

> While the content or knowledge one needs to encounter the events differ, the skills, risks and attitudes necessary for a successful outcome generally overlap. For example, the life events of beginning a new job and marriage differ in the content of events, but require related skills—decision making, risk taking, and so on.
>
> Danish et al (1981)

Danish & D'Augelli (1982) have put forward a programme designed to teach life-skills. It consists of six individual skills:

- goal assessment
- knowledge acquisition
- decision-making
- risk assessment
- creation of social support
- planning of skill development.

The main component of the programme is the goal setting component. In their scheme it is the individuals themselves who decide what is important to learn, what goals to attain and how to attain them. The role of the health professional is to act in an advisory capacity and to use her expertise to help individuals identify their goals and develop plans to attain them. Goal assessment is made up of three parts:

• goal identification
• goal importance
• goal attainment.

Rather than concentrating on what not to do, Danish & D'Augelli (1982) state that individuals should be encouraged to identify specific, positive behaviours so that they may have the opportunity to initiate action and then evaluate whether these actions are related to how they wish to behave. Goal importance seeks to distinguish between those goals that are important to the individual and those that are important to others. The authors suggest that the former are more easily obtained than the latter.

The final process of goal attainment is barred by what Danish & D'Augelli term a number of 'roadblocks'. The first roadblock is a lack of knowledge and refers to information or facts which are needed if the goal is to be achieved. The second roadblock is a lack of decision-making skills where individuals often know what to do but not how to do it. The third refers to worries about the risks involved in any action taken. Some individuals know what to do and how to do it but are afraid of the risks. If the costs outweigh the benefits, action may not be taken. The final roadblock is a lack of social support. Social support may be a crucial factor in maintaining new behaviour. Each of these roadblocks has been developed by Danish & D'Augelli into specific skills taught in a Life Development Intervention Programme. The last skill included in the programme is planning skill development, a process designed to help individuals learn how to design and implement their own skill programmes.

The ultimate goal of skill dissemination is that it becomes a self-help process. As most self-help materials, particularly self-help books, do not teach skills but disseminate knowledge, Danish & D'Augelli (1982) propose that skills should be taught using an educational approach. In other words, the intervenor becomes a teacher rather than a therapist and a medical–disease orientation is replaced by a learning one. The process of skill training consists of the following steps:

1. the skill is defined in behavioural terms
2. the rationale for the skill is presented and discussed
3. a skill attainment criterion is specified
4. a model of effective and ineffective skills is presented
5. the skills are practised under supervision
6. outside practice emphasising continued behavioural rehearsal
7. an evaluation of skill levels using a behavioural checklist and other evaluation tools (Danish 1977).

The format includes a conceptual understanding of the skills, seeing others demonstrate aspects of the skill and practising the skill while receiving feedback. This particular approach emphasises the role of the health professional as a teacher rather than a person involved in clinical treatment. As such there is a strong emphasis on prevention and 'growth' rather than treatment and rehabilitation.

LIFE EVENTS

Erikson's stages of development are 'normative life events'; meaning those events that are likely to affect all of us at some time during our lives. Further, in his theory, he gives an indication of when these events are likely to occur. However, there are life events which happen to only some people at totally unpredictable times during their lives. Kimmel (1980) refers to normative transitions as 'those changes that are expected according to the social norms for individuals at particular times of their lives,' whereas idiosyncratic transitions refer to 'those changes in life patterns that are unique to a particular individual'. Examples of normative transitions would be changing schools, marriage, parenthood and retirement. Examples of idiosyncratic transitions would be divorce, death of a child, a major illness and winning or losing a large amount of money.

Kimmel (1980) suggests that, whilst not all life events can be categorised neatly into normative and idiosyncratic transitions, the life events that are normative cause less stress than their idiosyncratic counterparts. Neugarten (1977) says that 'The normal expectable life events do not themselves constitute crises, nor are they trauma producing.' Normative transitions are turning points, and do call for changes in self-concept, sense of identity, new social roles and new adaptations, but 'they are not, for the vast group of normal persons, traumatic events or crises that trigger mental illness or destroy the continuity of the self.' For Kimmel and Neugarten, life events may be quantified in terms of whether they are anticipated or unanticipated; the anticipated life event is related to change, reorientation and transition; the unanticipated life event is related to trauma and major stress.

Classification of life events

An early attempt to go beyond a binary quantification of stress in life events was provided by Holmes & Rahe (1967). They attempted to obtain a quantitative index of the degree of stress experienced following exposure to a situation requiring some form of adjustment. Holmes & Rahe (1967) asked 394 subjects to rate the length of time it took them to adjust to various life events, the intensity of these events and the average amount of adaptation to the events. They were told that marriage had a value of 500, and were asked to rate 43 life events using marriage as a reference point. No event was found to be more than twice as stressful as marriage, however the majority of events (36) were rated less stressful than marriage. The relative stress values of the life events are given in Table 5.1.

The Social Readjustment Rating Scale (SRRS) was an early attempt to classify and describe life events. The main problem with the scale was

Table 5.1 Life events in order of stressfulness (Holmes & Rahe 1967)

Life event	Stress value
1. Death of spouse	100
2. Divorce	73
3. Marital separation	65
4. Jail term	63
5. Death of a close family member	63
6. Personal injury or illness	53
7. Marriage	50
8. Fired at work	47
9. Marital reconciliation	45
10. Retirement	45
11. Change in health of family member	44
12. Pregnancy	40
13. Sex difficulties	39
14. Gain of new family member	39
15. Business readjustment	39
16. Change in financial state	38
17. Death of a close friend	37
18. Change to a different line of work	36
19. Change in number of arguments with spouse	35
20. Large mortgage repayments	31
21. Foreclosure of mortgage or loan	30
22. Change in responsibilities at work	29
23. Son or daughter leaving home	29
24. Trouble with in-laws	29
25. Outstanding personal achievement	28
26. Wife begins or stops work	26
27. Begin or end school	26
28. Change in living conditions	25
29. Revision of personal habits	24
30. Trouble with boss	23
31. Change in work hours or conditions	20
32. Change in residence	20
33. Change in schools	20
34. Change in recreation	19
35. Change in church activities	19
36. Change in social activities	18
37. Small mortgage repayments	17
38. Change in sleeping habits	16
39. Change in number of family get-togethers	15
40. Change in eating habits	15
41. Vacation	13
42. Christmas	12
43. Minor violations of the law	11

that it utilised only one dimension—stress. As we have seen in the last chapter, people perceive the same stressful event in different ways; cognitive appraisal of life events does not feature in the scale. A further inadequacy is the tendency to treat positive and negative life events as being equally stressful. Johnson & McCutchen (1980) found that subjects who had experienced higher levels of negative change were found to be more anxious and more depressed than those experiencing the same levels of positive change.

Kanner et al (1981) constructed the 'Hassles and Uplifts' scale to take this into consideration, and have utilised the scale to assess the daily and cumulative impact of everyday demands. The most frequent 'hassles' over a 9-month period were:

1. concerns about weight
2. health of a family member
3. rising prices of common goods
4. home maintenance, inside
5. too many things to do.

The most frequent uplifts were:

1. relating well with your spouse or lover
2. relating well with friends
3. completing a task
4. feeling healthy
5. getting enough sleep.

This study was based on a sample of 448 white, middle-class adults aged 20 to 60 years (hassles) and 100 white, middle-class adults aged 45 to 64 years (uplifts). Scores on the Uplift scale were found to be positively related to psychological symptoms for women only. When importance of event was taken into consideration factors relating to work were by far the most troublesome.

Classifications of life events that use more than one dimension have been put forward by Reese & Smyer (1983) and Brim & Ryer (1980). Brim & Ryer (1980) describe life events using a three-dimensional classification. Their aim was to provide individuals with information about the likelihood that a particular event would occur, when it might occur and the likelihood that it might also happen to other people too. Hence the three structural characteristics of their taxonomy are:

- *Likelihood*—the probability that an event will take place
- *Age-relatedness*—the correlation of the event with age
- *Prevalence*—whether the event will occur for many people or just a few.

Reese & Smyer (1983) used two dimensions to classify life events. They identified 14 event contexts and 4 event types producing a total of 56 cells. When they classified 355 life events according to this taxonomy, they found a wide variation with respect to the categories used. Friendships, community and miscellaneous categories were used infrequently (less than 4% of the events), whereas others such as family, work, health and love/marriage accounted for nearly half of the events (48.8%).

Reese & Smyer (1983) suggest that these findings might be due to the fact that the heavily used categories have been too broadly drawn and the under-used categories too finely drawn. They also found a varied distribution of the events among the types:

- socio-cultural 48.0%
- personal-psychological 31.9%
- biological 16.1%
- physical-environmental 4.0%.

These results, and the findings with respect to the contexts, may be due to the respective interests of the researchers who formed the basis of the study. They tended to be social scientists as opposed to physical/biological scientists.

Reese & Smyer (1983) suggest that the taxonomy may be used to investigate the interrelationships between various dimensions, to look at how such factors as age, sex, culture and history affect the dimensional values of life events and whether the salient dimensions of a particular life event change as a function of age, sex, culture and history.

Life events and primary prevention

A major focus of research into life events has been the attempts to clarify the relationship between the events and the aetiology of mental and physical disorders. Following the work of Holmes & Rahe (1967), a number of studies have found significant associations between the occurrence of life events in the recent past and a wide array of physical and psychological disorders (McGrath & Burkhart 1983). Despite consistent significant associations between life events and disorders, the level of correlation in most cases is quite small (0.30). These somewhat disappointing results have led to a number of criticisms (some of which have already been mentioned) and attempts at reformulating the conceptual and empirical framework of life event research.

One set of assumptions underlying much of the research is that change in individuals' lives resulting from life events may be associated with heightened levels of psychosocial stress and, in turn, that such stress is an important factor in physical and psychological disorder (Dohrenwend 1978). Bloom (1979) in fact argues that one goal of health professionals is to try to prevent the undesirable consequences of stressful life events in as many people as possible. This is, however, just one of the primary major goals of prevention. Cowen (1980) has argued that the ultimate goals of prevention are 'to engineer structures, processes, situations, events, and programs that maximally benefit, both in scope and temporal stability, the psychological adjustment, effectiveness, happiness, and coping skills of large numbers of individuals'. Of equal importance to the prevention of pathology is the creation of competence, health and well-being, as well as the facilitation of mastery of one's environment.

Two different approaches to primary prevention can be identified: (a) the prediction and understanding of physical and psychological disorder in a population as a function of its association with life events; (b) the process by which life events facilitate adaptation, development and 'growth' in an individual. The former owes much of its emphasis to the epidemiological approach of Bloom (1979), whereas the latter is also derived from the 'crisis' theory of Caplan (1964).

An examination of life events recently experienced by an individual may be helpful in identifying those who may be at risk for the development of emotional or physical disorders prior to such difficulties actually being manifest. One focus of primary prevention is on programmes that operate before any damage has been done and thus reduce the incidence of any disorder. A careful assessment of the types and number of life events experienced by an individual or population can be important indicators of the need for such programmes.

Identification of those conditions which consistently predispose individuals to developing physical or psychological difficulties, such as experiencing life events, may be critical to the success of efforts to justify the need for the allocation of scarce resources to preventive services. Without such evidence it may be difficult to convince those professionals trained in the more reactive, rather than proactive, human service delivery system.

Felner et al (1985)

Unfortunately there are a number of problems with this approach:

- *Positive vs negative life events.* Some life event inventories do not distinguish between positive and negative life events. For instance Holmes & Rahe (1967) say that it is the change per se which is responsible for life stress. However, negative life changes have been consistently found to correlate significantly with adverse physical or psychological conditions, while positive events often do not (Sarason et al 1978).
- *Antecedent or consequent.* Billings & Moos (1982) have noted that much of the research on life events has assumed that their occurrence is random. People may have a propensity to experience negative life events due to pre-existing emotional or social problems. Sexual difficulties, divorce, losing one's job and arguing with one's spouse may be potential consequences rather than causes of pathology (Dohrenwend 1979).
- *Anticipation and perceived control.* Stressful life events cause the most problems when they are perceived as uncontrollable (Dohrenwend & Martin 1979).

It is clear that the adaptive impact of life events is a function not only of the number of events, but of the quality of the events as well. There seems to be a tendency to concentrate on ways to ameliorate the consequences of negative life events without investigating the 'positive' potential of such situations. Caplan (1964) has suggested that a key element of even the serious life crisis is the opportunity for positive growth.

Indeed a life crisis represents one of the best times for intervention. An individual is more willing to listen to health professionals when the content of the message refers to the individual's immediate concerns and experiences. Thus Caplan's (1964) 'crisis intervention' can be primary prevention if the health professional is able to facilitate adaptation, learning and growth to the extent that individuals are able to benefit from the experience and can face up to any future potential crisis using skills they have developed in previous ones.

Another difficulty with the work on cumulative stress from life events is the assumption that life events can be quantified in numerical terms. Do 10 traffic tickets represent the same degree of stress as death of a spouse? Holmes (1979) says: 'Essentially, worldwide, death of a spouse requires twice as much change in adjustment as marriage and 10 times as much change as a traffic ticket.' There may be some equivalence between death of a spouse and 10 traffic tickets if one were to receive all 10 traffic tickets at the same time, but the amount of readjustment and change resulting from each event is ignored in the SRSS taxonomy.

One way of resolving some of the above difficulties is to distinguish between two separate types of events. There are those that are limited both temporally and in their repercussions on people's lives, and there are those that 'are really better viewed as markers or precipitants of the unfolding of major changes in an individual's life which may engender new stresses and changes and demand adaptive effort for some time to come.' (Felner et al 1980).

Rather than seeing life changes such as marriage, parenthood, divorce, moving house, bereavement, retirement and chronic illness as discrete stressful events, a better approach would be to focus on the entire transitional period during which people are being called upon to utilise adaptive techniques during the process of change.

Felner et al (1985) suggest a possible modus operandi:

A life transition framework which recognises that some life events are potential precipitants or markers of transitional processes rather than more limited events makes it possible, indeed critical, to attempt to identify common defining characteristics of transitions which may have greater levels of adaptive significance. While transitions such as retirement, geographic relocation, divorce, loss of spouse, being disabled, marriage or remarriage, becoming a parent, and changing or completing school appear to involve divergent sets of issues to resolve, they may be quite similar in terms of the types of tasks or changes they engender for individuals. A transitional framework allows us to focus on such commonalities and to develop strategies for enhancing individual's adaptive abilities across a wide array of life changes.

Two such transitional frameworks will be discussed next.

TWO CONCEPTUAL FRAMEWORKS

The following conceptual models represent a guide to the process of experiencing life crises and transitions. Both models, one British and one American, attempt to illustrate the adaptive and coping mechanisms required by individuals during the period of crisis or transition. In Chapter 2 we discussed the techniques and skills that health professionals can use to help people through their transitional period or time of crisis. The skills themselves are useful in many different contexts. With respect to life crises and transitions, however, it is useful to have an idea of the sorts of emotions, thoughts and problems that individuals are likely to experience during the course of their time of difficulty.

Caregivers need to be conversant with knowledge of coping tasks and skills and to be sensitive to people's emotional reactions and needs. Coupled with their own empathy and understanding of crisis situations, this information can help them diffuse the negative impact of life's crises and nurture the potential for growth intrinsic in such situations.

Moos (1986)

Hopson's model

A body of research has developed indicating a predictable cycle of reactions and feelings that accompany life events and transitions. Hopson (1981) and Hopson & Scally (1991) present a seven-phase model of stages accompanying transition. The cycle is a general pattern rather than a rigid sequence of events. Progression through the cycle is not smooth and continuous. Some people will oscillate between stages, others may take differing amounts of time to complete the transition, whilst some will become 'stuck' in certain stages unable to progress any further. Similarly the extent of the swings in mood will vary from one circumstance to another. Some commentators have substituted other labels for this dimension, such as morale (Harrison 1976) and competence (Parkes & Lewis 1981). The following stages represent a sequence of responses accompanying a wide range of life events or transitions:

Stage 1: Immobilisation

If a person were to win a substantial sum of money in a lottery or if he were to arrive home one evening and find his house burnt to the ground, the first reaction would be one of disbelief, a sort of numbness that these things just could not be happening to him. This shock is proportional to the degree of crisis experienced by the individual.

Stage 2(i): Reaction—elation or despair

The shock gives way to a sharp swing of mood either elation or despair, depending on the nature of the transition. As has been suggested earlier, the degree of the swing in mood will depend on the specific circumstances of the event.

Stage 2(ii): Reaction—minimisation

The 'high' or 'low' will be followed by a period of reassessment. In the case of positive life events, a large win may be accompanied by a realisation that friends might tend to view one differently due to the money. Negative life events may be ameliorated by dissonance reduction. People adopt strategies to remind them that things could be worse, they might even consider themselves to be well off in comparison to other people.

Stage 3: Self-doubt

Originally Hopson & Adams (1976) called this stage depression, which might be appropriate in some negative life events. However, depression does not really characterise the mood of a person after a positive event such as winning a large sum of money in a lottery. The gift of a large sum of money would be associated with some sort of change in lifestyle and this change would engender an element of self-doubt as to whether one could cope with a lifestyle up until now, never experienced. With negative events the minimisation phase may not be noticeable and the individual may pass from despair to self-doubt without noticing any change. The emotions associated with this phase are anxiety, anger and sometimes sadness.

Stage 4: Letting go

This is the most important phase in the whole cycle as it marks the transition from the past to the future. Up until this point the individual has remained emotionally attached to the past. This attachment has to be broken in order to develop new affectional bonds. Letting go is a very traumatic time since the individual has to sever old bonds without any knowledge of what lies in store in the future. However, it represents the point where individuals can convert the tragedies and disasters in their lives into growth points.

Stage 5: Testing

This is an experimental period where the individual can try out new options, identities and affectional bonds. It is accompanied by mood swings as successes and failures are experienced. Gradually the individual starts to build on the low point of the cycle and move upwards.

Stage 6: Search for meaning

At some point the individual has to look back on the transition or crisis and try to make sense of what has happened to him. This stage in the cycle represents an attempt to learn from the experience. It is not a morbid attempt to remain in the past, but a genuine attempt to search for meaning in what happened. As such it is a healthy form of reflective thinking.

Stage 7: Integration

The final phase completes the process of transition. The individual now feels a sense of integration between the new lifestyle and the crisis itself. A disabled person has become a person with a disability in one area and skills in others. The progression through the whole cycle enables individuals to face up to prospective crises and transitions with self-confidence and also the knowledge that, having coped with one difficult situation, they can cope with another.

These crises and transitions are very much developmental stages. They should not be viewed like an illness that affects one for a time then, when it has gone, one reverts to one's old state. The process of experiencing a life crisis or transition causes people to view their lives in different ways; ways that preclude a reversal to the old perspective. The phase of letting go signifies a change from one state to another. The developmental aspect of life transitions are illustrated in Hopson's model by the fact that successful negotiation of the stages results in an end point higher up the scale of mood and self-worth. It may well be the case that crises as such are necessary for personal growth.

Hopson's model represents a simple attempt to map out the experiences of people undergoing life crises and transitions. There are one or two problems arising from the simplicity. It seems to work well for negative life events, less well for positive ones. A positive life event is rarely associated with a large lowering in mood due to self-doubt. Similarly, an individual who has suffered a serious illness may not come out of the process in a higher mood state than before it occurred. Further, it is by no means certain that people will progress all the way through the cycle. Whilst Hopson is aware of this it is not very clear what needs to be done to help them to

do so. Apart from these relatively minor points, the model will prove useful for all health professionals who are faced with providing care to a wide range of individuals experiencing a wide range of crises and transitions.

Moos's model

Moos (1986) suggests that a crisis sets forth adaptive tasks to which various coping skills can be applied. According to this model there are five major sets of adaptive tasks:

- Establish the meaning and significance of the situation
- Confront reality
- Sustain relationships with family and friends
- Maintain a reasonable emotional balance
- Preserve a satisfactory self-image.

Establishing meaning. The first task is to establish the meaning and to understand the personal significance of the situation. Moos says that there is a continual need to refer back to the crisis in order to 'assimilate the meaning' of each aspect of it. After the initial shock has subsided and the significance of the event becomes apparent, individuals should try to understand, accept and construct an explanation for their present situation. Children whose parents have just become divorced have to understand the reality of the separation, accept the loss of the pre-divorce family and finally construct an explanation of the event in the context of its permanence.

Confronting reality. During any crisis or transition there are a number of requirements external to the event itself that have to be dealt with. After a death there are funeral arrangements to be made, financial affairs to be managed and decisions on how to rebuild one's life to be made.

Sustaining relationships. This set of tasks refers to the difficulty of keeping communication lines open. After experiencing a crisis or transition, it is often difficult to speak to friends and relations who want to help. Social support must either be maintained or facilitated despite the individual's reluctance to engage in interaction. In many crises, adequate relationships need to be formed with health and community care professionals as well in order to create empathic communication channels.

Maintaining emotional balance. Both transitions and crises arouse powerful emotions. It is important to try to keep these emotions in perspective. The nature of the crisis will tend to determine the strength and type of emotion, but the management of upsetting feelings is an important stage in developing and sustaining hope even when circumstances seem particularly gloomy.

Preserving self-image. Individuals who have experienced a divorce may lack self-confidence in their ability to form new relationships. Victims of rape who experienced a marked reduction of self-esteem took longer to recover than those whose self-esteem was higher (Burgess & Holmstrom 1979). It is important to strike a balance between accepting help and taking control of one's life on one's own.

Whilst these five adaptive tasks are encountered in every transition and crisis, their importance varies according to the individual, the nature of the stressor and the circumstances surrounding the event. It may be particularly difficult to establish the meaning of the death of a young child; similarly maintaining emotional balance under these circumstances may be well nigh impossible. Also victims of incest may not only experience difficulty forming relationships but also hold a poor view of themselves. All of these adaptive tasks are difficult and, not surprisingly, individuals develop specific coping skills to deal with them.

The coping skills that are employed to deal with adaptive tasks can be either adaptive or maladaptive, that is, skills effective in one situation may not be in another. Similarly, those that may be effective for a small amount of time may prove harmful if practised over a long period. Moos (1986) puts forward three categories of coping skills that involve cognitive, behavioural and affective components:

- *appraisal-focused coping* refers to skills used to modify the meaning and comprehend the threat of a situation
- *problem-focused coping* tries actively to confront the problem and deal with the consequences
- *emotion-focused coping* deals with the skills used for the management of feelings.

Within these three categories there are nine types of coping responses:

Logical analysis and mental preparation. Although represented as one type of coping skill, it has two parts. Logical analysis refers firstly to the ability to pay attention to one aspect of the crisis at a time 'breaking a seemingly overwhelming problem into small, potentially manageable bits'. Secondly, it is sometimes helpful to place the experience into a long-term perspective. Mental preparation is a skill that is often practised before the event as well as after. It refers to recalling memories of past successes in similar circumstances or anticipatory mourning of an expected death.

Cognitive redefinition. This skill accepts the reality of the event but restructures it into a more acceptable experience. (The same sort of technique for the management of pain was discussed in the last chapter.) In the context of life crises and transitions it refers more to individuals comparing themselves to others who are less fortunate, attending to aspects of themselves that make them appear advantaged, constructing alternative scenarios that are much worse and finally trying to extract positive features from the event, such as increased self-esteem or personal maturity (Taylor et al 1983).

Cognitive avoidance or denial. The use of denial as a coping mechanism is often seen as maladaptive, but it can provide a 'breathing space' where people are protected from becoming overwhelmed and given time to consolidate other personal coping resources. The skills of cognitive avoidance and denial are sometimes described as 'defence mechanisms' because they are an immediate response to stress. Whilst this coping skill may be necessary in the short term, to continue to deny a crisis will inevitably result in an inability to work through the major maladaptive tasks.

Seeking information and support. This set of skills is split into two. Seeking information is formulated in three parts: obtaining information about the crisis, investigating alternative courses of action and predicting their probable outcome. Seeking support from family and friends and other helpful people in the community is a valuable source of strength in difficult times. However, there is a certain amount of tension between the need to seek support and the need to be on one's own. In cases of sudden death, the bereaved often withdraw and may become inaccessible. Health professionals in these situations often describe later how useless and helpless they have felt and how emotionally fragile they feel (Wright 1993). They find it difficult to accept the value of 'just being there'. For most people the need to be on one's own is supplemented by a need for social support from family and friends and occasionally from people not involved with the family. In some instances national self-help organisations provide the type of support the individual needs.

Taking problem-solving action. These skills refer to the ability to 'get things done'. If, for example, a couple has experienced the birth of a first child, there are plans to be made regarding care of the baby, performing household tasks, employment arrangements and developing new roles. After the death of a spouse, numerous arrangements have to be made regarding the funeral, financial problems and a new social role. The operation of these skills leads to the development of a sense of competence and self-esteem, which can prove a relief for relatives as well as the individuals themselves.

Pursuing alternative rewards. Changing activities and pursuing new sources of satisfaction are often necessary correlates of crisis and transition. After the sudden death of a child, there may be a decision to direct more energy toward one's work or become involved in a self-help group. Divorce may cause the individual to seek alternative activities, friends and social roles.

Affective regulation. Control of one's emotions can be crucial to maintaining hope for the future. Individuals may react quite calmly to a crisis. It might seem as if they were detached from the whole situation. This has been interpreted as denial but may in fact be skilled affective regulation. Other ways to regulate emotion are to work through one's feelings and progressively to desensitise oneself to the emotional stimulus. A recent widow may not be able to look at a picture of her husband at first, but gradually she becomes able to sort through his clothes and deal with his personal effects.

Emotional discharge. This is the opposite of affective regulation and refers to giving vent to one's feelings openly. It includes crying, becoming angry, despairing and even screaming in protest, but it also includes more inappropriate responses such as laughing and 'acting out', where the individuals engage in tension-reducing strategies like drinking, smoking and eating binges.

Resigned acceptance. Accepting the situation for what it is and realising that there is nothing that can be done to change it are the skills of resigned acceptance. This does not mean that the person is unable to engage in problem-solving skills; it simply represents a conscious decision to accept the circumstances as they are. When the death of a close friend is inevitable, it is important to accept the situation in order to promote disengagement and reduce distress.

Moos (1986) suggests that these nine sets of coping skills are seldom used singly or exclusively and cover the most common coping skills used by individuals during the course of their lives. He also puts forward three factors that determine why some individuals respond differently to crises and transitions than others:

- Demographic and personal factors help to define psycho-social crises as well as to resolve them. They include age, gender, ethnicity, socioeconomic status, cognitive and emotional maturity, self-confidence, religious commitments and prior crises and coping experiences.
- Event-related factors refer to the type of stressor. The numerous classifications of life events have been discussed earlier in the chapter. Variations among stressors define the

nature of the tasks individuals face. Events over which a person has a certain degree of control are more likely to elicit problem-solving coping strategies, whereas uncontrollable events tend to evoke cognitive and emotion-focused responses.

- Aspects of the social and physical environment affect the adaptive tasks of individuals. Social support is an important ingredient in the management of crises and transitions. In certain circumstances, social cohesion may prove counterproductive. Adjusting to the death of a child might be more difficult in a 'closely knit' family because it is seen as more of a loss. In most circumstances, however, social support leads to better adaptation and produces more positive outcomes of crises and transitions. Institutional resources in the community, such as child care facilities, play a significant role in reducing the stress of parents who work outside the home. Also self-help groups provide opportunities for individuals to share experiences, advice and gain confidence to face everyday life.

There are similarities between this model and the one presented by Hopson (1981). Firstly, they both emphasise the possibility of positive outcomes from crises and transitions. Secondly, they both attempt to map out the sorts of cognitions, emotions and behaviours that typically accompany crises and transitions. Thirdly, they present the role of the health professional as a prevention operator, in that they suggest the importance of developing appropriate adaptive and coping skills to deal with future crises and transitions. In trying to provide models that will fit all cases there are inevitable shortcomings; Hopson (1981) does not represent the self-actualising properties of the crisis particularly well; Moos (1986) sometimes confuses adaptive tasks with coping skills; and they both fail to consider the balance that has to be struck between 'old self' and 'new self' (Tedeschi 1987). Nevertheless, they both provide a conceptual guideline that can aid health professionals in caring for people who have emotional difficulties. A number of years ago, I asked a health visitor what aspects of psychology she thought

were most useful in her job. She said anything that gave her some idea of what to do in situations where there was a large degree of emotional difficulty due to a crisis. These models at least go some way in providing this information; just how far they go and just how well they work can be examined next with reference to two crises/transitions: parenthood and bereavement.

PARENTHOOD

Pregnancy is the fulfilment of a woman's deepest yearnings . . . it is a calm, partly dream-like period during which women can give up all other demands and pressures and devote themselves to the forthcoming child.

Deutsch (1947)

Two main issues concerning becoming a parent for the first time are:

- Is the event construed by parents as a positive or negative experience?
- Is it a time of crisis or transition?

Theories

Mothers

The views of Deutsch, a leading psychoanalyst in the 1930s and 1940s, might seem misplaced in the context of present-day attitudes towards pregnancy, yet they were not seen as anything strange at the time. Indeed it is true to say that her views are an accurate reflection of the society in which she lived and its attitudes towards women. Pregnancy and motherhood were seen as positive events in a woman's life. Unfortunately this 'idealisation' of motherhood denied women the right to express doubts and negative feelings towards the event. If they did exhibit conflicting emotions, then it was often assumed that they were not going to become 'good' mothers. A number of studies began to appear illustrating the period of pregnancy as a time of mixed feelings and doubts.

Bibring (1959) was so surprised at the amount of psychiatric problems experienced by women during pregnancy that she turned to Erikson's theory of normative developmental life crises. She suggested that pregnancy, childbirth and parenthood were times of 'normative crisis', where women could be expected to experience emotional disturbance and feelings of rejection. This view gave recognition to the difficulties that women experience during this period but implicit in Erikson's theory of normative life crises is the need to go through the crisis and resolve it in order to move on to the next stage. Thus women who do not experience emotional difficulties are 'abnormal' because they are either denying or repressing the underlying emotional trauma. They have to 'come clean' about their emotions in order to resolve the crisis and establish a stable female identity. So do women experience emotional difficulties during this period?

Caplan (1960) found that 85% of a sample of women having a baby for the first time (primiparous) admitted feelings of marked disappointment and anxiety when they found out that they were pregnant. Cobliner (1965) found that 47% of a sample of women in New York openly stated at the beginning of the pregnancy that they did not want the child. However, Cartwright (1976) conducted a survey of primiparous women in Britain and found that 67% were pleased that they became pregnant when they did. These different findings can be explained firstly by reference to the time during the pregnancy when the interview was conducted. Attitudes to the birth may change during the course of the pregnancy, particularly when the mother, and father, are able to feel the presence of the baby in the womb (quickening). Secondly, pregnancies that were planned might have different psychological correlates from those that were unplanned.

Wolkind & Zajicek (1981) conducted a longitudinal study of 96 primiparous women from the East End of London. They investigated attitudes towards the pregnancy, emotional and physical health and self-concept development.

Attitudes

The women were asked about their feelings towards the pregnancy: 68% had planned to

Table 5.2 The changing attitudes to pregnancy (Wolkind & Zajicek 1981)

	Positive	Not positive
Planned pregnancies		
Feelings first	52	13
Feelings at 7 months	46	19
Unplanned pregnancies		
Feelings first	15	16
Feelings at 7 months	23	8

become pregnant and 32% had not. Feelings that were felt at the beginning of the pregnancy were compared to feelings felt after 7 months.

The results (Table 5.2) indicate that only a small percentage of women who planned their pregnancies had changed their attitudes after 7 months, whereas a larger percentage of women who had not planned their pregnancies at first changed their attitudes at 7 months, largely in the positive direction. The authors suggest that these findings support the work of Caplan (1960) and Cobliner (1965) who found that negative reactions at the beginning of pregnancy are often transformed due to quickening. Wolkind & Zajicek (1981) summarise their findings on women's attitudes to their pregnancy as follows:

The data described thus far gives us a picture of a group of married women, most of whom welcomed the pregnancy and felt positive about it, who seemed to cope with the reality and the prospect of fairly major life changes in a calm, rational way, and who were preparing themselves, as far as possible, for the experiences to come.

In order to get a better idea of whether pregnancy is associated with any form of crisis it is necessary to look at emotional reactions and physical symptoms expressed by this sample of women.

Emotional and physical health

The women were given an extensive psychiatric examination after 7 months of their pregnancy. It was found that 75% showed no disturbance at all, 11% had only mild emotional difficulties and 14% were diagnosed as having disorders that would definitely handicap them in some way.

Table 5.3 Percentage of women who had the following symptoms (Wolkind & Zajicek 1981)

	Pregnant women	Non-pregnant women	Student nurses
1. Indigestion	43	14	11
2. Sickness	16	2	2
3. Headaches	21	35	2
4. Constipation	26	22	13
5. Poor appetite	11	16	17
6. Tired	68	59	1
7. Faintness	21	12	12
8. Out of breath	46	9	4
9. Thumping of heart	23	26	11
10. Tingling in fingers or toes	22	9	4
11. Cramps in legs	68	21	7
12. Backache	48	30	4
13. Tired legs	55	40	2
14. Aching in neck and shoulders	16	35	6
15. Dragging feeling in tummy	39	16	12
16. Tender breasts	32	19	19
17. Itching in the private parts	12	11	20
18. Needed toilet quickly	66	24	3
19. Itching on skin	22	33	17
20. Perspiration	17	12	12
21. Spots before eyes	17	12	12

The sorts of problems mentioned were tearfulness, anxiety and depression; but the authors state that there was no evidence of the 'full-blown psychotic disorder' described by Bibring (1959). Physically, the women seemed to be in good health. After 7 months of pregnancy, 68% had no physical problems, 11% reported minor difficulties and 20% had complaints that required medical treatment. The most common physical problem at 7 months into the pregnancy was pre-eclampsia which is a hypertensive disorder in pregnant primiparous women.

In order to gain some information regarding the sorts of physical discomfort pregnant women experience during their pregnancy, 21 common symptoms of pregnancy (described in an obstetrics textbook) were presented to the women and they were asked whether they suffered from them (Table 5.3). The 21 symptoms were also presented to a sample of non-pregnant women with children and a sample of student nurses. The most common symptoms were indigestion (43%), lack of energy (68%), breathlessness (46%), leg cramps (68%), backache (48%), tired legs (55%) and the need to go to the toilet quickly (66%). Many of the other 'symptoms' did not

seem to bother the pregnant women. Also, whilst 68% of the pregnant women complained of lack of energy, 59% of the non-pregnant women complained of the same. Other similar experiences were backache and tired legs. The nurses scored lower on just about all the measures (lack of energy 1%) except on items 5 and 17.

To get some idea of pregnancy as a crisis period it was decided to compare those women who had at first wanted to become pregnant (planned pregnancy + positive feelings first) with those who did not want to become pregnant (unplanned and not initially positive). At 7 months into the pregnancy, there were significant differences between the two groups. Those who had not wanted to become pregnant had not begun to make preparations, had not read any books, felt that their lives would not be positive and expected to have more financial problems. There were no differences between the groups on such things as physical problems, psychiatric problems and disrupted family background.

Since quickening has been found to be an influential factor in changing attitudes to pregnancy, it was decided to investigate those women who did not react positively to the pregnancy even after quickening had occurred. The authors found that women who were negative at 7 months were significantly more likely to have had psychiatric problems during the pregnancy and period problems in the past. They were also more likely to resent the restrictions imposed by pregnancy. Wolkind & Zajicek (1981) summarise their findings with respect to crisis as follows:

The conflict about being pregnant which occurs at the beginning of pregnancy results in lack of preparation for the birth and feelings that having the child will cause problems. However, many such women seem to resolve their conflicts by seven months of pregnancy and tend to react positively at that time. Conflicts about being pregnant which occur later during pregnancy are not related to whether or not the pregnancy was planned and whether the women originally felt pleased to be pregnant. They are conflicts which seem to arise directly from the psychophysical experiences of pregnancy which are perhaps linked to more general reactions to womanhood.

It is interesting to note that 61% of a sample of primiparous women questioned by the authors felt that they had been changed in some way by the pregnancy. This suggests that the process of pregnancy, childbirth and parenthood is a developmental stage marking a transition from adulthood to parenthood. However, only 8% of the women felt that the pregnancy was a significant milestone in their lives. This latter finding lends credence to the suggestion that pregnancy is not necessarily a period of crisis, but a transitional period involving some degree of upheaval and change.

Fathers

Although Wolkind & Zajicek (1981) examined the effects of pregnancy and childbirth on fathers, unfortunately they did not actually speak to the fathers themselves, but assessed the wives' perceptions of their spouses' attitudes. May (1981) interviewed 20 first-time expectant fathers about their involvement in their wives' pregnancies and their attitudes toward it. May (1981) identified three phases of 'father involvement': the announcement phase, the moratorium and the focusing phase.

The announcement phase. This is the period when the pregnancy is first suspected. The length of the phase varies according to individual circumstances; sometimes it is a few hours, sometimes a few weeks. It seems that men are not oblivious to early signs of pregnancy and typically report the time where the diagnosis of pregnancy is in doubt as stressful and uncomfortable, regardless of whether the pregnancy was wanted or not. After the pregnancy has been confirmed and starts to have a noticeable impact on the woman, the fathers in the sample reported that they seemed to be lagging behind their wives in experiencing the pregnancy.

The moratorium phase. This phase usually occurs between the 12th and 25th weeks of the pregnancy and is characterised by the expectant fathers becoming emotionally distant from the pregnancy. This period can be quite stressful since the man does not experience the physical changes of the woman and thus has a different perspective on the event. The emotional distance allows the man to 'work through' his feelings about the pregnancy and the changes in lifestyle that are likely to occur as a result. The man's ambivalence towards the pregnancy can result in problems between the expectant couple. The woman may feel that her partner does not care in the same way she does toward the new baby and the man may not give adequate support to the woman because he does not see that it is necessary.

The focusing phase. This ends the moratorium. One man described this realisation: '. . . it is like measles, you get exposed, but it takes a while before you catch on that you have got it.' The phase begins around the 25th to 30th weeks, although it may begin sooner if the man is particularly prepared for the pregnancy. The man focuses on his own experience of the pregnancy, redefines his role vis-à-vis future status and becomes much more sensitive to his wife's needs. Men report that they feel fatherly and start to have mental images of themselves with the prospective child. May (1981) concludes that preparation during the focusing phase may relate to 'constructive' parenting after the birth of the child.

Parents

Finally, Miller & Sollie (1986) looked at the experiences of both parents together during their transition to parenthood. The study consisted of 120 couples who were required to complete and return questionnaires when the wife was in mid-pregnancy, when the baby was about 6 weeks old and when the baby was between 6 and 8 months old. The questionnaire was concerned with measures of personal well-being, personal stress and marital stress. New parents reported higher personal stress scores after they had become parents than during the pregnancy period. Wives personal stress scores were lower than their husband's during the pregnancy, but considerably higher afterwards. Personal well-being scores declined steadily throughout the three time periods, indicating that the time when the baby was 1 month old was harder than the pregnancy and 8 months postpartum was more difficult than 1 month postpartum. Marital stress increased steadily from pregnancy to 8 months postpartum for the mothers, but there was no change in the fathers' marital stress scores with time.

Miller & Sollie (1986) suggest that becoming a parent for the first time involves a slight decline in personal well-being and some increase in personal stress over the first year of parenting. New mothers feel these changes more acutely than fathers, and wives are more likely than their husbands to view the marriage as changing in a negative way. Coping with the stress of a new baby puts a certain amount of strain on the parents' relationship. Adaptation to stress involves two major kinds of family resources. The first is internal, the second is external (community and social support). Levitt et al (1986) highlighted the importance of the husband in providing emotional support. They interviewed 43 mothers of 13-month-old infants about the degree of emotional support they received from family and friends. Mothers reported an average of 13 persons in their social networks, but support was provided primarily by the husband. It seemed to be the case that the mothers only turned to friends for support if the relationship with their husband was strained.

Much of the research indicates that becoming a parent is stressful and that the greatest stress occurs after the baby has been born. Many of the parenthood classes offered by organisations such as the National Childbirth Trust are really prenatal or childbirth preparation classes which fall short in helping prospective parents after the child is born. Whilst there are postnatal support groups, there is no tuition along the lines of the prenatal classes with husbands present. There are practical problems in bringing new parents together, but it would seem that postparenthood classes, with both parents present, could provide support after the birth of a first child.

BEREAVEMENT

On the death of infants:

The courage and the resilience of these parents is truly remarkable. In their pain they discover new truths about themselves. Sometimes these truths are not always attractive, but a resolve begins to grow that life is worth living, and happiness is possible.
DeFrain et al (1982)

It is important to distinguish between bereavement, grief and mourning. Bereavement literally means 'to take away from' and refers to a state of loss resulting from the death of a 'significant person'. Grief refers to the emotional expressions of those who have become bereaved. These emotions are common to all cultures. Mourning behaviour is the culturally prescribed means of expressing bereavement and grief. Mourning behaviour may vary from culture to culture, e.g. the Hindu practice of suttee and the Jewish practice of sitting Shiva for 7 days following the funeral.

Stages of grief

Parkes (1986) and Parkes et al (1991) have outlined four stages of the grief reaction to the death of a loved one:

1. *Numbness and denial.* Newly bereaved people may feel a sense of unreality, a suspension of time, immediately after the death of somebody significant in their lives. This feeling is often described as numbness. It sometimes feels as if

life itself will not be possible from now on. There is also a tendency to deny the event and believe that it is all a bad dream. This period of intense grief may last from a few days to weeks.

2. *Yearning or pining.* This phase is characterised by a need to try to recover or recreate the dead person. Often this need manifests itself in the dreams of the bereaved, and people sometimes report having seen the dead person in a crowd.

3. *Despair and depression.* When the bereaved person finally acknowledges the reality of the death, there is a feeling of intense despair and sometimes depression. This is a period when individuals experience a certain amount of disorganisation and feel that they are unable to cope with tasks that previously afforded them little difficulty.

4. *Recovery or reorganisation.* At some point most bereaved individuals realise that their lives must go on and they must try to find a new meaning to their existence. The degree of recovery and the time span vary from person to person. In some cases, years after the death, residual levels of emotion remain. During this period there is likely to be a certain amount of anger directed at medical staff, the dead person and the self. Similarly, guilt appears frequently throughout the recovery period, usually taking the form of the 'If only I had . . .' syndrome.

These stages, or phases, of bereavement were based on interviews with widows and widowers during the first year of bereavement and as such represent the sorts of reactions to grief that may typically occur during that period. However, the stages are not necessarily experienced one after the other and in the same order. There may be times when yearning or pining is felt along with despair and depression. Also, recovery can be progressing steadily when an event or an anniversary can trigger a repeat of the whole process of the grief reaction. Thus the stages should be seen merely as reflecting the sorts of grief reactions that can occur after a bereavement and not as a fixed sequence of responses that need to be followed in order to reach the final goal of recovery (Kalish 1989).

It is important, however, to be wary of making too many generalisations about the grief reaction since the impact of a person's death on survivors is mediated by such things as whether the death is sudden or prolonged and the relationship of the survivor to the dead person.

Sudden death

It is perhaps ironic that if we had a choice about our own death then we would usually choose to go quickly. Yet if we had a choice about how our loved ones should die, we would probably prefer to have some time to come to terms with the situation and 'work things through' with them. Sudden death is not only unexpected but leaves the bereaved unable to complete 'unfinished business' with the dead person. Health professionals are likely to be faced with sudden death particularly in the contexts of Intensive Care and Accident and Emergency.

Wright (1993) puts forward a list of the emotional responses to sudden death. Unlike some other researchers, he places them in order of coping difficulty. He bases his list on information gained from the coping experiences of health professionals working in Emergency Departments in Britain and America. The most difficult bereavement response to cope with is withdrawal.

Withdrawal. A period of withdrawal may be useful since it enables people to take in the information they have just received and allows them some time to assess their feelings. However, if withdrawal is accompanied by a strong denial, then difficulties may arise. No matter how much an individual may want to deny the death, it has to be made clear that the problem will not go away and there are things to sort out. The period of withdrawal varies according to individual and situation and it is extremely difficult for health professionals to sit and do nothing when they are used to active care. Yet, often, the mere presence of somebody is exactly what the bereaved person needs most. Thus unhealthy withdrawal should not be confused with the time people need to organise themselves to respond to communication from health professionals.

Denial. It is easy for both health professionals and the bereaved alike to slip into a state of denial, after all both groups are affected by the death and it is natural for health professionals to want to care for and protect the relatives. But the death 'is true', it 'is happening to them' and they 'do feel like this'. Going along with these responses might seem prudent in the short term but will prove counterproductive in the long term. Frankness and honesty communicated in a caring way are the appropriate responses to denial.

Anger. Anger may be directed at health professionals, the family of the bereaved and the bereaved themselves. When it is addressed to colleagues it is particularly difficult to avoid getting involved by immediately leaping to their defence. Rather than reacting to aggression in a suppressive fashion, it is important to empathise with the feelings of the bereaved. When a loved one dies, blame is often apportioned incorrectly. It is not a time for well thought out analysis, and 'easy' interpretations of what has happened will be adopted.

Isolation. This should not be confused with withdrawal. It refers to feelings of being totally alone, despite being surrounded by caring individuals. At this point, directing the bereaved's attention to friends and family who will care for them may be misplaced, since the individual is trying to work through her immediate loss. Diverting attention from this task may not be found to be useful.

Bargaining. Wright (1993) says that this response occurs mainly when dealing with the death, or imminent death of babies or young children. Parents will offer everything they have in order to get their children brought back or cured. It is an attempt to try to establish control over a situation where parents have no control whatsoever. A refusal to indulge in bargaining may evoke anger, particularly if the parents perceive themselves to be discriminated against.

Inappropriate responses. Sometimes the announcement of sudden death is met by laughter and there are a number of theories that have been put forward to explain this response. However, for the health professional, the important aspect of this inappropriate response is the bereaved's feeling of guilt that grief has not been expressed properly. There may also be statements such as 'We won't be able to go to that party now', which seem inappropriate at the time but are perfectly common. The death is a huge strain on the system; comments of this nature deflect the stress and provide a brief respite.

Guilt. As an initial response, most people will feel some form of guilt. Sometimes guilt is externalised to health professionals to get their impressions and it is necessary in these circumstances to be completely nonjudgemental. People need to be given assurance about the fallibility of human nature in general.

Crying, sobbing and weeping. Most people today recognise the value of crying and health professionals generally find this response easy to cope with. There are still some people who regard crying as a weakness, yet in many ways the presence of someone crying breaks down certain barriers and indicates recognisable responses on the part of the health professional. Many people will want to cry but can't. In some cases they may wish to do it in private, in others they may require some stimulus to initiate the grief process.

Unfinished business. Lastly, there are many things left unsaid and undone. It is important to spend some time listening to regrets about the many sorts of things that could have been done with the deceased 'if only'.

Having to deal with the relatives of the patient is an unpopular task, mainly because health professionals are confronted with powerful feelings and no guidelines on how to respond. Knowing what to expect and responding in an empathic, caring and positive fashion reduces the stress related to dealing with bereaved individuals.

Expected death

Knowing that someone close is about to die gives one a certain amount of time to 'work through' some of the problems relating to the impending death. Even though the 'primary caretaker' may be the most exhausted, both physically and mentally, after the death he or she may have the least guilt and the fewest feelings of unfinished business of anyone else in the family. On the other hand, the period of time between knowing that a loved one is going to die and the death itself (sometimes called the living–dying interval) is fraught with problems that relate to the dying person's own conception of his death. More people now than in the past are dying from degenerative diseases and are told of the prognosis fairly soon after diagnosis (Pattison 1977).

The psychological impact of this period was explored by Kübler-Ross (1989). On the basis of her clinical experiences with about 200 terminally ill patients, she put forward a theory of five stages experienced by the dying person:

1. *Denial and isolation.* Upon learning that they have a terminal illness, people deny impending death saying things like 'No, not me!'. Feelings associated with death become isolated.

2. *Anger.* Once death is admitted, anger is expressed at the fact that they have been chosen to die while others have not. The objects of the individual's ire are not predictable.

3. *Bargaining.* Dying people attempt to bargain for a cure or a postponement of the death sentence. Kübler-Ross (1989) describes this as 'trying to do a deal with God'.

4. *Depression.* At some stage it becomes impossible for the dying person to deny that he has a terminal illness due to gradual progression of the illness. The acknowledgement of death has been described as an overwhelming sense of loss.

5. *Acceptance.* Having worked through the process of dying, the individual becomes able to accept his death. Reminiscences become less painful and the dying person is no longer anguished by the prospect of death.

The theory rapidly became accepted as a 'manual' for dying. However, many health professionals dealing with the terminally ill noted that dying patients did not always follow the pattern proposed by Kübler-Ross. Many dying people did exhibit the behaviours of each stage, but any stage was found to occur at any time during the dying process; often denial and acceptance were found to alternate throughout the living–dying interval. Further her theory was not based on any systematic research programme and should not be accepted unequivocally. The stages of the dying process do give an indication of the sorts of problems experienced by the dying patient during the living–dying interval, but the order and strength of experience may vary.

The process of dying relates to those who are terminally ill and not to the bereaved. The astute reader probably has noted that there are similarities between the stages of grief proposed by Parkes (1986) and Parkes et al (1991) and the responses to dying outlined by Kübler-Ross (1989). It follows that if individuals are given the opportunity to work through the problems outlined by Kübler-Ross (with the dying patient) before the death, then they will experience less difficulty in coping with similar problems after the death.

Relationships

The relationship of the survivor to the dead person determines the nature of the bereavement response. To understand grief more completely, one must examine the effects of death on children, and the effects of the death of a child on parents, as well as the more common effects of the death of a wife or a husband on their spouses.

Whether children suffer the loss of a parent or a sibling, the response to the loss will depend largely on the developmental level of the child. One of the first systematic studies of children's concept of death was undertaken by Nagy (1948) in Budapest. She asked over 400 children aged between 3–10 years to write, draw and talk about death. She proposed that children think about death in different ways as they grow older:

- *Stage 1.* Children between the ages of 3 and 5 years tend to view death as a temporary state similar to sleep. There is no sense of finality and people can be brought back to life if certain criteria are met. One child is reported to have said that the reason you are not allowed to sing loudly at funerals is because you might wake the dead person.

• *Stage 2.* Children between the ages of 5 and 9 years view death in much more of a concrete fashion. Death is represented by a skeleton or the 'bogey man'. If you are clever you can escape the death man when he comes to take you away. Those people who are still alive have become adept at outsmarting death when he calls for them.

• *Stage 3.* After the age of 9 years, children view death as universal and irreversible. The children are able to see that death is the termination of life and there is nothing anybody can do to bring back the departed.

Research based on interviews with children has largely supported Nagy's findings that young children have a limited concept of death. However, the individual experiences of the child have been found to play a significant part in understanding death. The death of a pet, for instance, can promote an early sophistication of death comprehension. Similarly, children with a terminal illness are able to understand death as an irreversible, final process (Bluebond-Langner 1978). Thus some circumstances can, and do, contrive to force children to view death in an adult fashion, but usually young children do not have a correct conception of causality, confusing cause and effect. Children often link together two unrelated events because they occurred at the same time: 'I did well at school because I had my blue jumper on.' If a child does not brush his teeth on the day a death occurs in the family, it would not be unreasonable to suppose that he would connect the two events. Not brushing his teeth caused the death, it was his fault and he feels extreme guilt.

The death of a son or daughter is one of the most shattering forms of bereavement. Parents normally think that their children will survive them. Thus when a child dies it presents particular problems for the parents.

Sudden infant death syndrome (SIDS) or cot death requires special consideration since very often there is no apparent cause of death.

Parents may spend a long time examining the way they looked after their child and discussing the absence of any physical symptoms. This latter feature of cot death leads to very pronounced guilt feelings. In some circumstances the police will be involved, which may suggest to the parents that they are suspected of causing the death in some way. Parents need careful explanations concerning the reasons for the procedures involved in cot deaths. One of the most difficult aspects of cot death is the lack of any explanation for the death. Paediatricians may be able to explain that in some cases it just happens and 'we don't know why', but this provides little solace to people who are used to having reasons for everything. The lack of answers causes parents to invent their own.

If parents wish to hold the body of their baby when they come to view it, they should be given the opportunity to do so despite the emotional difficulties. If parents are prevented from holding their child it can cause problems later on. It is also a good idea to have the child photographed even if the parents do not wish to view the body. At a later date they may value this type of record of their child.

The effects of bereavement will depend on such factors as the dying trajectory, the relationship to the dead person and the previous experiences of the bereaved. It is not intended to provide a discussion of all the features of bereavement, nor parenthood, they should be viewed here only in the context of life transitions and crises. The question remains as to whether the models proposed earlier give an appropriate indication of the sorts of problems and difficulties individuals are likely to experience at these important times. In general, the answer to the question is a tentative 'yes'. Whilst each individual case is different from another, there are certain commonalities across life events.

Hopson (1981) and Hopson & Scally (1991) do provide a useful guide to the mood swings that typically accompany a crisis or transition and Moos (1986) gives practical information about the adaptive and coping tasks confronting people at these times. Thus a knowledge of both these models is an important supplement to the development of the interpersonal skills discussed in Chapter 1. Having in mind a cognitive framework that represents the likely course of events as well as a knowledge of the problems and difficulties that may be experienced by the individual, enables the health professional not only to empathise with the person but also to develop a positive approach to the resolution of the crisis or transition.

REFERENCES

Bee H 1992 The developing child, 6th edn. Harper Collins, New York

Bibring G L 1959 Some consideration of the psychological processes in pregnancy. Psychoanalytic Study of the Child 14: 113–121

Billings A C, Moos R H 1982 Stressful life events and symptoms: a longitudinal model. Health Psychology 1: 99–117

Bloom B L 1979 Prevention of mental disorders: recent advances in theory and practice. Community Mental Health Journal 15: 179–191

Bluebond-Langner M 1978 The private worlds of dying children. Princeton University Press, Princeton

Brim O G, Ryer C D 1980 On the properties of life events. In: Baltes P B, Brim O G (eds) Life-span development and behaviour. Academic Press, London, vol 3

Buhler C, Massarik F 1968 (eds) The course of human life: a study of goals in the humanistic perspective. Springer, New York

Burgess A W, Holmstrom L L 1979 Adaptive strategies from rape. American Journal of Psychiatry 136: 1278–1282

Buss A R 1979 Dialectics, history and development: the historical roots of the individual, society and dialectic. In: Baltes P B, Brim O G (eds) Life-span development and behaviour. Academic Press, London, vol 2

Caplan G 1960 Emotional implications of pregnancy and influences on family relationships. In: Stuart H C, Prugh D G (eds) The healthy child. Harvard, Cambridge

Caplan G 1964 Principles of preventive psychiatry. Basic Books, New York

Cartwright A 1976 How many children? Routledge & Kegan Paul, London

Cobliner W G 1965 Some maternal attitudes towards conception. Mental Hygiene 49: 4–10

Cowen E L 1980 The wooing of primary prevention. American Journal of Community Psychology 8: 258–284

Danish S J 1977 Human development and human services: a marriage proposal. In: Iscoe I, Bloom B L, Spielberger C C (eds) Community psychology in transition. Halstead, New York

Danish S J, D'Augelli A R 1980 Promoting competence and enhancing development through life development intervention. In: Bond L A, Rosen C (eds) Competence and coping during adulthood. University Press of New England, Hanover NH

Danish S J, D'Augelli A R 1982 Helping skills II: life development intervention. Human Sciences Press, New York

Danish S J, Smyer M S, Novak C A 1981 Developmental intervention: enhancing life event processes. In: Baltes P B, Brim O G (eds) Life-span development and behaviour. Academic Press, London, vol 3

DeFrain J, Taylor J, Ernst L 1982 Coping with sudden infant death. Lexington, Mass

Deutsch H 1947 The psychology of women. Grune & Stratton, London

Dohrenwend B P 1978 Social stress and community psychology. American Journal of Community Psychology 6: 1–14

Dohrenwend B P 1979 Stressful life events and psychopathology: some issues of theory and method. In: Barrett J E (ed) Stress and mental disorder. Raven Press, New York

Dohrenwend B S, Martin J L 1979 Personal versus situational determinants of anticipation and control of the occurrence of stressful life events. American Journal of Community Psychology 7: 453–468

Erikson E H 1980 Identity and the life cycle: a reissue. W W Norton, New York

Felner R D, Farber S S, Primavera J 1980 Transition and stressful life events: a model for primary prevention. In: Price R H, Ketterer R F, Bader B C, Monohan J (eds) Prevention in mental health: research, policy and practice. Sage, Beverley Hills

Felner R D, Farber S S, Primavera J 1985 Transitions and stressful life events: a model for primary prevention. In: Felner R D, Jason L A, Moritsugu J N, Farber S S (eds) Preventive psychology. Pergamon Press, New York

Harrison R 1976 The demoralising experience of prolonged unemployment. Department of Employment Gazette 1–10

Havighurst R J 1972 Developmental tasks and education, 3rd edn. David McKay, New York

Holmes T H 1979 Development and application of a quantitative measure of life change magnitude. In: Barret J E (ed) Stress and mental disorder. Raven Press, New York

Holmes T H, Rahe R H 1967 The social readjustment rating scale. Journal of Psychomatic Research 11: 213–218

Hopson B 1981 Response to papers by Schlossberg, Brammer and Abrego. Counselling Psychology 9: 36–39

Hopson B, Adams J 1976 Towards an understanding of transitions: defining some boundaries of transition dynamics. In: Adams J, Hayes J, Hopson B (eds) Transition: understanding and managing personal change. Martin Robertson, London

Hopson B, Scally M 1991 Build your own rainbow: a work book for career and life management. Mercury Books, Leeds

Johnson J H, McCutchen S M 1980 Assessing life stress in older children and adolescents: preliminary findings with the life events checklist. In: Sarason I G, Spielberger C D (eds) Stress and anxiety. Hemisphere Publications, Washington DC

Kalish R A 1989 (ed) Midlife loss, coping strategies. Sage, London

Kanner A D, Coyne J C, Schaefer C, Lazarus R S 1981 Comparison of two models of stress measurement: daily hassles and uplifts versus major life events. Journal of Behavioural Medicine 4: 1–39

Kimmel D C 1980 Adulthood and aging. Wiley, New York

Kübler-Ross E 1989 On death and dying. Tavistock Routledge, London

Levinson D J, Darrow D N, Klein E B, Levinson M H, McKee B 1978 The seasons of a man's life. A A Knopf, New York

Levitt M J, Weber R A, Clark M C 1986 Social network relationships as sources of maternal support and well-being. Developmental Psychology 22: 310–316

McGrath R E V, Burkhart B R 1983 Measuring life stress: a comparison of different scoring systems for the social readjustment scale. Journal of Clinical Psychology 24: 83–110

May K A 1981 Three phases of father involvement in pregnancy. Nursing Research 31: 337–342

Miller B C, Sollie D C 1986 Normal stresses during the transition to parenthood. In: Moos R H (ed) Coping with life crises. Plenum, New York

Moos R H 1986 Coping with life crises: an integrated approach. Plenum, New York

Nagy M H 1948 The child's theories concerning death. Journal of Genetic Psychology 73: 3–27

Neugarten B L 1977 Adaptation and the life cycle. In: Schlossberg N K, Entine A D (eds) Counselling adults. Brooks/Cole, Monterey California

Parkes C, Lewis R 1981 Beyond the Peter principle. Journal of European Industrial Training 5: 17–21

Parkes C M 1986 Bereavement: studies of grief in adult life. Penguin, Harmondsworth

Parkes C M, Stevenson-Hinde J, Marris P (eds) 1991 Attachment across the life cycle. Routledge, London

Pattison E M 1977 The experience of dying. Prentice Hall, Englewood Cliffs NJ

Reese H W, Smyer M A 1983 The dimensionalization of life events. In: Callahan E J, McCluskey K A (eds) Life-span developmental psychology: nonnormative life events. Academic Press, New York

Roazen P 1976 Erik H Erikson. Free Press, New York

Sarason I G, Johnson J H, Siegel J M 1978 Assessing the impact of life changes: development of the life experience survey. Journal of Consulting and Clinical Psychology 46: 932–946

Stevens R 1983 Erik Erikson: an introduction. Open University Press, Milton Keynes

Taylor S, Wood J, Lichtman R 1983 It could be worse: selective evaluation as a response to victimization. Journal of Social Issues 39: 1–40

Tedeschi R 1987 Personal communication

Wolkind S, Zajicek E (eds) 1981 Pregnancy: a psychological and social study. Academic Press, London

Wright B 1993 Caring in crisis: a handbook of intervention skills for nurses, 2nd edn. Churchill Livingstone, Edinburgh

RECOMMENDED READING

Fisher S, Reason J 1988 (eds) Handbook of life stress, cognition and health. Wiley, Chichester
A comprehensive selection of chapters that illustrates the diversity of life stress and transition. Some of the sections are easier to understand than others but this is a book well worth dipping into.

Hopson B, Scally M, Stafford K 1988 Transitions: the challenge of change. Lifeskills, Leeds
This is a practical book designed to help people manage their own life transitions. It is based on the Hopson model discussed in this chapter and provides a good account of how to develop a response to life events.

Niven C A 1992 Psychological care for families: before during and after birth. Butterworth-Heinemann, Oxford
No relation. This book is directed at health professionals and is to be recommended because it takes a longitudinal perspective on the process of pregnancy, childbirth and parenthood.

Wright B 1990 Sudden death: intervention skills for nurses. Churchill Livingstone, Edinburgh
Along with *Caring and crisis*, this book gives a good account of how to deal with sudden death. It is based on the author's extensive experience in Accident and Emergency departments.

Danish S J, D'Augelli A R 1982 Helping skills II: life development intervention. Human Sciences Press, New York

Felner R D, Jason L A, Moritsugu J N, Farber S 1983 (eds) Preventive psychology. Pergamon Press, New York

Moos R H 1986 Coping with life crises: an integrated approach. Plenum, New York

Parkes C M 1987 Bereavement, 2nd edn. International University Press, London

Wolkind S, Zajicek E (eds) 1981 Pregnancy: a psychological and social study. Academic Press, London

6

Health behaviour

A central issue in health psychology is why some people do not comply with the advice of health professionals. This chapter discusses some models of health behaviour and puts forward explanations of patient noncompliance. The psychological components of coronary heart disease and ways of preventing it are looked at as well as the definition and the distinction between feeling down and being clinically depressed. Finally, patients' perceptions of health and illness are examined as an integral part of psychosomatic disorder.

Health care professionals are beginning to recognize and are providing empirical evidence demonstrating that the major causes of death are ones in which behavioural pathogens are the single most important factor.

Feuerstein et al (1986)

There is little doubt that the way we lead our lives, directly and indirectly, affects our health. It is therefore incumbent on health psychologists to try to examine the relationship between our behaviour and our health. The first section of this chapter looks at models that have been put forward to explain why some individuals indulge in healthy behaviour and others do not. For instance, some people are keen to seek out advice from health care professionals, whilst others actively deny that there is anything wrong with them.

The second section analyses the reasons why some people will comply with therapeutic health regimens whilst others, even though they realise the importance of what is being asked of them, do nothing to implement the health regimen. Research into developing better health care is wasted if it cannot be implemented on account of patient noncompliance.

Although psychological well-being is difficult to define, one condition that contributes, in a negative way, to well-being is depression. It is perhaps one of the most pervasive of all psychological conditions and has affected us all in some way or another. Sometimes depression is just 'feeling down', sometimes it can destroy all motivation to do anything about one's circumstances. Because the term is used extensively in different health contexts, it is important to define the condition and discuss approaches that have been developed to try to treat it. This is the concern of the third section.

The fourth section discusses the psychological factors influencing coronary heart disease. The reduction of coronary heart disease is probably one of the most serious problems facing health professionals today. Each year thousands of individuals are affected by the disease. Improving the physical health of the population is one way of reducing the incidence of the disease, but attention to physical health is not enough. It seems that psychological factors, such as the pace at which we live our lives, are just as important as physical factors in the aetiology of the disease. Thus, an examination of the psychological factors that predispose individuals to be at risk from coronary heart disease bears some attention.

Finally, a main determinant of the extent to which we seek health care or not is whether we think that we are ill. Before seeking advice on health care we pay attention to the sensations of our body. How do we perceive our illness symptoms? What sort of mistakes do we make in deciding whether these sensations indicate that there is something wrong with us and we have to seek health care? Mistaken illness perception may be a major feature of hypochondriasis.

Firstly, let us consider the case of Mr A. (Case History 6.1).

There are many people like Mr A. who refuse to seek health care, despite the obvious need to do so. The aim of health psychology is to try to understand why.

A number of models have been put forward to account for people's health behaviour and some of the most prominent are now discussed.

CASE HISTORY 6.1 MR A.

Mr A. gets up in the morning, tired because he did not sleep very well last night due to a surfeit of drink, coffee and the children waking him up.

He sits down to a breakfast of sausage, bacon and eggs and after eating he feels slightly better. He has a cigarette with his coffee. He gets into his car and smokes another cigarette. While driving to work, he is aware of some pains in his chest. He puts these pains down to indigestion, although he has been experiencing them quite frequently just lately and wonders why.

He arrives at work, parks his car in the underground car park, with its concomitant fumes, and takes the lift up to his office. Despite the no smoking signs, numerous people are smoking in the lift. He starts work and is relieved when the mid-morning break comes round and he can indulge in his favourite snack—a jam doughnut and a cup of coffee. He feels more chest pains, knowing at the back of his mind that they might not be due to indigestion.

A 'pub lunch' follows, consisting of steak and kidney pie with a generous portion of chips and a few pints of beer to wash it all down. Then it's back to work. In the afternoon he again experiences chest pains, which he ignores.

After work, he gets into his car and drives home through the usual rush hour traffic, arriving home to meet a houseful of boisterous children, wanting attention and to be carried everywhere. Finally he sits down to his evening meal in front of TV, and finishes off with a piece of chocolate cake and a cup of coffee. He finally goes to bed (with an aching under his left arm and unable to sleep) at about 11.30 p.m.

The next day he follows the same pattern. Mr A. refuses to visit a doctor despite the recurring chest pains.

MODELS OF HEALTH BEHAVIOUR

Kasl & Cobb (1966) make a distinction between three different types of 'health behaviour':

- *Health behaviour*—an activity undertaken by a person believing himself to be healthy for the purpose of preventing disease or detecting it in an asymptomatic stage.
- *Illness behaviour*—any activity undertaken by a person who feels ill, to define the state of his health and to discover a suitable remedy.
- *Sick-role behaviour*—activity undertaken for the purpose of getting well, by those who consider themselves ill. It includes receiving treatment from appropriate therapists, generally involves a whole range of dependent

behaviours and leads to some degree of neglect of one's usual duties.

The models to be discussed are essentially concerned with understanding and predicting health behaviour.

Health belief model

This was developed by four psychologists—Hochbaum, Kegeles, Leventhal and Rosenstock (Rosenstock 1974)—to predict individuals' preventive health behaviour. It was subsequently modified by Becker & Maiman (1975) to incorporate sick-role behaviour and compliance with medical regimens. Readiness to take action and engage in health-related behaviours depends on a number of factors. The first two are concerned with the extent to which individuals feel vulnerable to a particular illness. This involves whether they feel susceptible to contracting the illness and their thoughts about how severe it is:

1. *Susceptibility*. An individual's beliefs about whether he or she is likely to contract an illness.
2. *Severity*. The degree to which an individual perceives the consequences of having an illness to be severe.

Together these two factors comprise what is known as the perceived threat of an illness, sometimes known as vulnerability. With respect to the case of Mr A. (Case History 6.1), vulnerability comprises the extent to which he believes that his lifestyle is likely to result in heart disease and also the extent to which he believes the consequences of contracting heart disease are particularly severe. If Mr A. perceives himself as vulnerable, then this represents the first stage in doing something about his condition.

The next two factors are concerned with the pros and cons of taking some action to combat the illness. 'What is to be gained? What do I have to pay?'

3. *Benefits*. This refers to the potential to be gained from a particular course of action that will reduce the health threat.

4. *Barriers*. Any decision to act will have a certain number of consequences. There may be a degree of physical, psychological or financial distress associated with any form of action.

In this next stage, Mr A. has to 'weigh up' the benefits that might accrue from a change in lifestyle against the cost to him in terms of the extent to which he may be 'put out' by such actions. After considering these four factors, Mr. A. may decide to take some form of action, but there are two further factors that may stimulate him to do something about his condition.

5. *Cues to action*. Cues are stimuli that trigger appropriate health behaviour. They can either be internal (perception of bodily states), or external, (stimuli from the environment such as the mass media).
6. *Diverse factors*. These include demographic, ethnic, social and personality factors that may influence health behaviour.

Mr A. may be spurred into action by abnormally severe chest pains, by listening to advice from his colleagues at work, or by the concern of his family and close friends about his condition.

Becker et al (1977) include a seventh factor in their revision of the model, which is the predisposition, or motivation, of people to engage in health-related practices. Becker et al (1977) state that the health belief model is a useful tool in predicting the degree to which individuals are likely to play an active role in their, and others', health care. They provide as an example of the model in action an attempt to predict whether mothers of obese children would keep their clinic appointments. The subjects of the experiment were 182 mothers of children newly diagnosed as obese. Over a 12-month period, the subjects were required to visit the clinic four times—this was a measure of their actual behaviour. They also measured the amount of weight change that occurred during this period.

A questionnaire was used to gain information about the mothers' health beliefs regarding such items as how easily the child became ill (susceptibility); the extent to which being overweight caused serious illness (severity); how attention to diet could help alleviate obesity problems (benefits); whether there were problems adhering to a diet when the children did not want to have anything to do with it; an assessment of the mothers' own concern about health care in general and the extent to which their willingness to engage in health-related practices affected compliance (motivation).

The results suggested that there was a relationship between the mothers' health beliefs and a reduction in obesity over the 12-month period. More than half of the correlations between the questionnaire items and the attendance at clinic plus subsequent weight loss were significant. However, the health belief model seemed to be better at predicting actual behavioural outcomes (i.e. weight loss) than behaviour per se (keeping appointments at the clinic).

There is no doubt that the health belief model can be a useful guide to health behaviour under certain circumstances (Rosenstock 1974; Rosenstock & Kirscht 1979), but there are a number of criticisms. Firstly, the reformulations proposed by Becker & Maiman (1975) make the theory unnecessarily unwieldy with 11 'readiness' factors and 23 'enabling' factors. This clearly constitutes more variables than can be included in any one study (Wallston & Wallston 1984). Secondly, the model treats people as rational decision makers. Janis (1984) says 'The important point is that the health belief model, like other models of rational choice, fails to specify under what conditions people will give priority to avoiding subjective discomfort at the cost of endangering their lives, and under what conditions they will make a more rational decision.' Finally, Wallston & Wallston (1984) think that combining the health belief predictors interactively may prove more fruitful than simply adding them together.

Locus of control model

Rotter (1954) proposed that behaviour was a function of the individual's belief that the behaviour will lead to a reinforcement (expectancy) and how much that reinforcement is liked (reinforcement value). The most important factor in determining generalised expectancies is locus of control. To measure these generalised expectancies, almost a dozen different locus of control measures have been developed (Lefcourt 1982), but the test that Rotter devised is known as the I–E Scale. Consider the following statements:

1. a. Many people can be described as victims of fate.
   b. What happens to other people is very much of their own making.
2. a. Most of the things that happen to me are a matter of luck.
   b. I am in complete control of my destiny.
3. a. The known world is ordered according to a grand design, but I just cannot work it out.
   b. The world is complicated, but I can usually work things out if I try hard enough.
4. a. It is stupid to think that you can change other people's beliefs.
   b. I know when I am right and can convince others.

If you agree with those statements marked 'a', then you have an external locus of control, that is, you believe that we are not masters of our own fate and are subject to the control of outside forces such as luck or destiny. If you agree with those statements marked 'b', then you have an internal locus of control. You believe that you have the ability to influence and determine the features that affect your life. If you have an external locus of control, then you are less likely to engage in behaviours that could have a positive effect on your life, believing that it does not matter what you do, fate has already decided for you. If, on the other hand, you have an internal locus of control then you are much more likely to do things for yourself, because you believe that you can have a significant say in how your life is run.

An increasing number of health researchers have measured locus of control beliefs and have attempted to relate these expectancies to a host of health-related behaviours (Oberle, 1991). Some of these studies used a scale where there was no mention of health factors (Levenson 1973), others have incorporated specific health items into their scale (Wallston & Wallston 1984). Some studies have found that a person is most likely to engage in health behaviour if he has a belief in internal health locus of control and a high valuing of health; others have found the opposite to be true.

Example. DeVellis et al (1980) asked people with epilepsy to fill in a form giving information about four items of behaviour: failure to take medication, frequency of driving, consumption of alcohol and willingness to engage in seeking out more information about epilepsy. They were also given the Multidimensional Health Locus of Control Scale. The experimenters found interesting correlations between those that had an internal locus of control and adherence to medical advice. People who had higher beliefs in internal control were less likely to adhere to medical advice, drove more, drank and were more likely to seek out information concerning epilepsy. It may be that people with internal beliefs have the freedom to decide for themselves when it is appropriate not to adhere. For example, if seizures are well under control, driving may be an appropriate risk. Therefore individuals who have an internal locus of control may be more motivated to take action concerning their health, but sometimes are less likely to adhere to medical advice.

There are a number of drawbacks to this approach. Firstly, its predictive value is not as reliable as the health belief model (Wallston & Wallston 1984). Secondly, the prediction of behaviour from attitudes requires a high degree of correspondence; it is doubtful whether the model can accommodate such difficulties. Stainton-Rogers (1991) thinks the model is totally inappropriate as an explanation of health behaviour; however, Oberle (1991) thinks that the main problem has not been with the concept of locus of control itself but with the standard of the studies that have used the model. Finally, it may be more profitable to investigate other constructs as well as locus of control that are defined by the specific situation.

Conflict theory model

This is a model of personal decision-making that attempts to specify the conditions under which individuals 'will give priority to avoiding sub-jective discomfort at the cost of endangering their lives, and under what conditions they will make a more rational decision by seeking out and taking into account the available medical information about the real consequences of alternative courses of action so as to maximise their chances of survival' (Janis 1984). Janis & Mann (1977) have described five different patterns of coping with realistic threats and five stages that individuals go through in order to arrive at a stable decision. The patterns were derived from observing individuals, analysing research data and monitoring public health messages. The five coping patterns of the decision maker are:

- *Unconflicted persistence.* Information about risks is ignored, and the person continues to behave in a complacent fashion.
- *Unconflicted change.* The adoption of whatever course of action has been recommended without question.
- *Defensive avoidance.* The issue is evaded by putting things off, shifting the responsibility to someone else or selectively attending to the sorts of information one wants to hear.
- *Hypervigilance.* Due to a feeling of impending doom, the person jumps at the first solution that appears to provide the answer, without considering other courses of action. This is sometimes construed as panic.
- *Vigilance.* The individual carefully considers alternatives in an unbiased manner before making a decision.

Janis & Mann (1977) consider the fifth pattern, vigilance, to be a prerequisite of appropriate decision-making. The other four all lead to maladaptive behavioural consequences. In order that the vigilance pattern can be put into operation, three conditions must be met: (1) awareness of the serious risks for whichever alternative is chosen; (2) hope of finding a better alternative; and (3) belief that there is adequate time to search and deliberate before a decision is made. If condition one (conflict) is not met, unconflicted adherence or unconflicted change is to be expected; if the second condition (hope) is not met, defensive avoidance will be the dominant coping pattern; if the third condition (adequate time) is not met, hypervigilance will be the dominant coping pattern.

Having satisfied all these criteria, the decision maker is now in a position to proceed through the stages of making a stable decision. These are:

1. *Appraising the challenge*. The individual has to consider whether the risks are serious if he does not change.

2. *Surveying alternatives*. The search for an acceptable alternative to deal with the problem.

3. *Weighing alternatives*. This stage refers to evaluating the pros and cons of each alternative and questions are asked concerning the selection of the alternative that meets the essential requirements of the individual. Based on this information, a decision is made and a course of action initiated.

4. *Deliberating about commitment*. A plan is developed to implement the decision and interested parties are informed about the person's commitment.

5. *Adhering despite negative feedback*. Any new threats or opportunities are discounted and the individual remains committed to implementing his decision.

The most important feature of the theory is the emphasis on the coping pattern of vigilance. If any of the other coping patterns are dominant then the 'decision maker will fail to engage in adequate information search and appraisal of consequences, overlooking or ignoring crucial information about relevant costs and benefits. Under these conditions, the outcome will not be correctly predicted by the Health Belief Model or by any other rationalistic model of decision making' (Janis 1984). The model has not yet been fully tested but Milner (1994) successfully used the model in a study of decision-making processes in self-help groups. Group structure was not only related to decision-making but to self-esteem as well.

Self-efficacy

Self-efficacy can be defined as the extent to which people believe they are competent to confront the challenges in life. Self-efficacy forms part of Bandura's social cognitive theory (Bandura, 1986) which holds that behaviour is learned through modelling, visualising, self-monitoring and skill training. Behaviour is determined by expectancies and incentives. Expectancies are categorised into:

- expectancies about environmental cues— beliefs about how events are connected
- outcome expectancies—beliefs about how behaviour is likely to influence outcomes
- efficacy expectancies—expectancies about one's own competence to perform the behaviour needed to influence the outcome.

Incentive is the value of a particular object or outcome (health status, approval of others, economic gain). Thus people with a weight problem will attempt to change their diet if they believe that their current eating habits pose a threat to any personally valued outcome such as health or appearance (environmental cues); that particular changes in eating habits will reduce the threats (outcome expectations) and they are capable of adopting new eating habits (efficacy expectations). Bandura (1989) says that expectations of personal efficacy determine whether coping behaviour will be sustained in the face of adversity. In the case of people with weight problems, a strong sense of self-efficacy will result in adherence to a particular diet regimen even though there is only a small change in weight. Those with a weak sense of self-efficacy, in the same circumstances, would be more likely to become discouraged and give up. Linn (1988) related the ability to tolerate pain to self-efficacy. Those subjects with high self-efficacy were able to tolerate more pain than those with low self-efficacy. Bandura et al (1988) say that self-efficacy enables people to cope with stressors because it activates the production of endogenous opioids that block the transmission of pain and allow the person to function more effectively.

Theory of reasoned action

The main contention of this theory is that intention is the best predictor of behaviour. Suppose you are in a restaurant with a friend who has just given up drinking alcohol. The waiter asks if your friend would like a glass of wine with her meal. You wonder whether she will accept. According to the theory of reasoned action (Ajzen & Fishbein 1980) you would ask what she intends to do. But what determines intentions? The theory indicates that intention to peform a behaviour is determined by beliefs and attitudes. Let's take the example of the person with a weight problem who wants to shed a few pounds. The behavioural intention is 'I would like to lose some weight'. The two attitudes influencing this intention are:

- The attitude regarding the behaviour of eating—'Eating certain foods would be a good thing to do.'
- The subjective norm of eating—'Eating certain foods is seen by many people as an appropriate act.'

In turn these attitudes are influenced by beliefs, so that the attitude regarding the behaviour of eating is affected by:

- Beliefs about the outcomes of eating—'If I eat well I will improve my health and be more attractive.'
- Evaluations regarding the outcomes of eating—'Being healthy and good looking are enjoyable, satisfying and pleasant.'

The subjective norm is influenced by:

- Beliefs about other's opinions—'My family and friends think I should eat certain foods.'
- Motivation to comply with other's opinions—'I would like to do what my friends and family want.'

Ajzen (1985) added another concept to the theory and labelled it the theory of planned action. He proposed that perceived control was an important factor in behavioural intention. Thus one of the best predictors of weight loss is the perceived control over one's weight. It involves beliefs about abilities, opportunities and obstacles to the behaviour. The theory has been applied to smoking (Fishbein 1982), losing weight (Schifter & Ajzen 1985) and breast self-examination (Lierman et al 1990).

The models and theories of health behaviour that have been presented represent a significant step forward in understanding why people do and do not seek health care. They also have been applied to a wide range of health topics from attitudes to safe sex to brushing and flossing teeth. However, there are two main drawbacks:

- Weinstein (1988) says that the theories assume that people think about risks in a detailed, rational fashion. In fact, people may modify their behaviour for vague, illogical reasons.
- With the various reformulations of the models and theories, the distinction between many of them has become blurred. Sogaard (1993) points out that both the health belief model and the social cognitive model are based on Lewin's field theory (Lewin 1951). Recently, the health belief model has been revised to incorporate self-efficacy (Rosenstock et al 1988). Similarly the notion of perceived control is close to Bandura's concept of self-efficacy (Ajzen & Madden 1986).

Although inroads have been made into the study of health behaviour it seems there is still quite a way to go before we are able to predict the circumstances under which people will, or will not, engage in healthy behaviour.

COMPLIANCE

Glidewell (1983) relates the interview he had with a 'hardworking mother of three' who was having to manage on her own. He asked her why she had not taken advantage of free polio injections for her children. She said that she would lose a day's pay from work if she had to queue up all day for injections for her children. He asked her if her children's protection from polio was not worth a day's pay and she replied, 'If I don't get them shot, what are the chances my children will get polio?' This was just the question he had been dreading. After a long painful pause, he replied, 'About one in a hundred thousand.' She then gave him a look of the most intense disgust that he had ever experienced and said, 'Shit, man get out of here!' As

Glidewell says, 'The trouble with prevention is that the threat is so rarely urgent and likely.'

Despite their good intentions, health professionals face many problems when trying to engage their patients' cooperation in adhering to medical advice. Even when the patient has invested considerable effort in seeking out health care, the chances are quite high that the advice offered will be ignored or misapplied. Dunbar & Stunkard (1979) state that patient noncompliance is considered by many to be one of the most serious problems facing the health profession today. Therefore it is important to examine the extent of noncompliance, the factors affecting noncompliance and ways of reducing noncompliance.

Extent of noncompliance

Sackett (1976) defines patient compliance as 'the extent to which a patient's behaviour coincides with the clinical prescription provided by a health professional'. The patient may not comply on purpose or may simply forget or misunderstand the instructions. Ley & Spelman (1967) and Ley (1988) state that 48.7% of patients fail to take their antibiotic tablets, 37.5% fail to take their antituberculosis drugs, and, even among those patients who attempt to comply with the instructions given to them, anything from one-quarter to two-thirds may be taking the wrong dose and up to 30% are making errors that are potentially dangerous.

The extent of noncompliance depends on a number of factors:

- complexity of the treatment procedure
- degree of change required in one's lifestyle
- length of time during which the patient has to follow the advice
- whether the illness is extremely painful
- whether the treatment is seen as potentially life saving
- severity of illness as perceived by the patient and not the health professional.

The degree of noncompliance varies according to whether the regimen is curative or preventive, long term or short term. Sackett & Snow (1979) found that adherence to a 10-day medical schedule was 70–80% when the aim was to cure the patient, and 60–70% when the aim was prevention. Failure to follow long-term programmes, where the condition is not acute, has even lower compliance rates (50%) and this gets worse with time.

Accurate assessment of those individuals who are predisposed to noncompliance is a difficult task (Cluss & Epstein 1984). Kasl (1975) found that health professionals are often unable to judge which of their patients are not following their advice and tend to overestimate the extent to which their patients will comply. It is also difficult to measure the level of compliance with any degree of precision. Gordis (1979) says that estimates of compliance by the health professional and self-reports by the patient are inaccurate. There has been some success in measuring compliance by investigating pill counts (how many pills are left in a bottle) and direct assay of a drug in a patient's body, but this is only useful where the treatment involves some form of medication and is inappropriate in behavioural programmes. Finally, despite overtures from all those people involved in health education to discontinue or reduce such behaviours as smoking, drinking, overeating and sedentary living, we still continue to 'fly in the face' of evidence we know to be true.

Factors affecting noncompliance

The factors affecting noncompliance may be grouped under four headings:

Understanding the instructions

No individual can comply with instructions if he or she has misunderstood what has been said. Ley & Spelman (1967) found that up to 60% of patients interviewed after their visit to their doctor had misunderstood the instructions given to them. Sometimes this is the fault of medical personnel providing incomplete information, using medical jargon and giving patients too much to remember.

Anderson (1986), in a study of doctor–patient communication in Hong Kong, found that patients were given an average of 18 items of information to remember at each consultation, with an overall recall level of only 31%. The provision of clear and explicit information is particularly important when antibiotic medication is prescribed as patients will often stop taking the tablets when the symptoms disappear rather than continuing to take them for the required period of time (Haynes et al 1979).

Practical approaches to increasing patient compliance are provided by DiNicola & DiMatteo (1984):

- Make written instructions unambiguous and easily interpreted.
- Give patients instructions about the treatment before explaining anything else. When people are given a list of items to remember there is a 'primacy effect'; they tend to remember those items that are presented at the beginning of the list. This primacy effect has been shown to be particularly strong for the retention of medical information (Ley 1972).
- Instructions should be presented in non-technical language and their importance stressed.

Quality of the interaction

The quality of the interaction between health professional and patient plays an important part in determining the degree of compliance. Korsch & Negrete (1972) observed the visits of 800 parents and their children to a children's hospital in Los Angeles. 14 days later they interviewed the mothers to ascertain whether they had implemented the doctor's instructions. They found that there was a close association between the mother's satisfaction with the consultation and the extent to which she carried out the doctor's advice; there was no correlation between the duration of the consultation and the amount of satisfaction expressed by the mother. Thus short consultations need not be counterproductive if attention is paid to improving the quality of the interaction. Some specific complaints were lack of interest shown by the doctor, excessive use of jargon, a lack of empathy and nearly half

the mothers were unclear about what had caused their child's illness, which sometimes leads to unnecessary anxiety. In Chapter 1 we saw that these faults can be easily remedied using interpersonal skill training. That there is a need for such training programmes is evidenced by the fact that most of the doctors in the Korsch & Negrete (1972) study thought that they had been friendly towards their patients, but less than half of the patients shared this impression.

On the basis of this research, Ley (1988) has drawn up a set of guidelines to produce satisfied and compliant patients in the paediatric context:

- Be friendly rather than businesslike.
- Engage in at least some conversation which is not directly connected with the problem.
- Spend time talking to the child.
- Discover the mother's expectations, and explain why these are not fulfilled, if they are not.
- Discover the mother's concerns and take appropriate action.
- Give information as well as ask questions.

The importance of interpersonal skills in facilitating compliance to medical regimens is highlighted by DiNicola & DiMatteo (1982):

Research on interpersonal factors as they affect cooperation with medical regimens suggests also that physicians' sensitivity to patients' verbal and nonverbal communications and their empathy with and understanding of patients' feelings may be critically important to patient compliance as well as related satisfaction with care.

The family and social isolation

The family can be very influential in determining a person's health beliefs and values and it can also determine what constitutes an acceptable treatment programme. Pratt (1976) has called attention to the role the family plays in developing health habits and teaching them to the children. The family also provides support and makes decisions regarding the care of the ill members.

The degree to which one is isolated from the company of other people, social isolation, is negatively correlated to compliance (Baekeland & Lundwall 1975). Members of an individual's 'social network' will often influence a person to seek health care. The 'lay referral network' consists of that group of people, usually family and friends, to whom the individual first describes any symptoms and from whom the patient seeks advice. (A detailed analysis of networks and their relationship to health care appears in Chapter 8.) However, in the context of compliance, it should be noted that the lay referral network is a significant determinant of the decision to seek and to follow medical advice.

Beliefs, attitudes and personality

Becker et al (1979) have proposed that the health belief model is useful in predicting noncompliance. They illustrate the usefulness of the model in a study by Hartman & Becker (1978) that predicted noncompliance with a prescribed regimen for chronic haemodialysis patients. 50 patients with end-stage renal disease had to follow a complex medical regimen of diet, fluid restriction, medication and dialysis. They were interviewed about their health beliefs using the model. Hartman & Becker found that measures of each of the major dimensions of the model were shown to be useful predictors of therapeutic compliance.

Other psychologists have looked at the relationship between measures of personality and compliance. Blumenthal et al (1982) gave 35 patients, who had recently experienced a myocardial infarction, the Minnesota Multiphasic Personality Inventory (MMPI) whilst measuring their compliance with an exercise programme. They found that personality data correctly distinguished between compliers and dropouts. Noncompliers were more depressed, anxious, concerned about their health, had lower ego strength and were socially introverted. Low ego strength was characterised by such things as deficits in self-restraint and poor environmental mastery. Social introversion was a measure of how comfortable people were in social situations. Blumenthal et al (1982) suggest that it was these personality

characteristics which led to certain individuals dropping out of the programme.

Therefore, there exists important research evidence that problems in the health professional–patient relationship, an individual's family and friends and finally his or her health beliefs and personality all contribute to determine patient behaviour in response to medical advice.

Reducing noncompliance

Unfortunately there is not always a correspondence between the factors that predict and explain compliance and the techniques that have been developed to decrease noncompliance. However, a number of different strategies have been advanced to try to provide a solution to the problem. DiNicola & DiMatteo (1984) propose a five-point plan for dealing with patient noncompliance:

- A prerequisite of any plan to establish compliance is the development of intention to comply (the theory of reasoned action). Many noncompliant patients never had any intention of adhering to medical advice in the first place. Simply stated, a person is likely to express an intention to go on a diet if he has positive beliefs about and attitudes toward dieting; and his family and friends are positively disposed toward dieting. A publicly stated commitment will enhance the probability that the patient will carry out the required behaviour. A written contract can also prove effective, but as we saw in Chapter 3, contingency contracting can be ineffective over long periods of time. Finally, whatever commitment is entered into by the patient, it must be self-initiated; coercion on the part of the health professional will have the opposite effect.

- Health behaviour is strongly influenced by habit, thus strategies have to be developed that will not only change behaviour, but maintain the change. Behavioural self-control requires the patient to self-monitor, self-evaluate and self-reinforce any new behaviour.

For instance, a weight loss programme requires individuals to be aware of exactly how much they are consuming, to evaluate how well they are managing to keep to their new eating programme, and continually to provide rewards for keeping to the programme.

- Behavioural control is often not sufficient on its own to change behaviour. Cognitive factors are important too. A programme can be totally ruined by the patient using self-defeating statements like: 'Oh, I'm a real pig when it comes to eating junk food. I can't stick to any diet. I'm doomed to be fat.' To avoid such statements it is important to develop in patients a sense of competence, self-control and a belief in themselves.

Janis & Rodin (1979) say that this may be accomplished using 'referent power'. Referent power refers to a situation where the health professional becomes a reference person for the patient. She becomes someone who is like the person in many ways and who advocates a particular healthy behaviour.

Another approach favoured by Meichenbaum (1977) is to make patients more aware of their own thoughts, to encourage them to use positive self-statements and to collect data that will refute negative self-statements. Behaviour modification often entails a high frequency of contact between providers and patients, and as this can prove expensive in terms of time and money, the use of cognitive factors may prove an effective adjunct to behavioural techniques.

- Social support in the form of emotional support from family and friends and physical assistance (money and time) is an important factor in medical compliance. Simple things like not having a babysitter, no transportation and an illness in the family can contribute to lack of compliance. Family and friends can help reduce anxiety caused by a particular illness; they can remove temptations to non-adherence; and they can often provide a mutual support group to enhance compliance.

- Support from health professionals is another factor which can affect compliant behaviour. Their support is particularly valuable when the patient views the new health behaviour to be of minor importance. Similarly, they can influence patient behaviour by transmitting their enthusiasm for a particular course of action and consistently applying reinforcements and encouragements for its adoption.

These five factors represent the supports for patient compliance; if they outweigh the barriers, compliance should follow. Feuerstein et al (1986) also provide a programme of action containing five elements:

- *Education.* Patient education can increase compliance as long as it is an active education such as the use of self-help books and tapes.

- *Accommodation.* An attempt must be made to deal with personality characteristics that impede compliance. For instance, the autonomous patient should be encouraged to feel that he is an active part of the treatment programme, whereas the anxious patient needs to have his anxiety levels reduced by reassurance or other techniques so that he is motivated to follow advice. Feuerstein et al (1986) say that if the anxiety level is too high or too low, the patient will be less likely to comply.

- *Modification of environmental and social factors.* This refers to the establishment of social support from family and friends. Groups can be designed to aid the compliance in programmes concerned with such things as weight reduction, stopping smoking, and reducing alcohol consumption.

- *Changes in therapeutic regimen.* The treatment programme can be made as simple as possible, and the patient actively involved in designing it. In this way simple components of the programme can be reinforced, leading to compliance with further elements of the programme as time progresses.

- *Enhancement of the health professional–patient interaction.* It is important to provide the patient with feedback after getting diagnostic information. Patients need explanations about the nature of their condition, how it was caused, and what may be done about it.

A migraine headache may lead a person to wonder whether he might have a brain tumour. An explanation of how migraines are caused and how they are treated can lead to a greater confidence in the consultative process and consequently facilitate compliance.

These two approaches illustrate that, despite certain minor differences, there is a broad consensus of opinion about what constitutes a practical clinical intervention programme to increase patient compliance. Unfortunately this knowledge does not seem to have been taken on board by many doctors.

Lorenc (1986) obtained responses from 174 GPs and 43 consultants in the North Staffordshire area to a questionnaire containing eight statements about medical compliance (Box 6.1).

One point was awarded for each correct answer. The average score for the GPs was 3.02 and the average score for the consultants 2.28. This difference was significant ($p < 0.05$). On the basis of these results it would seem that there is a need to increase doctors' knowledge about this area.

The quotation at the beginning of this section suggested that the fruits of medical research were inadequate if the patient did nothing about the medical advice given to her; it seems that the same criticism has to be levelled at psychologists, and others, who seem to have failed to communicate the research on compliance to those who could benefit from it.

DEPRESSION

Beck (1989) says that depression causes a person to have a problem performing even the most elemental and vital tasks such as eating and eliminating.

> The essence of the problem appears to be that, although he can define for himself what he should do, he does not experience any internal stimulus to do it. Even when urged, cajoled, or threatened, he does not seem able to arouse any desire to do these things.
>
> Beck (1989)

Beck termed the condition mentioned above 'paralysis of will'. Yet we have all experienced at some time or another a state of mind which has prohibited us from doing something that we know to be necessary: the feeling that one cannot be bothered to eat; or knowing that a visit to the doctor is important but the motivation to go is absent; or telling people to stop pestering one and stop getting on one's nerves. All these feelings, thoughts and behaviours are common enough, but would we label them as symptoms of depression? Is feeling 'a bit down' or 'blue' just a minor form of clinical depression, or is it a different condition altogether?

Classification

In order to answer these questions, it is necessary to define what is meant by depression. Unfortunately, as is common with other 'psychological disorders', the inability to come up with an adequate definition has resulted in continuing debate over the answers to these questions. There is, however, a reasonable agreement as to the sorts of symptoms that characterise the condition of depression. Becker (1974) lists the following as the most common signs and symptoms:

- sad, lonely, apathetic, or irritable mood
- an exaggeratedly negative, self-punitive self-concept
- disturbed bodily functioning, accompanied

Box 6.1   Statements in the Lorenc (1986) questionnaire

1. Compliance can be increased by using calendar packs rather than standard bottles.
2. Compliance can be increased by providing comprehensible information leaflets.
3. A patient's educational level has nothing to do with his/her likelihood to be noncompliant.
4. Patients on long-term treatment are less likely to comply than those on short-term treatment.
5. Satisfied patients are more likely to comply with a prescribed medical regimen.
6. Patients aged over 65 are more likely to be noncompliant than younger patients.
7. People who live alone tend to neglect their medicines more often than other patients.
8. More frequent dosage automatically means lower compliance.

by decreased appetite, poor sleep, constipation, and diminished sexual interest
- physical complaints of aches, weakness, fatigue
- altered activity level with slowing or agitation
- impaired thought processes with high distractibility, indecisiveness, disinterestedness, and preoccupation with hopelessness and helplessness.

These symptoms are sometimes present in other psychological disorders, but there is evidence that depression is a condition that is distinct from other disorders (Murphy et al 1974).

The next issue is whether there are different types of depression. It is important for health professionals to have a knowledge of the way depression has been classified as the terms used are often mentioned in the course of dealing with patients. A distinction is frequently made between endogenous and reactive (or exogenous) depression. *Endogenous depression* is produced by something that is thought to have gone wrong within the individual, such as a genetic predisposition to the disorder or some physiological dysfunction. *Reactive depression* results from psychosocial causes, such as death of a spouse or losing one's job, which are presumed to occur as a response to external events.

Another major distinction is between unipolar and bipolar depression. *Bipolar depression* occurs in patients who experience episodes of hypomania interspersed between periods of depression. Mania, and its lesser form hypomania, are in many ways the reverse of depression. They are characterised by feelings of elation and euphoria, the patients often commenting that they have never felt better in their lives. There is considerable overactivity, with little sleep taken. The patient with mania, or hypomania, does not think that anything is wrong and may do strange things in the mistaken assumption that his personal circumstances have never been better. These mood swings do not usually alternate like a 'big dipper', as, often, there are long periods of normal behaviour in between the abnormal behaviour. Other individuals, however, just experience bouts of depression with no

associated hypomania and these are regarded as having · *unipolar depression*. There are some difficulties with this classification, in that an individual is unable to be classified as unipolar until he/she has experienced sufficient episodes of hypomania-free depression to qualify (usually at least three; Perris 1982).

There are other subclassifications such as *psychotic vs neurotic, primary vs secondary* and *pure depression vs depression spectrum disorder.* These categories are not so ubiquitous as the major ones represented above, however, and a comprehensive description of them is provided by Andreason (1982).

The evidence for such subclassifications of depression is debatable. One of the problems lies in developing an appropriate methodology to test the distinctions. Miller & Morley (1986) found that a number of studies do give support to the notion of endogenous depression but there is considerably less support for the concept of reactive depression. They state that at best only one-half of the endogenous/reactive distinction is validated. Bakal (1979) questions whether endogenous depression might not reflect the outcome of years of poor life experiences. A housewife who suddenly becomes clinically depressed might not recognise that she became so largely because she was increasingly ignored by her family. Endogenous depression might sometimes be undetected reactive depression.

There is stronger evidence for a unipolar/bipolar subclassification. Again at first sight, it seems easy to distinguish between these two groups because bipolar depressives have hypomanic swings which unipolar depressives do not. However, it could be the case that unipolar depressives do in fact have mood swings, but they are not high enough to qualify as a significant variation in mood. Perris (1982) originally found that there was a genetic link between the different types of depression. If one's father or mother were classified as bipolar depressive, then it was likely that if depression occurred it too would be bipolar. Research since Perris's early studies has found the distinction to be not quite so clear cut. Where the affective disorder has been found to be unipolar, the link between parents and offspring has been established. The picture for relatives of bipolar cases is more confused. Sometimes parents with bipolar disorders will produce offspring with unipolar disorders.

Perris (1982) argues that one of the reasons why this might occur is due to the time one has to wait in classifying the disorder. Mistakes can easily be made during this period. He concludes that there is some degree of support for the distinction between unipolar and bipolar disorders and cites as further evidence age differences in onset. There is a fairly consistent trend for bipolar cases to have their first episode of disorder in their mid-20s. First episodes of unipolar disorder usually occur 15–20 years later. Lastly, response to treatment using lithium carbonate differs according to unipolar or bipolar affective disorder, with bipolar cases responding favourably and unipolar cases not responding very well at all (Mendels 1976).

Two reviews on the subclassification of depression (Perris 1982; Depue & Munroe 1978) concluded that the best support for distinguishing between different types of depression comes from the studies investigating unipolar and bipolar depression. There is too much confusion and contradiction, with respect to the studies of the endogenous/reactive distinction, to prove useful even as a working hypothesis.

Treatment

The treatment of depression may be divided into physical and psychological treatments. Herbst & Paykel (1989) divide physical treatments into antidepressant medication and ECT. The two most effective types of antidepressant drug are the tricyclics such as amitriptyline and the monoamine oxidase inhibitors such as phenazine. Usually the tricyclics are preferred since they are less prone to side-effects. Lithium is also used (especially for bipolar disorders), but administration of the drug requires careful monitoring since the therapeutic dose is very close to the toxic dose.

In the early 1930s it was observed that epilepsy and psychoses like schizophrenia seldom occurred together. On the basis of this observation, it was hypothesised that epileptic seizures in some way blocked the psychosis. Therefore it was proposed to create artificial seizures to see whether they would have the same effect. In 1938, electric shock was used in Italy for this purpose and became known as ECT. An electric current was passed between two electrodes attached to the patient's temples. When a current of 80–140 volts was reached, the patient had a seizure and became unconscious. The seizure was accompanied by violent muscle spasms which often caused the patients to injure themselves. However, the procedure did seem to be effective, particularly in the treatment of depression.

Unfortunately there were some rather unpleasant side-effects. Apart from the muscle spasms, which were controlled using muscle relaxants, there was memory loss, temporary confusion and interference with the desire to eat and drink. Added to this, nobody knew what the long-term result of passing large amounts of electricity through the brain would be. Under these circumstances a great deal of opposition developed to the practice of ECT. In its defence, it was effective in circumstances where other forms of therapy had failed.

In 1977, Norman Endler, a psychologist, suddenly became profoundly depressed. This totally disrupted his life at home and at work. He tried traditional treatments such as psychotherapy and antidepressants to no avail.

At that time I was so desperate that if Dr Persad had suggested that walking down Yonge Street (the main street in Toronto) nude would be beneficial to me, I would probably have tried it. Therefore, I agreed, although reluctantly, to ECT as a course of treatment for my depression.

Endler (1982)

The word 'reluctant' understates his feelings, since as a graduate student, Endler had seen ECT treatment break a patient's back. Over a 2-week period he received seven ECT sessions and reported afterwards that his 'holiday of darkness' was over. He became a firm believer in ECT, and refers to it as 'living better electrically'. However, its success with a limited number of severe depressives should not detract from what some would regard as a barbaric form of treatment. But in situations where all other forms of therapy have failed and the patient is suicidal, the option to use ECT is difficult to ignore.

Psychological approaches to depression are dominated by the theories of Seligman and Beck.

Seligman's learned helplessness theory

Seligman (1980) proposed that depressed people have learned helplessness from experiences and believe themselves unable to influence and control events. The concept of learned helplessness developed from experiments with animals, which have been described in detail on page 86.

Seligman (1980) argues that learned helplessness and depression have much in common and that one reason why individuals might become depressed is because they have learnt to become helpless. Over a period of time they have felt themselves to have no control over their circumstances, they have perceived themselves to have 'no way out'. Thus, even when presented with 'an escape route', they do not take it but 'crawl into themselves' and give up trying. This represents quite a conceptual jump from animal studies to a theory of depression in human beings; nevertheless there is a certain amount of evidence that some features of depression might be due to the learned helplessness phenomenon (Peterson & Seligman 1984).

One study that investigated the concept of learned helplessness in humans was carried out by Miller & Seligman (1975). They administered the Beck Depression Inventory to a number of students. On the basis of their scores, the students were assigned to 'depressed' or 'non-depressed' groups. Each group was then split into three and assigned to different conditions: (a) exposed to white noise—could terminate at will; (b) exposed to white noise—no escape; (c) no noise. All the students were then required to solve anagrams, which followed a standard letter pattern.

The 'non-depressed' group performed in the following way—those that had been exposed to inescapable noise were significantly worse at solving the anagrams than those with the option to turn it off and those with no noise at all. Meanwhile, the 'depressed' group gave the following results—those subjects who had no noise at all performed worse than their counterparts in the 'non-depressed' group. Also the introduction of inescapable noise did not further affect the performance of the subjects in the 'depressed' group. The researchers suggest that the 'depressed' subjects had already experienced learned helplessness before they came to solve the anagrams and this resulted in their poor performance. It should be remembered that these subjects were not depressed patients, but ordinary students who scored below average on the Beck scale.

Some psychologists have extended the concept of learned helplessness yet further and suggested that it can also apply to whole communities. Gibbs et al (1977) said that if the people in a community think that they have no control over their circumstances, then the entire community can become helpless. For instance, the residents of an area where there is high unemployment might feel that they have no control over what is happening to them, that no matter how much they try, they will never be able to get a job. Under these circumstances whole communities may develop learned helplessness.

There have been a number of criticisms of the learned helplessness theory. These will be dealt with briefly as the theory has been reformulated (Abramson et al 1978).

The first criticism refers to the predominant use of subjects who were not classified as clinically depressed. In the previous study the subjects were students who were classified as depressed on the basis of the Beck scale. The extent to which they represent a sample similar to clinically depressed patients has been questioned. A second criticism refers to the extent to which studies carried out in psychological laboratories are representative of 'real-life' circumstances. A final criticism of the work on human subjects was that the procedures designed to induce helplessness might have merely produced low motivation and not the changes in mood and cognition that Seligman claimed were present.

Abramson et al (1978) agreed that the theory as it stood was inadequate and revised it. The main feature of the revision was the emphasis on the perceptions of the subjects. For instance, it did not matter whether the person was in control of his/her circumstances; if individuals perceived themselves to have no control over events, then learned helplessness would ensue. The revision concentrated on the nature of these perceptions. Depression would occur if the perceptions of events were *internal, stable and global*. If an individual feels that he is the cause of what has gone wrong, and not some external factor, then the perception is internal. If the individual feels that what has gone wrong is a persistent characteristic of his behaviour and not just a 'one-off', then the perception is stable. If the individual thinks that his tendency to make a mess of things applies to all situations and not just what is happening at the moment, then the perception is global. If negative events are viewed in this way, and positive events have an external, almost accidental cause, then learned helplessness will occur. This reformulation, with its emphasis on how people interpret events, has been seen by some as quite a different theory altogether (Williams 1984a). Certainly the new 'cognitive' component is a significant departure from the 'behavioural' origins of the theory and is now perhaps quite similar to Beck's cognitive theory of depression.

Beck's cognitive theory of depression

The learned helplessness theory developed from experimental research into animal behaviour, whereas Beck's theory is based on clinical observation. The theory is based on the negative thoughts of the depressed person. Incorrect conceptions precede emotional feelings. Beck (1967, 1989) proposes that depression results from three sorts of negative thinking:

- The self—'I am a real failure.'
- The world—'The things that happen around here are really awful.'

- The future—'Life is always going to be bad.'

Depression also results from four sorts of incorrect thinking:

- *Selective abstraction*. The individual only thinks about the negative features of his behaviour.
- *Overgeneralisation*. Because one thing has gone wrong, everything else is going to go wrong.
- *Exaggeration*. Exaggeration of the significance of negative events and minimising the importance of positive ones.
- *Personalisation*. Negative events are related to oneself even where there are no grounds for doing so.

The third feature of Beck's theory concerns the concept of 'schema'. A schema is the habitual way in which an individual interprets his world and makes sense of his experiences. Instead of perceiving the world through 'rose-tinted spectacles', the depressed individual interprets events through 'depression-tinted spectacles'.

Beck (1989) gives a description of how faulty cognitions may start a chain reaction leading to clinical depression. A wife has deserted her husband. The effect that her desertion has on the husband will depend on the cognitions the husband has about his wife. His thoughts might consist of a series of positive associations that range from the realistic ('she is important to me') to the unrealistic ('I enjoy life only because of her'). The more absolute these positive associations, the greater will be the sense of loss. Thus, if the positive associations are exaggerated in nature, he might now begin to formulate exaggerated negative statements with respect to his self ('I am nothing without her; I can't go on without her').

The next stage might be that the husband starts to question his own self-worth ('if only I had been a better husband'). As the reaction develops, the husband's self-doubts expand into negative generalisations about himself, his world, and his future. The husband, now better described as the depressed patient, stops all activities that previously gave him pleasure. Life becomes meaningless, and he may begin to contemplate suicide. Physiological symptoms involving sleep disturbance and loss of appetite further aggravate the condition.

Williams (1988) has reviewed a number of studies examining Beck's cognitive theory and concludes that the evidence that depressive ways of thinking predispose people to become clinically depressed is not strong. Unhappy thoughts can lower mood, but not all low mood can be considered to be depression. It seems that clinical depression is a much more complicated phenomenon than any one theory supposed. However, the Beck approach does provide one of the most promising avenues for further research and it should be noted that his theory has proved more effective than other psychological theories in suggesting ways of treating depressed patients (Williams 1984b).

Cognitive therapy

Let us look at how a cognitive therapist might put the above ideas to work in a treatment programme. Consider Case History 6.2:

The first course of action to take is to discover Jackie's particular way of viewing the world. Often people are unaware of their biased views of events. Their reactions to these events are fast and unthinking, even automatic. Therefore it is important to detect these thoughts and reactions. This may be achieved by:

CASE HISTORY 6.2 JACKIE W.

Jackie W. is a health visitor. She was 38 years old when her husband died suddenly of a heart attack. They had no children, and she felt completely alone for the first time. Her colleagues at work understood this and had made allowances to support her in any way they could. They started to get worried when, long after most people would have stopped mourning, she continued to show little interest in her work and in her friends. When she got home from work, she would sit down in a chair and sort through old photographs of her husband. Jackie was convinced that she was in some way responsible for her husband's death. She was aware that she was not doing as much as she might at work and felt that her colleagues snubbed and rejected her because of this. After a friend had heard her casually mention suicide, it was decided to engage the help of a specialist.

- direct interviewing about specific problem situations
- the use of imagery to help recall 'difficult' events
- Jackie keeping a diary.

The latter course of action is guided by the instruction to pay particular attention to the thoughts that are going through her mind in known situations. In this particular instance, she may be 'selectively abstracting' information about her friends. She only recalls those instances where her friends have seemed cold and distant, ignoring all the times when they have been supportive and friendly. On the basis of these thoughts she may begin to 'overgeneralise' and conclude that nobody likes her.

Having established the presence of cognitive errors it is necessary to confront Jackie and challenge these thoughts. For each type of error there are alternative constructions of events. Thus Jackie would be encouraged to think of all the times her colleagues had been pleasant to her. Sometimes it might be difficult to face up to these alternatives, so there are a number of techniques to help her do so:

- *Distancing.* Events and situations are described in the third person. Thus Jackie is able to 'stand back' from events and view them more dispassionately.
- *Fact vs hypothesis.* Jackie should be encouraged to distinguish between facts and what she thinks to be facts. Also she should make guesses about what is likely to happen if her assumptions turn out to be valid.
- *Behavioural tests.* Finally, a series of behavioural tests of alternative views of the world should be set up. These tests should be graded, so that she receives repeated success over more and more difficult situations.

This represents a summary of Beck's approach to cognitive behaviour therapy. There are other cognitive behaviour therapies such as Ellis's Rational Emotive Therapy (1980) and Meichenbaum's Stress Inoculation Therapy (1977) (for a further analysis see Williams (1984a).

CORONARY HEART DISEASE

A World Health Organization (WHO) report in January 1987 placed Great Britain first in the league of deaths as a result of heart disease. According to the WHO's World Health Statistics Annual for 1986, Scotland and Northern Ireland had the highest figures for deaths from coronary heart disease at 298 per 100 000, followed by Czechoslovakia at 290, the Irish Republic 282, Finland 264, England and Wales 243, Hungary 238, and the United States 230. These statistics illustrate the extent of the problem throughout the world.

Coronary heart disease (CHD) occurs when the coronary arteries narrow to such an extent that they cannot take enough blood to supply the muscles of the heart with sufficient oxygen and nourishment. As a result the individual may experience intense pain in the chest and down the arm. This is called *angina pectoris* and occurs at the moment the heart suffers from a lack of oxygen. If this condition continues, and part of the heart muscle dies, *myocardial infarction* (MI) results.

Risk factors

Factors known to affect the incidence of CHD include high-cholesterol diet, smoking, obesity, high blood pressure, physical inactivity and family history. Although these factors are major determinants of heart disease, it is seldom mentioned that these physical risk factors are totally absent in nearly 50% of all new cases (Keys et al 1972; Russek & Russek 1976). These research findings have shifted the attention from the role of physical health behaviour in heart disease to an examination of the psychological risk factors.

In the 1950s two cardiologists Friedman & Rosenman noted that men had a higher incidence of heart disease than women, despite the fact that they both had the same amount of cholesterol intake. They concluded that there must be some other important factor involved in CHD. The women in the study suggested that stress at work was contributing to their husbands' demise. Accordingly, Rosenman & Friedman posted questionnaires to 150 San Franciscan businessmen asking them to indicate what habits had preceded a heart attack in a friend of theirs. About 70% of them said that things like excessive competition and meeting deadlines were the most common factors preceding a heart attack; only 5% reported that fatty foods, smoking and lack of exercise were involved.

On the basis of these and other observations, Friedman & Rosenman (1959) conducted a study comparing two groups of males matched on age, diet, and exercise. One group displayed the coronary-prone behaviour pattern, the other group did not. Friedman & Rosenman (1959) found an increased prevalence of clinical CHD in the group that exhibited the coronary-prone behaviour pattern in contrast to the group that did not. This behaviour pattern they called Type A.

Type A behaviour

The Type A behaviour pattern is a lifestyle that is characterised by extreme competitiveness, high need to achieve, aggression, impatience, restlessness, hyperalertness and the feeling of being constantly under pressure (Jenkins 1971). The individual who has a Type A behaviour pattern will wish to be in complete control over all features of his environment and thus will often have to increase his pace of life in order to maintain such mastery.

Western Collaborative Group Study

In order to confirm the connection between Type A behaviour and heart disease Friedman & Rosenman, along with psychologists and epidemiologists, set up a longitudinal study called the Western Collaborative Group Study (WCGS), (Friedman & Rosenman 1974). The study was started in 1961 and finished about 9 years later. Over this period of time they investigated a total of 3154 men aged between 39 and 59 years at intake. They were all employed by 10 California companies.

The data they collected on these men consisted of Type A or B behaviour patterns (a Type

B behaviour pattern has none of the Type A characteristics), education, medical history, physical activity at work, smoking habits, blood pressure, and cholesterol levels. After $2\frac{1}{2}$ years the researchers examined the Type A and Type B groups for the development of heart disease. The Type A men aged between 39 and 49 years had 6.5 times the incidence of coronary heart disease in Type B men. After $8\frac{1}{2}$ years, the incidence of clinical coronary heart disease was twice as high in Type A men as in Type B men.

This finding may be explained by the argument that the difference is simply because Type A men smoke more than Type B men, for example. However, this result held even after statistical techniques were used to control for the physical risk factors such as smoking. A matter for concern is the extent to which coronary-prone behaviour can be modified. Educating individuals to take more exercise, to stop smoking and to adopt a healthy diet is difficult but possible and well within the grasp of good health education programmes. Changing people's personality is a much more daunting task.

Measurement of Type A behaviour

Type A behaviour has been measured in different ways. Friedman & Rosenman (1974) used a structured interview technique. Jenkins et al (1971) favoured a questionnaire called The Jenkins Activity Survey. Haynes et al (1978) used the Framingham Type A Scales, a self-report measure of 10 items that evaluate the individual's competitive drive, time-urgency, and perception of job pressure.

The structured interview has been widely used in the assessment of Type A behaviour. An interesting feature of the technique is the observation of the individual's behaviour while he is responding to the interviewer's questions. Assessment is thus based on both the content of the individual's responses and the presence or absence of Type A behaviour displayed during the course of the interview. There are three basic themes that characterise the behaviour pattern:

- degree of drive and ambition

- degree of past and present competitive, aggressive, and hostile feelings
- degree of time-urgency.

While the interview is taking place, the interviewer also takes note of nonverbal behaviours such as gestures, facial grimaces, alertness, and speed of motion. This places quite a strain on the interviewer, who has to undergo rigorous training sessions in order to conduct the interview while concurrently evaluating the various patterns seen.

The problems with this approach are that it is difficult to train interviewers to an identical high standard in order to maintain reliability. The questions themselves are transparent and this may result in a response bias, where the expected responses are provided, for example:

When you are in your automobile, and there is a car in your lane going far too slowly for you, what do you do about it?

a. Would you *mutter and complain* to yourself? Honk your horn? Flash your lights?
b. Would anyone riding with you know that you were *annoyed*?

A final criticism is that individuals are categorised as either Type A or Type B; there is no indication of the pattern of behaviour within a particular type.

The Jenkins Activity Survey contains 50 items, 21 of which are weighted to differentiate between Type A and Type B behaviours. They may be divided into four main areas, whose importance is reflected in the number of items assigned to it in the inventory:

- 1 item—hostile feelings and behaviour.
- 5 items—hard-driving competitiveness.
- 7 items—continually working under pressure and not taking time off
- 8 items—doing things too quickly, such as eating.

The Framingham A Scales have three main scales of Type A behaviour:

- *Reaction-to-anger*. These scales measure the ways individuals express and cope with anger, internalising it, externalising it or talking it over with a friend.

- *Situational-stress*. Refers to stress at home and at work. It includes such things as lack of support at work and marital discord.
- *Somatic-strain*. This is an index of tension, anxiety and strain.

These three measures of Type A behaviour—the structured interview; the JAS; and the Framingham A Scales—have been evaluated by Matthews (1982). She says that there seems to be evidence of a reasonable amount of reliability in all the measures, but the extent to which they overlap is limited. Considering each one in turn, she states that the predominant behavioural characteristic of Type A men, as evaluated by the SI, is the way they react strongly to events that are frustrating, difficult and competitive. This reactivity takes the form of rapid, loud and explosive speech, in addition to cardiovascular arousal.

The characteristics of Type A individuals, as measured by the JAS, are aggression, competition and a determined need to achieve. There is some cardiovascular reactivity during competitive events. Finally, the Framingham A Scale characterises Type A behaviour as dissatisfaction and feeling uncomfortable with competition and job stress. In general, the Type A behaviour pattern consists of achievement orientation, time-urgency, and aggression.

Development of behaviour pattern

Most of the discussion so far has centred on the behaviours that make up the Type A pattern and how they are related to coronary heart disease. The next stage is to examine why people develop these behaviours, for if we have an idea of what constitutes the underlying psychological dimensions of the behaviour pattern, then we can obtain a better idea of how to stop it occurring. Matthews (1982) cites four approaches:

Component analysis

The emphasis of this approach is establishing the core psychological elements of Type A that are specifically related to heart disease. It implies that some components of Type A behaviour are more related to heart disease than others. Indeed, factor analysis of the Western Collaborative Group Study indicated that the two most important variables were competitive drive and impatience. Further studies indicated that characteristics of the voice were important too.

Unfortunately this approach does not give any real indication of the psychological basis of the behaviour pattern or why people are classed as Type A individuals.

Self-involvement

A study by Scherwitz et al (1978) found a relationship between the amount of self-referencing (referring to oneself all the time; me, my, mine) during an interview and levels of systolic blood pressure. The researchers argue that continuous self-involvement can create problems for people when their standards are very high and their performance is found wanting. The discrepancies are highlighted by the self-referencing, leading often to considerable striving, frustration, and a sense of helplessness. This in turn manifests itself in the form of increased blood pressure. Williams (1988) finds the results of the research on this approach to be equivocal. One reason for the lack of concrete evidence in favour of the approach is that a number of studies have assumed self-involvement on the basis of mere observations, without actually determining it experimentally.

Uncontrollability

Striving hard to succeed in life, denying that one is tired, and conducting affairs at a 'breakneck' speed are all attempts that the Type A person makes to maintain control over his or her environment. The Type A individual does not like uncontrollable events, and will do anything in his power to try to maintain the upper hand.

Glass (1977) proposed that this struggle to control events is characterised by hard-driving aggressiveness, quick annoyance, and competitiveness. When Type A and B individuals are placed in what is known as a 'failure situation' (a task whose solution is unattainable), they react to it in different ways. Type As attribute their failure to lack of ability and lose faith in their competence to exert environmental influence. Type Bs attribute their failure to external factors, such as bad luck and become passive, withdrawing from a situation they think uncontrollable. Because control over events is extremely important for Type A individuals, they have to accelerate the pace at which they live in order to maintain this control. Thus time-urgency is a central feature of their behaviour.

Burnham et al (1975) asked Type As and Type Bs to read a technical passage out loud and to stop after 1 minute had elapsed. The researchers proposed that, because Type A people have this time-urgency, they would underestimate the minute and time would pass very slowly for them. Type A individuals stopped after an average of 52.6 seconds, whereas Type B individuals stopped after an average of 75.0 seconds.

Ambiguous standards of evaluation

An example of what is meant by ambiguous standards of evaluation is provided by Matthews & Siegel (1983). A person is employed to do a particular job. However, the job specifications contain no method for evaluating how well the individual is performing in that job. There is ambiguity about the standard of his performance. Matthews & Siegel (1983) say that if this individual values productivity strongly and does not obtain appropriate feedback about how he is performing at his job, this will evoke Type A behaviours. It is argued that Type As prefer the company of other Type As because they are continually comparing their own behaviour with that of others and are able to elicit feedback more easily from individuals who are engaged in the same activity.

Recent research by Spielberger (1993) and Smith & Pope (1990) has suggested that anger is a crucial element in coronary heart disease. Also, anger is involved in other factors such as time-urgency. People with a Type A behaviour pattern who are concerned about using their time well find that they become very angry when other people slow them down by interfering with their work.

To summarise, the Type A individual is impatient, competitive, speaks loudly and quickly, continually refers to himself, likes to be in complete control of events and needs to have clearly defined, unambiguous rewards.

Gender differences

The majority of the research into coronary heart disease and Type A behaviour has concentrated on men. One reason for this is the fact that men are much more prone to CHD than women; in fact coronary heart disease strikes twice as many males as females. An explanation that has been put forward to explain gender differences in CHD relates to the assumption that female sex hormones reduce cholesterol levels in the blood and thereby reduce the risk of heart disease. Waldron (1976) suggests that the evidence for this theory is inconclusive. Another variable that could distinguish between the gender differences in CHD is smoking. Since cigarette smoking increases the risk of heart disease, and since more males than females smoke cigarettes, then it seems plausible that there might be some connection. However, there is evidence that whilst smoking is an important factor in heart disease, non-smoking males still suffer more coronary heart disease than women.

Waldron (1976) proposes that the reason males show more heart disease than females is because more males than females have a coronary-prone pattern of behaviour. She provides evidence that Type A females suffer less heart disease than Type A males, but they show more heart disease than Type B males. Further, males with a low risk of contracting CHD are no more likely to contract the disease than low risk females. An analysis of the components of Type A behaviour reveals that the characteristics such as aggression and competition are traits that are actively rewarded in men. Yet women who possess these same traits in business are described in a derogatory fashion.

Waldron (1976) suggests that women are

socialised to avoid developing these traits and hence develop less heart disease. She also thinks that, with more women becoming employed in full-time occupations, the gender-ratio differences will decrease, although there is no evidence at the moment to suggest that Type A women will contract heart disease at the same rate as Type A men.

Work environment

Davidson & Cooper (1980) reviewed the research in this area and put forward a model relating Type A behaviour to the work environment which emphasised the following five factors:

The susceptible Type A individual

Research in this area has found that time urgency decreases with age; stress itself at work does not necessarily lead to increased Type A behaviour; more Type A behaviour is associated with higher occupational status, and there is a tendency for women who work to be Type A.

The work environment

There is a relationship between work load and anxiety in Type A individuals; Type A people tend to be dissatisfied with subordinates, feel misunderstood by managers and like to work alone when under pressure; Type A people are not necessarily satisfied with their job although they are very involved in their work; Type A individuals select jobs that involve exposure to a lot of stress.

Control conflict

Type A workers need to feel more in control than Type B workers. When challenged by a system already well structured and organised, the Type A individual will experience frustration in the form of control conflict and seek to reduce the influence of external control.

Chesney et al (1981) proposed that an extremely controlled environment would present a threat to the Type A manager, who if placed in such an environment, would experience more control conflict than in a work environment that he could control.

Maladaptive coping behaviours

The temporal perception of Type A individuals is often distorted. They tend to underestimate the time needed to complete a task and thus put themselves under pressure. Disproportionate emphasis on time-urgency can lead to hostility towards the Type A person, particularly if the people involved are Type A individuals. Type As suppress symptoms of such things as feelings of tiredness, which is one example of maladaptive coping behaviour.

Symptoms

The symptoms include coronary heart disease, high cholesterol levels, hypertension, smoking, lack of exercise and poor family relations.

The advantage of the model proposed by Davidson & Cooper (1980) is that it provides a useful framework for an analysis of Type A behaviour and the work environment, which is the prime context for such behaviour. Control conflict can also be a particular problem for Type A individuals who have become unemployed. They may be faced with living in a home environment where they have little control, and attempts to exert influence on the family circumstances may be met with considerable role confusion as well as conflict. The factors discussed by Davidson & Cooper (1980) also apply in many instances to the unemployed individual facing long periods of time in new, and sometimes alien, circumstances.

Changing Type A behaviour

There have been numerous attempts at changing or modifying Type A behaviour. The main difficulty for prospective intervention programmes concerns the degree of change. Is it necessary to change all Type A behaviour or just those elements that have been associated with coronary heart disease? The problem with programmes designed to change all Type A behaviour is that certain components of the behaviour pattern may be necessary for career advancement. With this caution in mind, let us examine some of the approaches that have attempted to change Type A behaviour.

In order to reach as many 'at risk' individuals as possible, the media have been engaged to transmit knowledge about the relationship between Type A behaviour and heart disease. Brody (1980), in the New York Times, published details of how some relatively simple changes in one's lifestyle could make a significant difference in health risks. Tips for the Type A individual were:

- Evaluate yourself. 'What is really important in my life?'
- Don't turn your life into a numbers game. 'How important is it to count my accomplishments?'
- Forget about being a superperson. 'Do I have to be best at everything?'
- Spend some time alone. 'Do I have to be busy every minute?'
- Take time for relaxation. 'Can't I find time each week to go to the cinema or read a book?'
- Forget about constantly hurrying. 'Do I have to look at my watch all the time?'
- Overcome your feelings of hostility. 'Is this thing worth getting mad about?'

Merely providing people with information about how they might change is no guarantee that they will do so. However, Maccoby & Alexander (1979) claim that media programmes can be effective in changing behaviour. They compared providing information via the mass media and providing information via the mass media plus face-to-face intervention. They claim to have achieved substantial changes in behaviour sufficient to achieve substantial reductions in cardiovascular risk in communities as a whole. The mass media alone were slower to achieve comparable results than were the mass media plus face-to-face intervention. However, at the end of 2 years, they were equally effective.

Suinn (1974, 1980) has developed a cardiac stress management programme. It consists of two phases. Firstly the individual is taught to reduce his exposure to stress-eliciting situations associated with deadlines, rapid-paced activities, and competitive activities. This need not result in a loss of productivity, if activities are re-scheduled appropriately. The second phase is concerned with reducing the anxiety engendered by the discontinuation of habitual, rapid-paced activities. This may be achieved using relaxation training techniques to reduce anxiety and the stress response.

There has been a great deal of interest in the use of beta-adrenergic blocking drugs (beta blockers) such as propranolol to control Type A behaviour. Schneider et al (1984) tested the effect of beta blockers on Type A behaviour and cardiovascular reactivity. The patients treated with beta blockers showed significant changes in Type A speech characteristics, lower blood pressure and reduced heart rate.

Another approach emphasises the potential benefits of physical fitness in the prevention of coronary heart disease. Blumenthal et al (1980) assessed Type A and Type B individuals on physiological and psychological variables related to CHD, before and after a 10-week exercise programme. They found that, in comparison to Type B subjects, Type A subjects were able successfully to reduce the physiological cardiovascular risk factors, in addition to lowering their scores on the Jenkins Activity Survey.

Roskies (1989) has developed a multimodal treatment approach to modifying Type A behaviour that utilises a combination of techniques. Progressive muscular relaxation is used to reduce tension and also to train individuals to monitor tension as well. Second, rational emotive therapy is presented to practise control of negative emotions such as anger, anxiety, guilt, and depression. Both these techniques can produce an immediate increase in a sense of well-being. Third, communication skills training helps individuals send and receive messages that are clear and better formulated. Also there is an emphasis on directing one's attention to the problem rather than the individual. Fourth, problem-solving skills are provided to enable individuals to treat each situation independently and investigate all possible solutions, appraising the positive and negative benefits of each course of action. Finally, stress inoculation is used to increase awareness of the physical and cognitive cues of stress. Following a 14-week course of treatment using this approach, Type A individuals showed significant reduction in blood pressure, cholesterol, time pressure and a number of psychological symptoms. Niven & Johnson (1989) reviewed studies on stress management techniques and concluded that the most successful programmes included cognitive, behavioural and emotional components and were introduced to clients over a suitably long period of time. Also, those that had realistic goals in terms of behaviour change were the ones most likely to succeed.

Finally, Friedman et al (1984) compared two counselling programmes for modifying Type A behaviour in postmyocardial-infarct patients. Cardiac counselling consisted of 24, 90-minute sessions that occurred over a period of 3 years. During this time patients were given information on:

- the mode of development of myocardial infarction
- how to modify standard coronary risk factors like hypertension and smoking—it did not include information on Type A behaviour
- recent advances in the surgical and drug management of coronary heart disease
- the avoidance of daily activities known to precipitate cardiac events.

The behavioural counselling was given in addition to the cardiac counselling and consisted of sessions designed to:

- teach patients how to identify instances of the Type A behaviour pattern
- recognise excessive responses to stressful situations and develop mastery over these responses
- discuss patients' beliefs about themselves, attitudes to others and their beliefs about life in general: if necessary, implement cognitive restructuring.

The results indicated that those patients who received behavioural counselling in addition to cardiac counselling showed a significant reduction in Type A behaviour (43.8% of the 592 patients). Of this sample, 17.6% showed marked reductions in Type A behaviour as compared to 7.2% of the group that received cardiac counselling alone.

These diverse approaches represent a positive attempt to modify Type A behaviour. However, Western society generally admires and rewards this sort of behaviour to the extent that certain features of Type A behaviour are actively sought in individuals who desire high-status employment. If, as Suinn (1980) suggests, the maintaining factors of Type A behaviour are primarily cultural in origin, it is important to strike some compromise between reducing the incidence of Type A behaviour and continuing to maintain cultural values that emphasise high levels of productivity.

Other areas such as diabetes have significant psychological components and are just as important as CHD. Unfortunately there is not room to discuss them in sufficient detail to do them justice. However, the interested reader is referred to Surwit et al (1983) for a review of the relationship between diabetes, behaviour and health psychology.

ILLNESS PERCEPTION

A number of years ago a textile mill in the United States was closed because a large number of workers all fell ill at the same time with a mysterious disease, which was said to have been caused by a 'June bug' because of the month when it happened. The bug was said to have been infesting the materials with which the employees worked. However, on close examination, nobody could find any evidence of exactly what was causing this mysterious disease.

Could the answer to the 'June bug' be psychological? Some researchers have estimated that 30% of the complaints seen by doctors in general practice have a psychological origin (Bakal 1979). Psychological factors not only produce illness symptoms, they can also take them away. Many people have experienced the situation where they felt ill and decided to go to see a doctor, only to arrive at the doctor's surgery feeling remarkably better. All the symptoms that originally convinced them to go to the doctor have disappeared. What would you do under these circumstances? You might decide to press on and in response to the physician's opening remarks, say something like, 'I hope I'm not bothering you for nothing doctor . . . .' Or you might decide to pretend that you still have the symptoms that brought you there in the first place. Either way, you are in a most embarrassing position, wishing for once that you possessed the symptoms that brought you to the doctor in the first place.

Lynch et al (1974) cite the case of a woman who had an intermittent AV block (the heart misses one ventricular beat for every two atrial beats). This totally disappeared whilst a nurse was taking her pulse, and reappeared as soon as the nurse had left the coronary care unit. Clearly, psychological factors play a significant role in the way we experience and perceive illness symptoms.

In the past, the traditional view of illness was that it was either psychosomatic, a conversion reaction, or an organic disorder.

Psychosomatic disorders

Lachman (1972) defines psychosomatic disorders as 'physiological dysfunctions and structural aberrations that result primarily from psychological processes rather than from immediate physical agents like those involved in the organic disorders.' Note that organic changes do take place; the symptoms are real. For instance the belief that bronchial asthma triggered by psychological factors is in some way not real asthma has been found among both relatives and doctors of patients suffering from this disorder. The belief that 'it is all in the mind' is a common explanation of a disorder where there is no known organic basis. This leads to a feeling that psychological variables are not quite as significant as physical variables when it comes

to understanding the causes of illness. The problem with the concept of psychosomatic illness is that it presupposes that some illnesses have a psychological cause and some have a physical cause. In fact the majority of illnesses have both psychological and physical causes. Thus the term 'psychosomatic' is not particularly useful in describing the causes of illness.

Conversion reaction disorders

These are sometimes referred to as hysterical disorders and usually result in the person experiencing the loss or alteration of a sensory or motor function. An arm, or a leg, may suddenly become paralysed; hearing or vision may suddenly be lost; and the individual is usually unaware of how it happened. Conversion reaction disorders often occur during times of intense strain and stress. As the term 'conversion' implies, it refers to an unconscious process whereby some unacceptable impulse is converted into bodily sensation or feeling. In the case of one person who suddenly went blind for no apparent reason, a psychiatrist thought her blindness represented an unconscious desire to be free from her mother's continual scrutiny.

Two factors were thought to distinguish between psychosomatic and conversion reaction disorders:

- Conversion reaction disorders were assumed to involve only sensory and motor systems, whereas psychosomatic disorders were assumed to involve only the autonomic nervous system.
- Motivational factors, considered central to conversion reaction, were thought unimportant in psychosomatic disorders.

However, recent research has provided evidence that nausea, fainting and vomiting, symptoms mediated by the autonomic nervous system, have been observed in conversion reaction disorders. Further, motivational variables are not always present in conversion reaction disorders nor are they necessarily absent in psychosomatic disorders (Nemiah 1975).

Organic disorders

There are problems defining an organic disorder. Some researchers believe that the term refers to pathological agents such as parasites and toxic substances; others include asthma and hypertension in their list. Despite the problems of definition, it was thought that psychological factors played no part in organic disorders. This is not the case. Most disorders are susceptible to psychological influences, even cancer may be influenced by psychological variables.

There is little evidence to support the continued use of the terms psychosomatic, conversion reaction and organic as labels for the causes of specific illnesses. Illness is determined by an interaction of environmental, psychological and physiological factors and it is the nature of this interaction that will provide information concerning the aetiology of numerous illnesses.

Illness behaviour

Mechanic (1978), a sociologist, concluded that illness could be thought of in two ways: illness can refer to 'a limited scientific concept or to any condition that causes or might usefully cause an individual to concern himself with his symptoms and to seek help.' He concentrated on how cultural influences and social learning directly affect the illness behaviour an individual will engage in. From a psychological point of view, one major drawback to his approach is the way he uses the term symptom. For Mechanic, symptom refers to some organic dysfunction. However, many individuals react with illness behaviour when there is no sign of any organic malfunction. The perception of illness where there is no obvious organic cause has been termed *abnormal illness behaviour*.

Pilowsky (1978) developed a useful questionnaire that distinguished between various patterns or styles of abnormal illness behaviour. The Illness Behaviour Questionnaire (IBQ) was developed over a 2-year period and was based on a sample of 100 chronic pain patients. The subjects were an average age of 49.1 years, the pain was experienced for an average of 7.4 years, and all

the subjects had not responded to medical treatment. On the basis of their scores, the following clusters were observed:

- *General hypochondriasis.* Patients have a general anxiety about their health and a distinct fear of contracting disease.
- *Disease conviction.* There is a conviction that disease is present rather than a fear of contracting it. Patients reject medical advice and are abnormally preoccupied with their bodily functions.
- *Psychological perception of illness.* Patients are willing to attribute the cause of their disorder to psychological factors or their own behaviour.
- *Affective inhibition.* A reluctance to express negative emotions, such as anger, to other individuals.
- *Affective disturbance.* Patients are anxious and depressed (dysphoric).
- *Denial of problems.* Patients tend to deny any financial or family problems and think that their illness is the only difficulty in their lives.
- *Irritability.* There is a tendency to be quick to anger, which often places a strain on interpersonal relationships.

Pilowsky (1978) cluster analysed the scale profiles of the 100 patients and was able to classify six types of patients, three were adaptive forms of illness behaviour and three were maladaptive forms of illness behaviour.

Adaptive

- Capacity for using denial adaptively.
- Use of denial, but less effective in employing strategy.
- Irritability and interpersonal friction with denial of problems other than physical health.

Maladaptive

- Somatic preoccupation and rejection of reassurance.
- High disease conviction and many life problems.
- Anxious hypochondriacal concern with health.

The questionnaire provides a useful classification of abnormal illness behaviour, but does not make any predictions about how illnesses are likely to be perceived by different individuals.

Symptom perception

It was suggested at the beginning of this section that a psychological explanation of the 'June bug' could provide a solution to the mystery. This must be distinguished from a psychoanalytical explanation. Psychoanalysts label 'June bug' behaviour mass hysteria or hysterical contagion, and describe it as a conversion reaction, that is, people's unexpressed stresses are converted into physical symptoms. A less descriptive analysis of the behaviour is provided by Pennebaker (1982) and Colligan et al (1982).

All the employees at the mill were suffering from high levels of psychological and physical stress because it was the height of the production season. This stress manifested itself in a variety of unpleasant bodily sensations. With the collapse of the first few workers, the remaining employees searched for a reason to explain what was happening. They formed an illness hypothesis linked to presumed insect infestation. Their stress-related bodily sensations now had a legitimate interpretation—the June bug virus. This interpretation was reinforced by rumours passed from one person to the next and the vivid evidence of workers collapsing everywhere. This condition is known as Mass Psychogenic Illness (MPI) and is caused by individuals misperceiving illness cues.

Pennebaker (1984) says that the most fundamental assumption concerning symptom perception is that 'the perceptual processes that have traditionally been invoked in dealing with the perception of external environmental stimuli represent the same perceptual processes that are involved in the perception of internal sensory information'. This means that one is able to use the recent research into cognition, perception and information processing for understanding the perception of internal symptoms of illness. There are two main issues of special interest. The first concerns why we attend to certain

feelings and not to others. The second concerns how individuals organise and selectively search for information about their physical condition.

The stimuli that impinge on our senses can be said to come from two sources. There is information about our external environment and information about our internal environment. External environmental and internal sensory information compete for our attention. When the external environment is lacking in information, there is an increased probability that we will notice internal sensory information. Similarly, when our attention is taken up by a great deal of external information, we take less notice of our internal sensations. Thus, people are far more likely to report a variety of physical symptoms and sensations when the external environment is boring or lacking in information, than when they must pay particular attention to the environment. Pennebaker (1984) presents evidence that people are more likely to notice itching or tickling in their throats when the external environment is dull. They also state that people emit more coughs during boring parts of films. People who think that their job is boring or who live alone report more physical symptoms, take more aspirin and sleeping pills, report more days of little activity due to poor health than do people with interesting jobs or who live with one or two others. On the other hand, many of us have been in a situation where we have ceased to notice, say, the pain of a toothache because we have become totally involved in concentrating on a particular task. A person is most likely to notice subtle sensations and symptoms when the environment is lacking in information, and less likely to notice sensations when the perceptual system is overloaded with external information.

A second aspect of the perceptual process concerns the way in which people develop hypotheses about what is wrong with them, then pay attention to those sensations that support this hypothesis and neglect those sensations that do. The sort of hypotheses generated are determined by our general outlook on life or more specifically our cognitive perspective. This perspective is built up from a number of 'schemes' and only those sensations or symptoms that 'fit' these schemes will be attended to by the individual. There are large individual differences in the sorts of perspectives people have about illness, which leads to different people interpreting the same symptoms in totally different ways.

A useful analogy is the story about the man on a bridge peering over the side, looking at the water below. There are a number of people viewing this scene. The artist sees it as a set of colours and textures, the insurance salesman sees it as a bad risk, the physicist sees it as the force of the man acting against the force of the bridge and the policeman sees it as a potential suicide case. The perceptual stimuli are the same, but interpreted in different ways by people with different cognitive perspectives.

An experiment by Anderson & Pennebaker (1980) illustrated the role of 'selective schemata' in the perception of pain and pleasure. Subjects were asked to place their middle fingers on a vibrating emery board for 1 second. Prior to the experiment the subjects were required to sign a consent form. They were divided into three groups. The first group were given a consent form with the following statement on it: 'I understand that I will come into contact with a stimulus which has been found to produce a degree of pain' (pain group). The second group had exactly the same statement on the form, but the word 'pleasure' was substituted for the word 'pain' (pleasure group). The third group were not presented with a statement about pain or pleasure (control). Thus the experimental groups were presented with different schema for interpreting the same stimulus.

After touching the emery board, they had to rate the stimulus on a 13-point pain–pleasure scale. Minus scores indicated that the stimulus was painful. There were significant differences between the responses of all three groups. Pain group produced a mean rating of –1.00; the pleasure group +1.01; and the control group +0.13. Interviews with the subjects revealed that the pain subjects did not believe the stimulus could have felt pleasurable, and the pleasure subjects did not believe it could have hurt. In this particular instance, the individuals are

presented with a cognitive framework before they experience the sensations.

Often sensations occur in the absence of any immediate interpretive framework. Schacter & Singer (1962) injected subjects with adrenaline that caused certain physiological responses such as mild hand tremor, increased heart rate and a flushed feeling in the face. When some subjects were told that the injections would have these effects, there was no problem. Other subjects did not receive that information and had to work out for themselves what was going on. The experimenters manipulated these interpretations by having a confederate behave in a hostile, angry manner or in a happy, silly fashion. Subjects used these cues supplied by the confederate to interpret their own feelings. Those with an angry confederate decided they were angry themselves, while those with a happy confederate reported that they were very happy. Those who had been told that the reactions had been caused by the injections were not influenced by the confederate at all. Schacter & Singer (1962) concluded that we can easily misinterpret what we feel and thus look for information from the external environment to help us interpret our feelings.

A further illustration of the role of cognitive factors in the perception of symptoms is provided by Ruble (1977). 44 women were selected because they menstruated on the same day. They underwent a simulated electroencephalographic (EEG) examination which supposedly identified a woman's location in the menstrual cycle with a high degree of accuracy. A third of the subjects were informed that they were within 1–2 days of beginning menstruation (premenstrual group), another third were told not to expect the onset of menstruation for 7–10 days (intermenstrual group) and a final third received no information whatsoever. None of the groups actually differed in the day of menstruation onset. Subjects completed a questionnaire on the physical, psychological and behavioural symptoms associated with menstruation. Women in the premenstrual group rated themselves as experiencing more water retention, pain, changes in their eating habits and different levels of sexual arousal than women who believed themselves to be intermenstrual. Ruble (1977) did not deny the physiological components of menstrual complaints, but argued that an individual's beliefs concerning the association between cycle location and symptoms must also be taken into consideration.

There is a wealth of research illustrating the difficulty people have in interpreting their feelings. Dutton & Aron (1974) showed that fearful emotions can often be misperceived as attraction. We have seen in the experiment carried out by Anderson & Pennebaker (1980) that individuals can interpret a stimulus as either painful or pleasurable according to their cognitive perspective. Some might argue that the stimulus was not particularly strong and therefore open to misinterpretation. However, one might think that the feelings of fear and physical attraction are quite distinct.

Dutton & Aron (1974) tested the prediction that fearful feelings can be misperceived as attraction. The subjects were males who were interviewed when they were walking across either of two bridges in Vancouver. One of the bridges was a narrow suspension bridge that tilts, sways and wobbles 230 feet above a rocky canyon. Walking across this bridge was assumed to be an arousing situation. The other 'non-arousing' bridge was a solid, wide one that was only 10 feet above a shallow river. Either a male or a female interviewer approached each subject, asked a few questions, requested the subject to write a brief story in response to a picture and left the subject a phone number to call later if there were any questions. It was found that there were sexual references in the stories written by subjects who were on the arousing bridge with a female interviewer. Subjects on the same bridge with a male interviewer did not write sexy stories. Nor did those on the safe bridge, regardless of the interviewer's sex. More impressive, perhaps, was the fact that later telephone calls showed exactly the same pattern. The most telephone calls by the male subjects were to a female interviewer who had interviewed them on the frightening bridge.

An experiment by Valins & Ray (1967), report-ed earlier, illustrates a similar point. They showed snake-phobic individuals a series of slides of snakes and other anxiety-arousing stimuli. The subjects were led to believe that they were hearing their own heartbeats while viewing the slides. In fact, they heard heartbeats manipulated by the experimenters so that the subjects' heart rate increased when shown the anxiety-arousing slides, and decreased for the snake slides. This false feedback of autonomic functioning resulted in the snake-phobic subjects approaching real snakes more closely than did snake-phobic subjects who viewed the same series of slides while listening to the same sounds, but believed them to be meaningless. Such results were interpreted as providing support for the hypothesis that an individual's beliefs concerning the state of her internal environment, irrespective of actual state, are the primary determinants of emotional responses. These findings have particular relevance to the study of hypochondriasis.

Hypochondriasis

Barsky & Kierman (1983) define hypochondriasis as 'an unrealistic interpretation of one's bodily sensations as abnormal, leading to the fear and belief that one has a serious disease'. One explanation of the disorder emphasises the role of perceptual and cognitive processes. Barsky & Klerman (1983) suggest three possible mechanisms responsible for the disorder:

• Patients amplify and augment normal bodily sensations. A group of students who scored high on a hypochondriasis scale tended to report heightened arousal and heightened perceptual sensitivity to bodily sensations.

• Patients misinterpret bodily symptoms of emotional arousal and normal bodily function. Normal bodily sensations such as indigestion, increased heart rate and stomach flutter are misinterpreted as representing serious disease. The misattribution can increase emotional arousal, which, in turn, exacerbates the symptoms and continues the cycle.

• The constitutional predisposition to thinking and perceiving in physical and concrete terms, sets the stage for symptom preoccupation. This abnormality in awareness of emotion, observed in patients with classic psychosomatic disorders, is alexithymia. The innate nature of this disorder is, however, unsubstantiated.

A *perceptual* defect is the primary underlying disorder, not the illness behaviour itself. Therefore an appropriate treatment programme has to be based on helping the patient to identify the perceptual defect and irrational thoughts. Cognitive therapies such as rational emotive therapy (RET) and cognitive behaviour therapies such as stress inoculation training are ideally suited to confront this sort of problem.

Rational emotive therapy states that irrational thoughts or beliefs are empirically false or cannot be empirically verified. Thus when patients are confronted with tests and challenges of their irrational beliefs in therapy sessions, their self-defeating thoughts are changed.

Stress inoculation training has been particularly effective in the management of pain experiences. Typically, a patient would initially be given information to enhance his or her understanding of the pain and the stressors that accompany it. The patient would then be trained in a variety of coping strategies, such as relaxation, distraction and imagery techniques. Finally, the patient would be asked to rehearse these strategies while conceptualising the pain and stress at each phase of the pain experience.

CONCLUSION

On the one hand, a large number of people either interpret potentially dangerous symptoms as benign or actively try to suppress or distract themselves from these symptoms. Clearly health education has a significant role to play in setting up programmes to try to reduce the incidences of this sort of thinking.

A different kind of problem exists for the person who is prone to interpret benign sensations in illness-related ways. The hypochondriac is a persistent problem for health care professionals. Doctors, for instance, are likely to refer such patients to someone else or simply tell them that nothing is wrong. But first it must be realised that these patients honestly believe that they are sick. They have adopted a hypothesis about certain physical sensations. Further, the hypothesis is probably confirmed in that there are certain sensations that are present that substantiate the patient's interpretation. Rather than dismissing the patient as crazy, the health professional must provide alternative explanations for the sensations and adopt the psychological perspective espoused by the therapies mentioned above. When a health professional is confronted by a patient who says 'I hope I'm not wasting your time but ...' the appropriate reply ought to be 'I hope that you are.'

REFERENCES

Abramson L Y, Seligman M E P, Teasdale J D 1978 Learned helplessness in humans: critique and reformulation. Journal of Abnormal Psychology 87: 49–74

Ajzen I 1985 From intention to actions: a theory of planned behaviour. In: Kuhl J, Beckmann J (eds) Action-control: from cognition to behaviour. Springer, Heidelberg

Ajzen I, Fishbein M 1980 Understanding attitudes and predicting social behaviour. Prentice-Hall, Englewood Cliffs NJ

Ajzen I, Madden T J 1986 Prediction of goal directed behaviour: attitudes, intentions and perceived behavioural control. Journal of Experimental Social Psychology 22: 453–474

Anderson I L 1986 Patients' recall and satisfaction in an

outpatients clinic in Hong Kong. Paper presented to 'The doctor, the patient, the illness conference.' University of Durham

Anderson D B, Pennebaker J W 1980 Pain and pleasure: alternative interpretations of identical stimulation. European Journal of Social Psychology 10: 207–212

Andreason N C 1982 Concepts, diagnosis, and classification. In: Paykel E S (ed) Handbook of affective disorders. Churchill Livingstone, Edinburgh

Baekeland F, Lundwall L 1975 Dropping out of treatment: a critical review. Psychological Bulletin 82: 738–783

Bakal D A 1979 Psychology and medicine. Tavistock, London

Bandura A 1986 Social foundations of thought and action: a social cognitive theory. Prentice-Hall, New Jersey

Bandura A 1989 Perceived self-efficacy in the exercise of personal agency. The Psychologist 10: 411–424

Barsky A J, Klerman C L 1983 Overview: hypochondriasis, bodily complaints, and somatic styles. American Journal of Psychiatry 140: 273–283

Beck A T 1967 Depression: clinical experiments and theoretical analysis. Hoeber, New York

Beck A T 1976 Cognitive therapy and emotional disorder. International Universities Press, New York

Beck A T 1989 Cognitive therapy and the emotional disorders. Penguin, Harmondsworth

Becker J 1974 Depression: theory and research. Wiley, London

Becker M H, Maiman L A 1975 Sociobehavioural determinants of compliance with health and medical care recommendations. Medical Care 13: 10–24

Becker M H, Haefner D P, Kasl S V, Kirscht J P, Maiman L A, Rosenstock I M 1977 Selected psychosocial models and correlates of individual health-related behaviours. Medical Care 15: 27–46

Becker M H, Maiman L A, Kirscht J P, Haefner D P, Drachman R H, Taylor D W 1979 Patient perceptions and compliance: recent studies of the health belief model. In: Haynes R B, Taylor D W, Sackett D L (eds) Compliance in health care. Johns Hopkins University Press, Baltimore

Blumenthal J A, Williams R S, Williams R B, Wallace A G 1980 Effects of exercise on the Type A (coronary prone) behaviour pattern. Psychosomatic Medicine 42: 289–296

Blumenthal J A, Sanders W, Wallace A G, Williams R B, Needles T L 1982 Physiological and psychological variables predicting compliance to prescribed exercise therapy in patients recovering from myocardial infarction. Psychosomatic Medicine 44: 519–527

Brody J E 1980 Rushing your life away with Type A behaviour. New York Times, Oct 22

Burnham M A, Pennebaker J W, Glass B C 1975 Time consciousness, achievement striving, and the Type A coronary prone behaviour pattern. Journal of Abnormal Psychology 84: 76–79

Chesney M A, Eagleston J R, Rosenman R H 1981 Type A behaviour: assessment and intervention. In: Prokop C K, Bradley L A (eds) Medical psychology: contributions to behavioural medicine. Academic Press, New York

Cluss P A, Epstein L H 1984 A riboflavin tracer method for assessment of medication compliance in children. Behaviour Research Methods Instruments and Computers 16(5): 444–446

Colligan M J, Pennebaker J W, Murphy L 1982 (eds) Mass psychogenic illness: a social psychological analysis. Erlbaum, Hillsdale NJ

Davidson M J, Cooper C L 1980 Coronary-prone behaviour in the work environment. Journal of Occupational Medicine 22: 375–383

Depue R A, Munroe S M 1978 The unipolar–bipolar distinction in the depression disorders. Psychological Bulletin 85: 1001–1009

DeVellis R F, DeVellis B M, Wallston B S, Wallston K A 1980 Epilepsy and learned helplessness. Basic and Applied Social Psychology 1: 241–253

DiNicola D D, DiMatteo M R 1982 Communication, interpersonal influence, and resistance to medical treatment. In: Willis T A (ed) Basic processes in helping relationships. Academic Press, New York

DiNicola D D, DiMatteo M R 1984 Practitioners, patients, and compliance with medical regimens: a social

psychological perspective. In: Baum A, Taylor S E, Singer J E (eds) Handbook of psychology and health. Erlbaum, Hillsdale NJ

Dunbar J M, Stunkard A J 1979 Adherence to diet and drug regimens. In: Levy R, Rifkind B, Dennis B, Ernst N (eds) Nutrition: lipids and coronary heart disease. Raven Press, New York

Dutton D G, Aron A P 1974 Some evidence for heightened sexual attraction under conditions of high anxiety. Journal of Personality and Social Psychology 30: 510–517

Ellis A 1980 Rational-emotive therapy and cognitive behaviour therapy: similarities and differences. Cognitive Therapy and Research 4: 325–340

Endler N S 1982 Holiday of darkness: a psychologist's personal journey out of his depression. Wiley, New York

Feuerstein M, Labbé E E, Kuczmierczyk A R 1986 Health psychology. Plenum Press, New York

Fishbein M 1982 Social psychological analysis of smoking behaviour. In: Eiser J R (ed) Social psychology and behavioral medicine. Wiley, Chichester

Friedman M, Rosenman R H 1959 Association of specific overt behaviour pattern with blood and cardiovascular findings: blood cholesterol level, blood clotting time, incidence of arcus senilis and clinical coronary artery disease. Journal of the American Medical Association 169: 1286–1296

Friedman M, Rosenman R H 1974 Type A behaviour and your heart. Fawcett Books, New York

Friedman M, Thorensen C E, Gill J J et al 1984 Alteration of Type A behaviour and reduction in cardiac recurrences in postmyocardial infarction patients. American Heart Journal 108: 237–248

Gibbs M, Lachenmeyer H, Sigal N 1977 (eds) Community psychology. Gardner Press, New York

Glass D C 1977 Behaviour patterns, stress, and heart disease. Erlbaum, Hillsdale NJ

Glidewell J C 1983 Afterword: prevention—the threat and the promise. In: Felner R D, Jason A J, Moritsugu J N, Farber S S (eds) Preventive psychology. Pergamon, New York

Gordis L 1979 Conceptual and methodologic problems in measuring patient compliance. In: Haynes R B, Taylor D W, Sackett D L (eds) Compliance in health care. Johns Hopkins University Press, Baltimore

Haefner D P 1974 The health belief model and preventive dental behaviours. Health Education Monographs 2: 420–432

Hartman P E, Becker M H 1978 Noncompliance with prescribed regimen among chronic hemodialysis patients: a method of prediction and educational diagnosis. Dialysis and Transplantation 7: 979–985

Haynes S G, Levine S, Scotch N et al 1978 The relationship of psychosocial factors to coronary heart disease in the Framingham study. 1. Methods and risk factors. American Journal of Epidemiology 107: 362–383

Haynes R B, Taylor D W, Sackett D L 1979 Compliance in health care. Johns Hopkins University Press, Baltimore

Herbst K R, Paykel E S 1989 Depression: an integrative approach. Heineman Medical, Oxford

Janis I L 1984 The patient as decision maker. In: Gentry W D (ed) Handbook of behavioral medicine. Guilford, New York

Janis I L, Mann L 1977 Decision making: a psychological analysis of conflict, choice, and commitment. Free Press, New York

Janis I L Rodin J 1979 Attribution, control, and decision making: social psychology of health care. In: Stone G C, Cohen F, Adler N E (eds) Health psychology. Jossey Bass, New York

Jenkins C D 1971 Psychologic and social precursors of coronary disease. New England Journal of Medicine 284: 244–255, 307–317

Jenkins C D, Zyzenski S J, Rosenman R H 1971 Progress toward a validation of a computer-scored test for the for the Type A coronary-prone behaviour pattern. Psychosomatic Medicine 33: 193–202

Kasl S V 1975 Issues in patient adherence to health care regimens. Journal of Human Stress 1: 5–17

Kasl S V, Cobb S 1966 Health behaviour, illness behaviour, and sick role, behaviour. Archives of Environmental Health 12: 246–266, 531–541

Keys A, Aravanis C, Blackburn H et al 1972 Probability of middle-age men developing coronary heart disease in five years. Circulation 45: 815–818

Korsch B M, Negrete V F 1972 Doctor–patient communication. Scientific American 227: 66–74

Lachman S J 1972 Psychosomatic disorders: a behaviouristic interpretation. Wiley, London

Lefcourt H M 1982 Locus of control: current trends in theory and research. Erlbaum, Hillsdale NJ

Levenson H 1973 Multidimensional locus of control in psychiatric patients. Journal of Consulting and Clinical Psychology 41: 397–404

Leventhal H, Meyer D, Nerenz D 1980 The common-sense representation of illness-danger. In: Rachman S (ed) Medical psychology. Pergamon Press, Oxford, vol 2

Lewin K 1951 Field theory in social science. Harper, New York

Ley P 1972 Primacy, rated importance, and recall of medical information. Journal of Health and Social Behaviour 13: 311–317

Ley P 1977 Psychological studies of doctor–patient communication. In: Rachman S (ed) Contributions to medical psychology. Pergamon, Oxford

Ley P 1988 Communicating with patients: improving communication, satisfaction and compliance. Croom Helm, London

Ley P, Spelman M S 1967 Communicating with the patient. Staples Press, London

Lierman L M, Young H M, Kasprzyk D, Benoliel J Q 1990 Predicting breast self-examination using the theory of reasoned action. Nursing Research 39(2): 97–101

Linn M W 1988 Psychotherapy with cancer patients. In: Goldberg R J (ed) Psychiatric aspects of cancer. Karger, Basel, vol 18

Lorenc L 1986 Doctors' knowledge of compliance related issues. Paper presented to 'The doctor, the patient, the illness' conference. University of Durham

Lynch J J, Thomas S A, Mills M E et al 1974 The effects of human contact on cardiac arrhythmia in coronary care patients. Journal of Nervous and Mental Disease 158: 88–99

Maccoby N, Alexander J 1979 Reducing heart disease risk using the mass media: comparing the effects on three communities. In: Muñoz R E, Snowden L R, Kelly J (eds) Social and psychological research in community settings. Jossey Bass, New York

Matthews K A 1982 Psychological perspectives on the Type A behaviour pattern. Psychological Bulletin 91: 293–323

Matthews K A, Siegel J M 1983 Type A behaviours by children, social comparison, and standards for self-evaluation. Developmental Psychology 19: 135–140

Mechanic D 1978 Medical sociology, 2nd edn. Macmillan, London

Meichenbaum D E 1977 Cognitive-behaviour modification: an integrative approach. Plenum Press, New York

Mendels J 1976 Lithium in the treatment of depression. American Journal of Psychiatry 133: 373–378

Miller E, Morley S 1986 Investigating abnormal behaviour. Erlbaum, Chichester

Miller W R, Seligman M E P 1975 Depression in humans. Journal of Abnormal Psychology 84: 228–238

Milner S 1994 Evaluation of a drop-in health centre. Unpublished PhD Thesis, University of Northumbria

Murphy G E, Woodruff R A, Herjanic M, Fischer J P 1974 Validity of the diagnosis of primary affective disorder: a prospective study with a fiveyear follow up. Archives of General Psychiatry 30: 751–756

Nemiah J C 1975 Hysterical neurosis, conversion type. In: Friedman A M, Kaplan H I, Sadock B J (eds) Comprehensive textbook of psychiatry. Williams & Williams, Baltimore, vol 1

Niven N, Johnson D 1989 Taking the lid off stress management. European Management Journal 17: 14–17

Oberle K 1991 A decade of research into locus of control: what have we learned. Journal of Advanced Nursing 91: 800–806

Pennebaker J W 1982 The psychology of physical symptoms. Springer, New York

Pennebaker J W 1984 Accuracy of symptom perception. In: Baum A, Taylor S E, Singer J E (eds) Handbook of psychology and health. Erlbaum, Hillsdale NJ

Perris C 1982 The distinction between bipolar and unipolar affective disorders. In: Paykel E S (ed) Handbook of affective disorders. Churchill Livingstone, Edinburgh

Peterson C, Seligman M E P 1984 Causal explanations as a risk factor for depression: theory and evidence. Psychological Review 91: 347–374

Pilowsky I 1978 A general classification of abnormal illness behaviours. British Journal of Medical Psychology 51: 131–137

Pratt L V 1976 Family structure and affective health behaviour: the energised family. Houghton-Mifflin, Boston

Rosenstock I M 1974 The health belief model and preventive health behaviour. Health Education Monographs 2: 354–386

Rosenstock I M, Kirscht J P 1979 Why people seek health care. In: Stone G C, Cohen F, Adler N E (eds) Health psychology. Jossey Bass, New York

Rosenstock I M, Strecher V J, Becker M H 1988 Social learning theory and the health belief model. Health Education Quarterly 15: 175–183

Roskies E 1989 Stress management for the healthy Type A: theory and practice. Guilford, New York

Rotter J B 1954 Social learning and clinical psychology. Prentice-Hall, Englewood Cliffs NJ

Ruble D 1977 Premenstrual symptoms: a reinterpretation. Science 197: 291–292

Russek H I, Russek L G 1976 Is emotional stress an etiological factor in coronary heart disease. Psychosomatics 17: 63–67

Sackett D L 1976 The magnitude of compliance and noncompliance. In: Sackett D L, Haynes R B (eds) Compliance with therapeutic regimens. Johns Hopkins University Press, Baltimore

Sackett D L, Snow J C 1979 The magnitude of compliance and noncompliance. In: Haynes R B, Taylor D W, Sackett D L (eds) Compliance in health care. Johns Hopkins University Press, Baltimore

Schacter S, Singer J 1962 Cognitive, social and physiological determinants of emotional state. Psychological Review 69: 379–399

Scherwitz L, Berton K, Leventhal H 1978 Type A behaviour, self-involvement, and cardiovascular response. Psychosomatic Medicine 40: 593–609

Schifter D E, Ajzen D E 1985 Intention, perceived control and weight loss: an application of the theory of planned behaviour. Journal of Personality and Social Psychology 49: 843–851

Schneider R, Friedrich G, Neus H, Rdel H, von Eiff L R 1984 The influence of beta blockers on cardiovascular reactivity and Type A behaviour pattern in hypertensives. Psychosomatic Medicine 45: 417–423

Seligman M E P 1980 Helplessness: theory and applications. In: Garber J, Seligman M E P (eds) Human helplessness. Academic Press, London

Seligman M E P, Maier S F 1967 Failure to escape traumatic shock. Journal of Experimental Psychology 74: 1–9

Smith T W, Pope M K 1990 Cynical hostility as a health risk: current status and future directions. Journal of Social Behaviour and Personality 5: 77–88

Sogaard A 1993 Theories and models of health behaviour. In: Schou L, Blinkhorn A S (eds) Oral health promotion. Oxford Medical, Oxford

Spielberger C D 1993 Type A behaviour and heart disease. The Psychologist 6: 266–267

Stainton-Rogers W 1991 Explaining health and illness: an exploration of diversity. Harvester Wheatsheaf, London

Strickland B R 1978 Internal–external expectancies and health related behaviours. Journal of Consulting and Clinical Psychology 46: 1192–1211

Suinn R M 1974 Behaviour therapy for 5 cardiac patients. Behavior Therapy 5: 569–571

Suinn R M 1980 Pattern A behaviours and heart disease: intervention approaches. In: Ferguson J M, Taylor C B (eds) The comprehensive handbook of behavioural medicine. Spectrum, Jamaica NY, vol 1

Surwit R S, Feinglos M N, Scovern A W 1983 Diabetes and behaviour: a paradigm for health psychology. American Psychologist 38: 255–262

Valins S, Ray A 1967 Effects of cognitive desensitisation on avoidance behaviour. Journal of Personality and Social Psychology 7: 345–350

Waldron I 1976 Why do women live longer than men? Journal of Human Stress 2: 2–13

Wallston B S, Wallston K A 1984 Social psychological models of health behaviour: an examination and integration. In: Baum A, Singer S E, Singer J E (eds) Handbook of psychology and health. Erlbaum, Hillsdale NJ

Weinstein N D 1988 The precaution adoption process. Health Psychology 7: 355–386

Williams J M G 1984a Cognitive-behaviour therapy for depression: problems and perspectives. British Journal of Psychiatry 145: 254–262

Williams J M G 1984b The psychological treatment of depression. Croom Helm, Beckenham

Williams J M G 1988 Cognitive psychology and emotional disorders. Wiley, Chichester

RECOMMENDED READING

Ley P 1988 Communicating with patients: improving communication, satisfaction and compliance. Croom Helm, London
Examines the link between communication and compliance in an easy to read fashion. It collates the author's research in this area over many years and examines the contribution of other major researchers in this field.

Roskies E 1987 Stress management for the healthy type A: theory and practice. Guilford Press, New York
I think this is the best book on stress management not just because it takes a multimodal perspective but because it provides a practical guide on how to set up stress management programmes that really work.

Sarafino E P 1994 Health psychology: biopsychosocial interactions 2nd edn. Wiley, New York
There are more and more books being written on health psychology these days. This one is, I think, the best because of its extensive coverage of many important health psychology issues. The biopsychosocial perspective is most useful.

Williams J M G 1988 Cognitive psychology and emotional disorders. Wiley, Chichester
This author has written a number of books in this area. This one examines the contribution cognitive psychology can make toward understanding a number of emotional disorders.

Feuerstein M, Labbé E E, Kuczmierfczyk A R 1986 Health psychology. Plenum Press, New York

Gatchel R J, Baum A 1983 An introduction to health psychology. Random House, New York

Haynes R B, Sackett D L 1976 (eds) Compliance with therapeutic regimens. Johns Hopkins University Press, Baltimore

Pennebaker J W 1982 The psychology of physical symptoms. Springer, New York

Stone G C, Cohen F, Adler N E 1979 (eds) Health psychology. Jossey Bass, New York

Models

SECTION CONTENTS

7

Developmental model

It is not proposed to provide a detailed examination of child psychology or the psychology of ageing, merely to highlight some of the differences associated with the behaviour of the young and old alike. Hence, the topics that are dealt with include the sensory acuities of the neonate, infant temperament, crying and feeding, parent–child interaction, intellectual decline and disease in old age, maternal deprivation, children's conception of health and illness, social isolation and disengagement of old age.

Thus far, it has been assumed that the individuals who are the subjects of health psychology are, for the most part, adults. However, in many circumstances health professionals deal with children and old people as their patients. The purpose of the developmental approach is to map out some changes in human development that occur during childhood and old age. The majority of changes in behaviour occur during childhood, therefore it is necessary to determine in what ways children's behaviour differs from that of adults.

The first section of the chapter investigates the extent to which the newborn child possesses the ability to make sense of the world via her sensory faculties and also looks at the degree to which sensory acuities are affected by age. The second section tries to determine whether babies are born with different temperaments and discusses the attempts to distinguish between 'difficult' and 'easy' babies.

Parent–child interaction forms an important sequence of events in the child's cognitive and emotional development. The ways that young children develop attachments to adults can affect subsequent emotional development. In many instances parents are separated for varying degrees of time from their children; therefore it is necessary to find out whether separations have any effect on the developing child. The last section about the child discusses whether children think in totally different ways from adults and examines the implications for health professionals who have frequent contact with children.

Finally, the degree to which there is intellectual decline in old age is examined; then the relationship between disease and intellectual functioning and whether old people wish to remain isolated and apart from the rest of the community are explored. The purpose of this chapter is not to provide health professionals with an exhaustive account of old age or child development, but to determine the extent to which these stages in human development represent significant departures from adult human behaviour.

THE SENSES

The very first sensation which an infant gets is for him the outer universe . . . . The Object is one big blooming buzzing Confusion. That Confusion is the baby's universe . . . .

William James (1961)

The idea that babies emerged into the world with no ability to comprehend what was going on around them did not originate with the early functional psychologists like James but with the British empiricist philosophers such as John Locke. He proposed that the mind of the neonate was a *tabula rasa* or blank slate and that what was etched on that slate would be determined by the nature of the environment that ensued. Many years later, we now know that this is in fact not the case. Neonates are born with some quite sophisticated sensory acuities that have been developing in the mother's uterus for a number of months.

Vision

At birth, the eye of the neonate is about half the size of an adult's eye, and will not reach full size until the infant is 12–14 years old (Smart &

Smart 1982). However, the eyes of the newborn infant are anatomically complete and have been so since the 7th month after conception. The neonate is capable of avoiding bright lights and the pupillary reflex is functional, which means that the amount of light getting into the eye can be controlled. The optic tract that transmits messages from the eye to the brain is partially myelinated, indicating that the speed and efficiency of the conduction of impulses is not as efficient as in adults, but nevertheless operational (Bremner 1988).

The shape of the neonate's eye is also different from that of an adult. Due to the lens, cornea and retina maturing faster than the iris and the ciliary muscles, the eyeball is less rounded than normal and takes on a 'squashed' appearance known as a *short eyeball*. This leads to a shortening of the distance between lens and retina causing some distortion of the visual image.

The inability of the ciliary muscles to operate efficiently also affects the visual image. Because these muscles are unable to manipulate the lens correctly, the neonate is unable to focus correctly. This leads to an optimum focal point of approximately 20 centimetres or 8 inches, so that anything presented to the newborn infant outside this range will appear relatively blurred (Haynes et al 1965). Thus placing mobiles and other crib toys too far away will not stimulate the child very much because they will appear blurred.

Infant visual acuity, or how well the infant can see, is estimated to be about 20/150. This means that an infant can see an object at 20 feet as well as an average adult can see the object at 150 feet and is thus far-sighted (has difficulty focusing on close up objects). By the age of 2 years, the visual acuity has improved to 20/100; at age 4, it is 20/40 and at the age of 6 or 7, it has reached 20/20. (The system for measuring eyesight is different in the United Kingdom.) The ability to track a moving object is inefficient at birth, but improves rapidly and at the age of 3 months is the same as in an adult (Dayton et al 1964).

The visual system of the neonate is far from inactive at birth. Therefore it is important that health professionals realise the need for reasonable levels of stimulation. Sensory and perceptual deprivation can occur in newborn babies as well as adults. In the previous chapter we saw the consequences of deprivation for adults; at least they are able to alter their circumstances to gain access to reasonable levels of stimulation. The neonate is not capable of doing this and is thus dependent on adults for 'upholstering' his visual environment. Care must be taken not to overload the system, but there is a need for the provision of stimulation very soon after birth, and therefore it is important for health professionals dealing with newborn babies to take this into consideration.

The visual system continues to change as the individual grows older, the most significant changes occurring after the age of 50 years. The lens becomes increasingly dense and develops a yellow tinge. The ciliary muscles lose their efficiency and decrease in size. Finally there is a decrease in pupil size and the retina becomes less sensitive. Not surprisingly these changes result in a loss of visual acuity. For instance, the closest point at which the eye can see an object without blurring gets farther and farther away, necessitating the use of spectacles when this 'near point' is beyond the distance at which one would hold a book or newspaper (Fozard 1990). Another feature of ageing is the development of cataracts, where the lens becomes cloudy. Approximately 90% of cataract sufferers may be described as elderly. This does not mean that getting cataracts is a necessary consequence of ageing, for only about 10% of people in their 60s, 20% of people in their 70s and a third of people in their 80s, develop cataracts (Paton & Craig 1974).

Taken together, all the structural age changes in the human visual system conspire to impair visual functioning gradually, and the impairment is particularly noticeable in the elderly. The deterioration in the functioning of the visual system with age should be a major consideration of all concerned with care of the elderly. For instance, people with poor vision can have great difficulty finding their way around the hospital, both inside and out. They are often unable to see signs or other cues to finding their way. Cataracts may be a specific problem, causing sensitivity to the glare sometimes present on signs. Since the hospital admission of elderly people is three times higher than that of younger people, these issues are of considerable importance to the patients and health care professionals alike (Schumaker & Reizenstein 1982).

Audition

Like the eye, the ear is fairly well developed at birth. The outer ear and the auditory canal will continue to grow until adolescence, but the middle ear achieves functional capacity a few months after birth. Even at birth, the middle ear becomes quickly capable of responding in a functional manner. Keith (1975) found that the middle ear was free from mucus and amniotic fluid a few hours after birth and thus able to operate as well in newborns as it does in older children. Lastly, the inner ear has attained all its gross structures, and whilst its responsiveness is initially limited, this is soon rectified in the first few months.

There are, however, certain limitations in the functioning of the auditory system at birth. The ability of the newborn to discern intensity or loudness of sound is not quite the same as adults. Accredolo & Hake (1982) have reviewed a number of studies and report that the median threshold for neonates is between 20 and 30 decibels, whereas adults have a median of about 5 and 10 decibels.

With reference to the frequency or pitch of sound, newborns seem to be more sensitive to higher-pitched sounds in the vicinity of 4000 hertz (Bremner 1988). (The lowest note on the piano is around 27.5 hertz and the highest 4180 hertz.) This sensitivity to the top end of the spectrum might lead adults to speak to babies in high-pitched tones because they get a greater response by doing so. A great deal of the research on infant hearing has concentrated on their receptivity to human speech. By the age of 1 month the infant can distinguish between the sounds *pa* and *ba*; by four months he is able to distinguish between consonant and vowel sounds (Fogel 1984).

Some recent studies have suggested that even very young neonates are able to recognise specific adult voices. DeCasper & Fifer (1980) found that 3-day-old infants would regularly vary their normal patterns of sucking in order to be rewarded by their mother reading them a story. The same babies, however, would not alter their sucking patterns if they were read to by another woman reading the same story. The implications of this and other studies are that the hearing system of neonates is remarkably well developed at birth, and that they are able to respond to, and distinguish between, sounds well within the spectrum of adult audition.

During the later years of adulthood, there are some noticeable changes in the receptiveness of the auditory system. Whilst there are structural changes in the outer and middle ear over the years, those most associated with hearing loss occur in the inner ear. These are degeneration of the sensory receptor cells, loss of auditory nerve cells and a decrease of flexibility in the cochlear partition, which is responsible for the transmission of vibrations from one chamber to another. The result of these changes is a progressive inability to hear high frequency tones, known as *presbyacusis*.

There are also changes in the threshold of sound perception that result with ageing. The ability to hear sounds in old age decreases, particularly if they are towards the high-frequency end of the sound spectrum. The consequences of hearing loss have been found to affect social interaction (Corso 1987) and have proved a significant factor in measures of intellectual competence (Granick et al 1976). When communicating with an individual who has a hearing impairment it is important to take these factors into consideration.

An easy way to get an idea of what it might be like to suffer from an age-related hearing deficiency is to turn the treble down and increase the bass on a hi-fi system. The muffled sound that results is not improved by increasing the volume. Similarly, speaking very loudly does little to improve one's intelligibility for a person with a hearing dysfunction; it may only cause frustration. Patience and persistence are essential in dealing with communication problems due to hearing difficulties. The following guidelines might prove useful:

- Do not shout at a patient—this may actually distort what you are saying. Speak at your normal rate, being as articulate as possible.
- Place yourself about 1–2 metres from the listener and in a good light so that he can view your lips. Do not cover your mouth with your hand.
- If he does not seem to be able to hear what you are saying, repeat the message using short, simple sentences.
- Never talk about a person with hearing difficulties in his presence. Always include him in your conversation.

Smell

The olfactory system begins to appear in the embryo about 30 days after conception. By the 6th month after conception, the fetus should begin to respond to odours (Accredolo & Hake 1982). The ability of the newborn to detect different odours is relatively weak at birth, but it develops during the first 3 days of life (Lipsitt et al 1963). The ability of the neonate to discriminate between smells was demonstrated by MacFarlane (1977). He presented babies with their own mother's breast pad and another mother's breast pad. He used head turning as an indicator of preference and found that neonates of 2 days did not differentiate between the two breast pads, but neonates of 10 days turned significantly more towards their own mother's breast pad. This finding also applies to bottle-fed neonates (Makin & Porter 1989). Finally, Steiner (1979) found that infants made positive or negative facial responses to a variety of odours, even though they could not possibly have had any previous experience of the odours in question.

One might suppose that the sense of smell deteriorates with age, since this seems to be the case with respect to seeing and hearing. The evidence, however, does not wholly support such a supposition. Engen (1982) reviews the research and concludes that there is little or no age decline in the sense of smell. Indeed, Rovee et al (1975) tested people ranging in age from 6–94 years old and found that there was no difference in the ability to judge the subjective intensity of the smell of different solutions of alcohol. They conclude that there are no age changes in the sense of smell throughout the life span and that the sensitivities that develop the earliest, such as smell, last the longest.

Yet Strehler (1977) says that there is an increase in the threshold for smell, similar to the threshold increase found for vision and hearing. Thus, higher levels of stimulation of smell receptors are required for older persons than is the case for younger persons. A possible resolution to this difference of opinion is provided by Engen (1982) who exhorts us to consider other, perhaps more important, factors that can affect the sense of smell such as disease and smoking.

The data on smell thresholds have two important implications. Firstly, whether due to age, disease or other factors such as smoking, the elderly may be less sensitive to certain odours than younger people. This means that they may be more susceptible to life-threatening events such as leaking gas. However, the research also indicates that some old people have sensory acuities equivalent to much younger individuals and it should not be assumed that because of age they are impervious to particular smells.

Taste

The two most frequently used measures of taste discrimination in infants have been sucking frequency and quantity of ingestion. Neonates ranging from 1 day to 4 months old have been found to suck faster and swallow more when presented with sweet solutions than with any others. They can even discriminate between glucose and the slightly sweeter taste of sucrose (Engen et al 1974). Newborns seem to respond differentially to at least three of the basic flavours—sweet, sour, and bitter.

Steiner (1979) and Ganchrow et al (1983) conducted a series of studies investigating the sensation of taste in newborns. Babies who had never been fed had flavoured water placed in their mouths. Steiner varied the flavour of the water and observed the response of the babies. He found that babies responded to the sweet

liquid with a relaxed expression, not unlike a smile. The response to the sour liquid was pursed lips, whilst to the bitter liquid, the baby responds with an arched mouth with sides turned down and an expression of disgust. Steiner said that the very fact that babies showed different expressions in response to the various flavours, indicated that they tasted different to the baby.

Cowart (1981) has reviewed the research on the development of taste throughout the life span. She distinguishes between being able to discriminate flavours that are present in a substance (sensitivity), and preferring some flavours to others (preference).

This developmental perspective is particularly relevant because it addresses the following important questions:

- Do neonates have an innate ability to distinguish between certain flavours?
- Does one's taste sensitivity decline in old age, leading to disinterest in certain foods?
- Do neonates prefer certain tastes, if so which ones?
- Do children like salty foods or do they have a sweet tooth?
- Does taste preference change during adulthood?

It seems that neonates are capable of making quite sophisticated discriminations between different flavours, particularly sweet solutions. Taste sensitivity remains stable throughout childhood and adulthood, but declines slightly in old age. The most substantial changes are reported to occur after the age of 60 years. This decline in sensitivity may be a factor in decreased food intake, which may affect the nutritional status of the old person.

There is definitely a preference for sweet tastes in neonates. However, the preference for strong sweet tastes declines during late childhood and early adolescence and may extend to old age. The developmental profile for salty taste preferences is not so clear cut. Neonates find weak salty tastes to be either neutral or mildly unpleasant. By the time they have become toddlers they frequently prefer salty foods but reject salt water. In late childhood a definite preference for salt water has developed, but tends to decline from this point onwards to old age.

Salt and sweet taste preferences have particular relevance for the promotion of healthy eating habits. It seems that by middle to late childhood, children like salty and sweet tastes, both of which can be bad for their health. Are these preferences due to an innate predisposition to like certain tastes at certain times or are they due to the sorts of foods parents give their children? Cowart suggests the need for more sophisticated research in what she terms a neglected area to answer these sorts of questions. Also a greater attention needs to be given to the taste preferences of different cultural groups. Moskowitz et al (1975) looked at cultural preference for sour and bitter tastes and found that there was a trend towards a decrease in aversion with continued exposure in certain cultures.

The sense of taste has received scant attention considering its importance for the eating habits of the elderly. Some old people can lose all motivation for eating because food has lost its attractiveness. Under these circumstances health professionals must realise that imploring the person to eat more is ineffective, and that a greater attention to increasing the quality and taste of food is just as important as maintaining its calorific value.

Touch

The sense of touch is present in the neonate and probably in the fetus too (Accredolo & Hake 1982). The sophistication of the tactile system is evidenced by the neonate's reflex behaviour; even the slightest touch on the palm of the hand will elicit the grasp reflex. The evidence for changes in sensitivity to touch with age is inconclusive. Kenshalo (1977) says that although some studies have shown decreases in sensitivity thresholds as people pass the ages of 50 and 60 years, others have not. Certainly any decreases are not inevitable and perhaps only occur in a minority of cases.

The major proportion of studies on the sense of touch have investigated its development in

association with other senses. Meltzoff & Borton (1979) illustrated that newborn infants of 29 days were able to make associations across the sensory modalities of touch and vision. They gave the infants one of two pacifiers, either a smooth round one or one with bumps on it. After sucking on these pacifiers they were given two large, styroform models of the pacifiers to look at. Meltzoff & Borton found that they spent much more time looking at the model of the pacifier that they had mouthed than the one which they had not touched at all. They suggested that not only were infants able to differentiate the objects with respect to touch but were also able to link this to their visual system.

If there are these connections between the senses, then the question arises as to whether infants are able to use information from one sense to replace information from another. Bower (1989) conducted a series of experiments using ultrasonic devices to help blind babies locate objects. The ultrasonic equipment emits waves which bounce off objects. The waves are picked up by the device which transmits them to the infant's ear. The pitch of the sound tells the baby how far away the object might be. The loudness of the sound tells the baby how big the object is. The clarity of the sound gives information concerning the texture of the surface of the object. The right/left source of the sound gives an indication of where the object may be located in space.

The babies were aged between 5 and 16 months. Bower found that even the very young babies were able to reach accurately for objects using this apparatus and, perhaps surprisingly, adapted to it much quicker than the older ones. Bower argues that the younger infants are not treating the information they receive as 'sound' at all, but are responding to it in much the same way as sighted infants perceive light. Older infants and adults have more difficulty in adapting to the system because they treat sound and sight as distinct sources of information; they are less likely to treat the sources in an interchangeable fashion.

Thus there is little doubt that the sensory acuities of the neonate are reasonably well developed at birth. In general these acuities become better developed with time until individuals reach old age. At this point the threshold of responsiveness to various stimuli tends to increase causing more difficulty in detecting and differentiating images, sounds, smells, tastes and perhaps objects too. But the equivocal nature of the research data with respect to studies of sensory acuities of old people may be due to the presence of more important factors than the ageing process itself.

INFANT TEMPERAMENT

Observe the newborn at a hospital nursery. In one cradle rests a passive, still infant, while the child beside her kicks and squirms; one baby is easily distracted by surrounding noise, another seems oblivious to it . . .

Gardner (1982)

So far, the emphasis has been on the ways in which infants are alike in terms of their sensory acuities. There are, however, certain differences between babies with respect to the variety and patterning of behaviour, which may be labelled temperament. Thomas et al (1970) conducted a large-scale study of infant temperament that was concerned with:

- establishing whether infants could be categorised accurately in terms of their temperamental qualities
- establishing whether these temperamental qualities remain consistent throughout the life span.

Categorisation

Thomas et al (1970) interviewed 141 parents about the behaviour of their babies, starting when the infants were aged 2 months. They also made on-site observations to support their interview data. When they analysed the data, nine characteristics of temperament emerged: activity level, rhythmicity, distractibility, approach/withdrawal, adaptability, attention span and preference, intensity of reaction, threshold of responsiveness and quality of mood.

The infants were rated either low, medium or high on each of these variables at the ages of

2 months, 6 months, 1 year, 2 years, 5 years and 10 years. The nine temperamental qualities were found to be consistent and reliable throughout this period of time. A further analysis of the data revealed that there were patterns of inter-relationship between the characteristics. Some of the traits were found to cluster together, that is, the vigorous baby was often less 'cuddly', more irritable and restless, whereas the placid baby was often 'cuddly' and less irritable. From this they identified 3 basic clusters which they said would prove useful in counselling new mothers:

Easy babies

About 40% of the infants in their sample fell into this category. They were regular in their natural functions; had a positive approach to new objects and events; were mild in their intensity of reaction and adjusted easily to change.

Difficult babies

Difficult babies had irregular sleeping and eating patterns; experienced more than average difficulty in negotiating new events; were intense in their reaction to stimuli and had a 'fussy' quality of mood. Approximately 10% of babies fell into this category.

Slow to warm up babies

They had a relatively low activity level; showed a kind of 'passive resistance' to new things and people; had a low threshold of responsiveness (stopped sucking on a bottle when approached) and although they were largely indifferent to new situations, once they had adapted, their response was largely positive. About 15% of babies were slow to warm up.

Such a categorisation was intended to make mothers, fathers and caregivers more aware of the inborn differences in the temperaments of infants. Perhaps knowing that some babies are born 'difficult' may lead to fewer feelings of inadequacy in parents and caregivers.

There are, however, one or two problems with a categorisation of this sort. Firstly it should be noted that some 35% of the babies were unclassifiable. If such a large proportion of the sample is unclassifiable, then it calls into question the relevance of these clusters. Secondly, as we shall see in the next section, the behaviour of infants should be seen as a reaction in part to the temperament and behaviour of the parents. A study of the nature of parent–child interaction may prove a more useful guide for parents and caregivers (Weber et al 1986).

Despite reservations about the clusters, there does seem to be a degree of unanimity with respect to the dimensions of temperament themselves. Since the work of Thomas et al (1970) there have been a number of attempts to classify temperament (Chess & Thomas 1984; Buss & Plomin 1984; Bohlin et al 1981; Rothbart 1981, 1986). They all seem to have delineated behaviour into similar temperament categories. Although Hubert et al (1982) argued that choice of temperament differs too greatly across investigations to make conceptually guided research possible, a review of the literature by Goldsmith & Campos (1982) found considerable overlap between temperament dimensions.

Consistency

There is little doubt that there are differences between infants with respect to temperament, but do these temperamental qualities remain consistent throughout childhood and adulthood? Thomas et al observed the children between the ages of 2 months and 10 years. They claim that there was remarkable consistency of temperamental traits throughout that period of development. The infant of 2 months who was found to wriggle when his nappy was changed could not sit still long enough to do his homework at the age of 10. This appears to be reasonably consistent, but they also stated that the infant of 2 months who 'did not move very much when being dressed' would be likely to grow up into a child of 10 years old who 'liked chess and reading'. Whether not liking being dressed in infancy, and a penchant for chess and reading in later childhood represent the same temperamental quality is not quite so obvious.

The main difficulty with the longitudinal assessment of temperamental characteristics is the stability or instability of the environment. In a relatively stable environment, behaviour is apt to remain consistent. However, in many cases, children experience an environment that is far from stable, and it is these environmental changes that are responsible for the significant differences in the child's and the infant's behaviour.

Unfortunately the approach of Thomas et al is limited to those instances where stability prevails, so it cannot quantify the environmental effects. They do admit that the interaction between parents and children is important but do not provide any guidelines for measuring it. Rutter (1987) found that children's temperaments affect the way people respond to them. 'Difficult' children are punished more which makes them frustrated and thus more difficult to handle. A cycle of mistreatment ensues.

Parents are very concerned about the temperament of their children. Therefore it is important that health professionals working with parents are aware of the implications of the research data. Some babies are more difficult than others. This may be due to genetic factors or it may be due to the child's response to the parent. In behavioural terms the cause is unimportant and it should be stressed to the parents that they have a significant role to play in the child's development. It can be dangerous to label a child as difficult and resign oneself to accept this fact. It is up to the health professional to show parents how they can interact appropriately with their children. In these circumstances an analysis of the interactional nature of behavioural development may prove more beneficial for the health professional than the ability to categorise infants as temperamentally easy or difficult.

Feeding and sleeping

One of the main concerns of parents during the first few months of their baby's life is feeding and sleeping. Wright et al (1983) found that night feeds disappeared more slowly in breast-fed babies than bottle-fed babies. One of the reasons put forward for this finding was that 'night waking is more probable in a setting in which mother (and father) are less likely to perceive its occurrence as a problem.' In other words, parents of breast-fed babies tended to accept night waking as the norm and not bother about it, whereas parents of bottle-fed babies viewed night waking as unusual, requiring some action. The authors suggest that their findings have implications for the advice given to parents by health professionals. Advice to delay the introduction of solid food until the infant is 3–4 months old is entirely compatible with the behaviour of breast-fed babies but not with bottle-fed babies who may have developed a pattern of sleeping through the night by the age of 3 months. The authors also found that the problem of night waking both in the first year of life and at nursery school were associated with earlier breast feeding. A good review of this area is provided by Boakes (1987).

PARENT–CHILD INTERACTION

Two words often associated with the interaction between parents and children are 'attachment' and 'bonding'. They refer to the emotional relationship that exists between parents and children during the first months of life. Bowlby (1969, 1973, 1980) has described attachment as 'an affectional bond' between the child and the adult. However, it is important to distinguish whether attachment or bonding refers to the parents' attachment to the child or the child's attachment to the parent. Let's start by looking at the ways in which parents form their bond to the baby.

Research by Klaus & Kennell (1976) showed that it was extremely important for mothers to have early contact with their babies. They said that there was a 'critical period' for the mother's development of an attachment to her child in the first hours after birth. Therefore it was necessary to provide immediate contact between mother and baby because failure to do so would result in weak attachments. As a result of this research, hospital practices have changed with mothers and fathers encouraged to hold their babies immediately after delivery.

This early contact between parents and their babies is very often reported to be an extremely happy occasion, but Klaus & Kennell (1976) went further and said that such contact was imperative for the development of appropriate attachment behaviour; recent research suggests that this is not quite the case. There does seem to be some evidence that mothers who have handled their babies immediately after birth show more tenderness towards them in the first few weeks of life than mothers who did not have the opportunity to interact with their babies until later (Grossman et al 1981). O'Connor et al (1980) also produced findings which suggested that early contact may help prevent later parenting problems among mothers who may be at high risk for abuse. However, for the majority of parents, the long-term effects of being separated from their babies for a few hours after birth are not critical (Grossman et al 1981).

A disruption of the interactive process between parents and their children over long periods of time can be a significant factor in child abuse or neglect. Difficulties may occur if there is a lack of response from either party in the interactive sequences. Premature infants are particularly 'at risk' since they are usually separated from their parents for the first weeks or months and are then unresponsive after they return home from hospital. Whilst many parents work extra hard to stimulate and become involved with their children, eventually they withdraw somewhat due to the lack of appropriate feedback (Barnard et al 1984). Parents may also disrupt the interaction process, especially if they lack the 'attachment skills', are self-centred or are under a lot of stress at the time (Kempe & Kempe 1981).

Attachment behaviour

The process of children becoming attached to their parents begins with what Schaffer (1971) terms 'social signalling systems'. The two most important social signalling systems or attachment behaviours are crying and smiling.

Crying

In order that some form of interaction can take place, it is necessary to bring the parent into close proximity with the child. In terms of parent–child interaction, the function of crying is to initiate the interaction process. Wolff (1969) identified three distinct patterns of cry: the basic cry, the 'mad' or angry cry and the pain cry. He found that mothers very quickly learn to distinguish between the different patterns of crying and can detect even the smallest deviations from the norm. Similarly, Gustafson & Harris (1990) found that a sample of mothers were better at guessing the exact cause of cries than a sample of non-mothers. Initially crying is an automatic response to physical stimuli, but the child soon learns that certain consequences follow on from his crying and the 'attention please' cry develops.

There has been an interesting debate over the past few years between those psychologists who think that to pick up the baby immediately every time she cries will reinforce the crying behaviour and she will do it more, and others who think that if the baby is crying then it is in need of something and not to respond would be cruel.

My own opinion is that one should respond to the child's cries where and when one can, but it may be difficult to go to the child each and every time she cries. However, the child should not be left to cry in the belief that it is doing her good in some way. The idea that she must learn that she cannot get everything she wants in life is misplaced, as she cannot entertain such concepts at this age. However, a small amount of crying will do no psychological harm and the parent need not feel guilty for not going to a child immediately, and every time she cries.

The amount and duration of crying varies from individual to individual. Korner et al (1981) monitored all the crying behaviour of a group of babies in the first 3 days of life and found that they cried only 2–11% of the time. The importance of crying behaviour in the development of appropriate attachment behaviour between parents and children was illustrated by a series of interviews conducted by Schaffer (1971)

with mothers of autistic children. It emerged that, with one exception, there was a complete absence of the ability to cry in situations where the response could normally be expected to occur. They never cried when hungry, and after the feed did not indicate when they had eaten enough. They never cried for attention during infancy, even when left alone for long periods of time. They remained utterly passive. It seems that some crying at least is necessary to initiate a reasonable amount of interaction.

Smiling

If the purpose of crying is to initiate an interaction, then the function of smiling is to maintain the interaction. Smiling is usually initiated by the presence of a person, but can be elicited by changes in brightness of the physical environment (Salzen 1963) or by a familiar object (Piaget 1953). A number of studies have sought to determine which features of the human face are responsible for eliciting the smiling response in infants.

Ahrens (1954) found a relationship between the age of the infant and the presence of key features of the human face. From the first month, the infant will smile at two dots on a piece of cardboard just as much as his mother's face. At this age, the eyes, or stimuli which look like eyes, are the features that the baby finds significant. Then, as the child grows older, more and more of the face is required to elicit a smile, until at around 3 months of age the baby will only respond if all the facial features are present. At about 5 months of age, he will respond equally to a smiling and a scowling face but thereafter will differentiate between the various expressions. At 6 months two-dimensional models are no use; a solid model face is required. Finally at the age of 7 months smiling is only elicited by certain familiar faces. Gewirtz (1965) summed up the process by saying that initially there is reflex smiling which is followed by social smiling and then selective social smiling.

Often the baby will initiate a sequence of interaction by using the greeting response (Bell 1974). This is where the child opens his eyes and mouth in a distinctive shape, makes a sort of cooing sound and smiles. This expression inevitably results in a response from the parent such as smiling, touching and talking. Thus a schedule of mutual conditioning is set up with the child conditioning the parent and the parent conditioning the child. The parent is rewarded by the infant's smiling response and is therefore encouraged to stimulate the child more by touching, talking and cuddling; the baby finds this rewarding so will respond with more smiling—and so on. It is this mutual stimulation that forms the basis for the development of a bond or attachment between the parents and the child.

The attachment bond

How do we know that a bond has developed? One way to find out is to separate the parent from the child and observe the response. Schaffer & Callender (1959) studied the effects of short-term hospitalisation on a sample of 76 infants aged between 3 and 51 weeks. When various indices of separation upset, such as amount of crying and degree of responsiveness to the mother (during her visit) and to the nurses, were plotted over age, a break was found to occur at about 7 months of age:

- *Above 7 months*—a separation picture characterised by protest during the initial period of hospitalisation, negativism towards staff, intervals of subdued behaviour or withdrawal and after returning home, a period of readjustment occurring in the form of insecurity with the mother.
- *Below 7 months*—no protest and strangers were accepted as mother substitutes. On return home there was a brief upset but this referred more to a change in environment than to the mother's renewed presence.

On the basis of these results, Schaffer & Callender concluded that some form of bond had developed between the children and their mothers at about 7 months of age. They also found that the intensity of attachment was as great at 7 months as at later ages.

In order to avoid the upset engendered by hospital separation it is necessary to provide more facilities for mothers to stay with their children during the time that they are in hospital. Where this is impracticable parents should be encouraged to get their children used to short-term separations by occasionally leaving them with relations or 'baby-sitters'. Under these circumstances the child becomes used to the parents going away, and more importantly, always coming back.

Schaffer & Emerson (1964) found further evidence for a bond developing at about 7 months. Their sample of 60 infants were looked at every month until they were 1 year old and then at 18 months. Mothers were asked to observe their infants' separation responses in a variety of everyday separations such as when they were left alone in a room, when they were left with other people or when they were put down after being held. In the first half of the year the children were not very worried when left with other people, but after about 7 months, were upset by strangers approaching them. Thus separation anxiety and fear of strangers were found to be two characteristics of the attachment bond and the *average* age for its development was when the children were 7 months old.

The next question refers to the number of individuals to which the child can become attached. Schaffer & Emerson (1964) found that most (71%) of their sample formed primary attachments to one person, but after 3 months the percentage having only one attachment figure was reduced to 41 and by 18 months it had been reduced to 13%. This 'breadth' of attachment to mothers, fathers, grandparents, aunts, uncles, siblings and even neighbours ensures that should anything go wrong with the primary attachment figure, another member of the family could take her place with a minimum of fuss, provided the quality of the relationship is the same.

Theories

The age of onset, intensity and breadth of the attachment bond have been established, but there still remains the question of why it occurs.

One explanation that has been put forward is the 'secondary drive theory' of attachment (Dollard & Miller 1950). This theory states that the reason the child becomes attached to the mother is because she provides the physical gratification of the child's basic drives such as hunger and thirst. Since the child is unable to satiate these drives herself, she becomes attached to the organism that can. This explanation of bonding appears reasonably plausible but unfortunately does not explain the findings of more recent research.

Harlow (1958) investigated attachment behaviours in infant rhesus monkeys. He took eight newborn rhesus monkeys and placed them in contact with two artificial surrogate mothers. One of the surrogates was designed to appear 'cuddly' to the infant monkeys (a cylinder of wood covered with terry cloth), the other was constructed of a cylinder of wire and thus relatively devoid of contact comfort. Nourishment was only provided by the 'wire mother'. Secondary drive theory would predict that the baby monkeys would spend more time with the surrogate mother who provided the food; this was not the case. The monkeys spent much more time with the cloth monkey, indicating that warmth and creature comfort were more important for attachment bonding than the gratification of physical need.

Schaffer & Emerson (1964) found that one-fifth of their sample formed strong attachments to individuals who rarely took part in gratifying the physical needs of the children. Often the primary attachment figure was the father, who played no part in the feeding process and was not present for the majority of the working day. Under these circumstances, on returning home, the father would engage in intensive, stimulating interaction with the child and it was this quality of interaction that proved significant in determining the primary attachment figure, not feeding the child or spending the most time with it during the day.

On the basis of such evidence, Schaffer (1991) proposes that we view attachment as essentially a perceptual or cognitive process. Children become attached to their parents because they find them stimulating. Stimulating play with babies is exciting and the individual who provides this excitement will command the greatest attention. Schaffer cites as evidence for his theory the behaviour of fathers who were primary attachment figures and also the fact that there is a great deal of stimulating information in the mother's face. It might not be the physical gratification of hunger that is responsible for the attachment bond, but the stimulation provided by the mother's face during feeding.

An alternative view of attachment is provided by the ethological approaches of Bowlby (1969) and Ainsworth et al (1978). They state that the purpose of attachment is to ensure proximity to the caretaker. The origins of this behaviour lie 'buried in the evolution of the species' and have developed to ensure that in case of danger the infant is predisposed to seek the closeness of the parent.

Ainsworth (1967, 1982) provided evidence of the universality of the attachment process by illustrating the presence of attachment behaviour in the infants of Uganda. She found that most children were clearly attached by the age of 6 months and began to fear strangers during the last quarter of their first year. However, the most important finding was that a few youngsters were insecurely attached. This no doubt provided the impetus for a later study of the nature of the attachment bond itself.

Ainsworth et al (1978) devised a procedure called 'The Strange Situation Procedure', which has been widely used to measure the strength of attachment between the infant and its caretakers. The procedure involves a sequence of eight episodes in which the behaviour of mother and infant can be assessed (Box 7.1).

Ainsworth et al (1978) identified three major types of infant attachment to the mother:

Group A. The infants in this group showed behaviour characterised by avoidance and anxiety. When the mother returned, the baby avoided closeness to her. Typically the babies would either ignore the return of the mother or casually greet her. Most show no distress when the mother leaves the room and the stranger is present. About 23% of the sample were classified as 'anxious-avoidant'.

Group B. These babies treat the mother and

Box 7.1 The Strange Situation Procedure (Ainsworth et al 1978)

Episode 1: duration 30 seconds
Observer introduces mother and baby to experimental room, then leaves.

Episode 2: duration 3 minutes
Mother is nonparticipant while baby explores. If necessary, play is stimulated after 2 minutes.

Episode 3: duration 3 minutes
Stranger enters room. Stranger silent. Stranger converses with mother. Stranger approaches baby. After 3 minutes mother leaves unobtrusively.

Episode 4: duration 3 minutes; less if baby is distressed
First separation episode. Stranger's behaviour is geared to that of the baby.

Episode 5: duration 3 minutes or more
First reunion episode. Mother greets and comforts baby, then tries to settle him again in play. Mother then leaves saying 'bye-bye'.

Episode 6: duration 3 minutes or less
Second separation episode.

Episode 7: duration 3 minutes or less
Continuation of second separation. Stranger enters and gears her behaviour to that of the baby.

Episode 8: duration 3 minutes
Second reunion episode. Mother enters, greets her baby, then picks him up. Meanwhile stranger leaves unobtrusively.

stranger very differently and were described as 'securely attached'. When the mother leaves the room they are distressed and may or may not be comforted by the stranger. When the mother returns, they give her more than a casual greeting and either move toward her or cry and smile. They rarely resist contact with the mother and protest when put down. About 65% of the sample were classified as 'securely attached'.

Group C. Of the three types, these babies cry the most frequently and explore the least. They are called resistant because they actively resist the ministrations of the stranger and also are somewhat unresponsive to the mother on her return. About 12% of the sample were classified as 'anxious-resistant'.

This classification system has proved a reliable assessment of attachment behaviour in infants (Vaughn et al 1979; Thompson et al 1982; Weber

et al 1986). Ainsworth et al (1978) and also Clarke-Stewart (1973), in contrast to Thomas & Chess (1977), place a greater emphasis on the behaviour of the parent in determining the reaction of infants to separations and strangers. They say that mothers who are affectionate and responsive to their babies' needs and desires, have securely attached babies. Mothers who tend to be rejecting, emotionally indifferent, and insensitive to their babies' needs have anxiously attached infants. There is no doubt in the minds of these researchers that parents play a significant role in determining the nature of the attachment bond, particularly with respect to Type A mother-avoidant infants.

The extent to which a secure or insecure attachment persists into later childhood depends upon the stability of the child's family circumstances, but Egeland & Sroufe (1981) found that a child who had become insecurely attached at 12 months might become more securely attached when levels of stress went down or in one instance when the grandmother had come to live with the family. Therefore it would appear that even a very poor early environment need not destine a child to a permanently insecure attachment.

MATERNAL DEPRIVATION

Bowlby (1951) was among the first to call attention to the concept of maternal deprivation. He argued that the lack of opportunity to attach oneself to a mother could result in the development of 'affectionless psychopathy'. This condition is characterised by the inability of the individual to form any kind of relationship with other people. These people are often described as cold, manipulative individuals who, as a result of receiving little or no affection from their mothers, are unable to form affectional ties with anybody else.

Bowlby's report for the World Health Organization was based on the early studies of institutionalisation by Spitz (1945) and Goldfarb (1943), and resulted in the practice of trying to ensure that all infants had a 'mother' as soon as possible after birth. However, the effects of institutionalisation (Spitz called the syndrome 'hospitalism') are by no means as simple as these early studies would have us believe. Firstly, Pinneau (1955) pointed out some basic methodological flaws in Spitz's research. Secondly, a number of studies have found that:

- Infants brought up without personalised mother love can remain well within the normal range of scores on developmental and intellectual tests (Rheingold 1956).
- Children may develop all the symptoms of hospitalism without ever leaving home. Mother-reared children can be just as deprived as institutionally reared children (Provence & Coleman 1957).

Rutter (1981) suggests that the concept of maternal deprivation is at best misleading. Does the word maternal refer only to the mother? Clearly, as we have just seen, this need not be the case. Further, does Bowlby mean deprivation or privation? In other words it is important to distinguish between having no mother at all and the lack of her presence at certain times. Rutter (1981) feels that a more useful approach is to investigate the effects of:

- short-term separations such as hospitalisation and 'working' mothers
- long-term separations such as divorce, death and institutionalisation.

Hospitalisation

We have seen that the short-term effects of hospitalisation can prove distressing for children who have formed an attachment bond with their parents (Schaffer & Callender 1959). There has been a great deal of discussion about the long-term effects of such separations. Douglas (1975) challenges the view that hospital admission in the preschool years is seldom followed by persistent disturbance. His report was based on a large-scale, national sample of individuals who were born in 1946. He investigated such items as number and length of hospitalisations and the effects on behaviour in later adolescence. His conclusions were that there was a significant correlation between number of admissions and duration of admission in the preschool years and 'troublesomeness', 'poor reading', 'delinquency' and 'unstable job history' in later adolescence.

This body of research has been analysed by Quinton & Rutter (1976) who found a number of methodological limitations. In their replication of the Douglas study, they found that there were no long-term psychological consequences following single hospital admissions of less than a week, but multiple or recurrent admissions were linked with later disorders. Care must be taken before concluding that even two admissions in the preschool years increase the risk of psychiatric disorder. The association might reflect the adverse effects of poor home conditions rather than anything directly related to hospital admissions per se.

Clarke & Clarke (1976) make a similar point by suggesting that the associations found by Douglas do not constitute a causal relationship between multiple admissions and disorder. Hospitalisation in the early years might be a product of many factors, including 'disadvantaged' homes. It is these factors that may be responsible for later adolescent disorders rather than recurrent hospital admission.

Working mothers

This term refers to mothers who do not choose to stay at home with their children or cannot afford to do so. Of course all mothers work, whether they do it outside the home, inside the home or both, but for those who have to leave their children with someone else for the majority of the day there is the worry that they might not be providing the required amount of 'mothering' necessary for the best development of their child. This anxiety stems from the child-care books of the 1950s and 1960s like that of Dr Spock who assumed that it was essential to be reared by a loving mother at home.

Since that time there has been a wealth of research indicating that short-term separations per se have no psychological consequences whatsoever. It should be remembered that a number of the primary attachment figures in Schaffer & Emerson's (1964) study were fathers, who only saw their children when they returned home from work. Kagan (1979) found that even though children may form attachments to the adults who care for them during the day, they show an overwhelming preference for their mothers. There is some evidence that children from 'unstimulating' families may actually benefit intellectually from going to daycare nurseries (Andrews et al 1982). What makes a significant difference to the child's development is the quality of care outside the home. Some child minders and daycare nurseries provide excellent facilities, others leave a lot to be desired. It is these factors that contribute to the child's emotional and intellectual development, not the separation itself. Tizard (1991) says: 'The evidence briefly summarised here suggests that young children are unlikely to suffer psychological damage if their mothers go out to work, although they may suffer initial distress. Indeed, they will benefit from a greater variety of social contacts outside the family.'

Divorce and death

According to Bowlby's hypothesis, there should be no difference between separations due to divorce and separations due to death; both involve separation from an attachment figure. He suggested that disorder in the child arises from a disruption of the affectional bond with his mother. Rutter (1981) cites evidence that shows no correlation between death of a parent and deviant personality. There is a correlation, however, between divorce and the development of personality disorders, but only divorce that is preceded by marital disharmony. For Rutter, it is the presence of marital discord that is responsible for any psychological damage that might occur. Those divorces that are undertaken amicably may prove less damaging than intact marriages with a high degree of marital strife. There was an association between separation from both parents and antisocial disorder in boys, but this applied only in homes where there was a poor marriage relationship between the parents. It has been shown that the delinquency rates are significantly higher for boys whose parents have been divorced or separated. The delinquency rate was only slightly higher for boys who had lost a parent by death. Rutter (1976) says:

The conclusions on 'broken homes' are surprisingly straightforward. Although parental death may play a part in the pathogenesis of some disorders, delinquency is mainly associated with breaks which follow parental discord rather than with the loss of a parent as such . . . . The present findings suggest that separation as such is of negligible importance in the causation of delinquency.

The child's life is often disrupted by the death of a parent. Firstly, death can often follow a long illness. Secondly, the grief of the surviving parent may affect the child more than the death of the other. Thirdly, there may be economic difficulties resulting from the death of a parent, particularly in families where the father dies. These factors can have greater psychological consequences than the death itself.

Institutionalisation

Tizard (1977) conducted a longitudinal study of the effects of institutionalisation on emotional and cognitive development in young children. She looked at 25 residential nurseries run by three large British voluntary societies. The standard in the nurseries was high, therefore generalisation to all sorts of institution is limited. On average, there were 15–25 children in each nursery and they were usually situated in the country or close to seaside towns. This made visiting by parents awkward. The children were divided into family groups of six, with a mixed age range until they were about 5 years old. They were allowed to have pets, there were home-style furnishings, the diet was good, so were the clothes. They were taken for walks and also had pocket money. There was no doubt that the physical environment, play equipment, diet, and attention to health were excellent, and probably better than that of many British children living at home.

Each nursery was a training centre for nursery nurses who stayed for about 3 years to complete their training. This system of staffing ensured a generous supply of staff at low cost, but inevitably resulted in poor continuity of care. For

2 days a week, 3–4 weeks a year, and nights, a particular nurse would not be there. Experience was widened by moving the student nurses from unit to unit within the nursery. This meant that after 2 years in the nursery, each child had been looked after by about 24 different adults for a week or more; after 4½ years the number had increased to about 50 different adults.

In all nurseries, close relationships with the children were actively discouraged. Close attachments to one nurse made it difficult for another nurse to handle the child, and if the child were subsequently to be adopted, then any attachment to a member of staff would make the process of transition from one environment to another extremely difficult.

The nurseries thus provided an environment for the children which was very different from that found in any private family. While considerable attention was given to the children's health and education, their care passed through the hands of large numbers of rather young girls, who attempted to remain emotionally detached from them.

Tizard (1977)

The results of living in such an environment may be summarised as follows. At 2 years, the children were found to be both more clinging and more diffuse in their attachments than children brought up in ordinary families. Their mean Cattell mental age was 22 months and they were slightly retarded in language development. At 4½ years, it was decided to investigate those children that were still in the nursery, those that had been adopted, those that had been restored to their parents and those in the 'working class' control group. The experimenters found that children who had been institutionalised at some time during the first 2 years of life were still more clinging and less likely to show deep attachments than the control group; in addition they showed more attention-seeking behaviour and were likely to become overly friendly with strangers. The mean IQ scores were as follows:

- Adopted   114.9
- Institutional 104.88
- Restored   100.07
- Control   111.47

The implications of these results are that:

- Any deficit in intellectual performance during the early years of development can be reversed (Adopted IQ 114.9).
- Explanations of intellectual deficit of the institutionalised children due to genetic inferiority are unfounded (Adopted IQ 114.9).
- Irrespective of environmental changes, both adopted and restored groups still showed attention-seeking behaviour.

Tizard & Hodges (1978) found that, at age 8, the children's emotional behaviour and IQ scores had remained unchanged, except for the institutional group whose IQ scores had decreased slightly.

The conclusions with respect to the effects of institutionalisation on cognitive development are that any deficit in performance can be reversed. However, there does tend to be a long-term consequence of early institutionalisation, in that all the children in the experimental groups were assessed by their teachers as being more attention-seeking, restless, disobedient and unpopular. It seems that the attachment behaviour of the nursery children is unable to be realised by forming a bond with a reliable, stable adult figure. The consequences of persisting attachment behaviour manifest themselves in later life as attention-seeking behaviour.

CHILDREN'S CONCEPTIONS OF ILLNESS

Researcher:	Now what does the doctor use the stethoscope for?
Jenny (age 5):	He puts this thing on your heart so it will help you breathe properly and so you are not going to die.
Mary (age 5½):	He listens to your heart.
Researcher:	And why does he do that?
Mary:	To see if it has stopped.
Researcher:	Is it important?
Mary:	Uh-huh, very important to your whole body—do you not know about this?

Parmelee (1986) states that in the age period from 1–3 years, children are likely to have an average of 8–9 illnesses a year, from the ages of 4–10 years 4–6 illnesses a year, and for the rest of their lives about 4 per year. The most common illnesses are respiratory illnesses such as the common cold. Since these illnesses spread sequentially throughout the family, this means that a family of two adults and two children will experience an average of 28 illnesses a year. These common illnesses form an integral part of a family's life in early years.

In communicating with children about illness and health, it is extremely important to establish whether their powers of comprehension differ from that of adults. The young child's apprehension of the stethoscope may not be due to the fact that it feels cold on the skin; it may be due to the belief that the purpose of the instrument is to determine whether they are alive or not. Under these circumstances no amount of warming the stethoscope up will reassure the child. So do children think in different ways to adults about such things as health and illness? A Swiss researcher, Piaget, suggested that children do not simply possess weaker cognitive abilities than adults; they actually seem to think and reason in sharply different ways (Piaget 1970).

Stages of illness cognition

For Piaget then, children think in qualitatively different ways to adults. But are these differences apparent in their conceptions of health and illness? A study by Bibace & Walsh (1979) suggests that they are. They gave 180 children aged between 3 and 13 years a series of 12 questions about various features of health and illness (see Box 7.2).

The children's answers to the questions were analysed and it was found that their responses could be categorised in terms of Piaget's stages of cognitive development.

Preoperational responses

Bibace & Walsh (1979, 1980) identified 3 types of explanation in this stage:

Incomprehension. The child evades the question or gives irrelevant answers.

What is a heart attack? 'A heart attack is on vacation.'

Box 7.2 Questions used by Bibace & Walsh in their study of children's concepts of health and illness

1. What does it mean to be healthy?
2. Do you remember anyone who was sick? What was wrong? How did he or she get sick? How did he or she get better?
3. Were you ever sick? Why did you get sick? How did you get sick? How did you get better?
4. What is the worst sickness to have? Why? What is the best sickness to have? Why?
5. What happens to people when they are sick? What happens to people when they are very sick?
6. What is a cold? How do people get colds? Where do colds come from? What makes colds go away?
7. What are the measles? How do people get the measles? Where do measles come from? What makes the measles get better?
8. What is a heart attack? Why do people get heart attacks?
9. What is cancer? How do people get cancer?
10. What is a headache? Why do people get headaches?
11. Have you ever had a pain? Where? What is pain? Why does it come? Where does it come from?
12. What are germs? What do they look like? Can you draw germs? Where do they come from?

Why is a heart attack on vacation? 'Can I have the pencil?'

Phenomenism. Illness is defined in terms of a single external symptom, usually a sight or sound that the child has, at some time, associated with the illness.

What is a heart attack? 'A heart attack is falling on your back.'
Why do people get heart attacks? 'A heart attack is from the sun.'

Contagion. Again illness is defined in terms of a single external symptom, but here the source of the illness is usually either a person or object that is near to, but not touching, the ill person, or an activity that occurs prior to the illness.

What are measles? 'Measles are bumps all over you.'
How do people get measles? 'From other people.'

How do people get measles from other people? 'When you walk near them.'

Concrete operational responses

At this stage, the child can only understand events in the real world in contrast to hypothetical events. There are two substages:

Contamination. The child at this stage does not distinguish between the mind and the body, so bad or immoral behaviour, just as contact with dirt or germs, causes illness.

> What is cancer? 'Cancer is when you are very sick and you have got to go to hospital and you throw up a lot, and stuff.'
> How do people get cancer? 'From smoking without their mother's permission. You shouldn't do it, it's bad.'

Internalisation. Illness is described as being within the body. The source of illness is described as some external factor such as germs or unhealthy body state such as high blood pressure.

> How do people get colds? 'From germs in the air, you breathe them in.'
> How does this give you a cold? 'The germs, they get in your blood.'

Bibace & Walsh (1979) state 'While the child is able to mention an internal organ, he or she cannot articulate how it operates physiologically.'

Formal operational responses

The child is now no longer bound by concrete reality and is able to include possibility.

Physiological. The child describes illness in terms of internal body organs and functions. The cause of an illness is clearly thought to be due to the malfunctioning of some internal part of the body. In this stage, the child perceives herself as being in control of the onset and cure of an illness, insofar as there are multiple causes and cures.

> What is a heart attack? 'A heart attack is when the heart stops pumping blood to the rest of the body. A person faints, stops breathing, and collapses.'

How do people get heart attacks? 'The valves keep the blood from getting to the heart so the heart stops and you get a heart attack.'

The child can now describe structures and functions that are not external or visible.

Psychophysiological. The child perceives an additional or alternative cause of illness, namely, the psychological cause. They are able to understand that thoughts or feelings can affect the way the body functions.

> What is a heart attack? 'It's when your heart stops or doesn't work right.'
> How do people get heart attacks? 'A heart attack is from being all nerve racked and weary.'

Support for this categorisation of children's thoughts on illness comes from the work of Perrin & Gerrity (1981) and Fielding (1985). It is easy to see the advantages of such a classification system. At a glance, the health professional is able to determine what a child of a particular age will understand and what he will not. This in turn will determine, not only the level of communication, but also the educational limits to understanding, for it is an implicit feature of Piaget's theory that if a child has not reached a particular stage of cognitive development, then no amount of teaching will accelerate her development because she does not possess the cognitive ability to do so. This latter point has important implications for health education. If the above authors are correct, then health education must be pitched at the child's level of cognitive understanding, otherwise he will be unable to comprehend the issues involved.

Cognitive development

Unfortunately children's cognitive development does not proceed in such a predictable fashion. Since the rise in popularity of Piaget's theory, there have been a large number of studies that have questioned the psychological validity of his approach (Vuyk 1981; Donaldson 1978).

For instance, with respect to Piaget's assertion that children below the age of 6 or 7 years are egocentric, Hughes & Donaldson (1983) have found that if the task is explained carefully to them and if it makes sense to them, then children as young as 3 and 4 years possess the ability to see things from another person's point of view. Similarly, when Borke (1975) replicated Piaget & Inhelder's (1956) famous 'mountains task', she found that 3- and 4-year-old children could de-centre. The only difference between her study and Piaget & Inhelder's study was that her task was introduced and explained in ways that were appropriate for 3-and 4-year-olds.

Data from the present study and from previous investigators exploring perceptual role-taking skills in 4- to 6-year-olds (Fishbein et al 1972, Flavell et al 1968) raise considerable doubt about the validity of Piaget's conclusion that young children are primarily egocentric and incapable of taking the viewpoint of another person. When presented with tasks that are age appropriate, even very young subjects demonstrate perceptual role-taking ability.

Borke (1975)

These and many other studies have demonstrated one important feature of children's cognitive development, namely that if what is being asked of the children 'makes sense' to them then they can understand more than Piaget would have us believe. Those studies of children's conception of illness that use a Piagetian framework and attempt to limit the child's understanding of illness according to his developmental stage are underestimating the cognitive capacity of the child. Clearly statements by Fielding (1985) such as 'an understanding of illness as a complex, multifaceted process only emerges at approximately 12 years of age' need careful investigation.

A study by Niven (1986) attempted to replicate the study of Bibace & Walsh but, like Borke (1975), used a methodology appropriate to the child's age. He looked at 122 children aged 5, 6, 8 and 9 years. He found that 5- and 6-year-olds were perfectly capable of giving quite sophisticated responses to questions like 'How do you get a cold?' Many replied that colds come from germs and whilst some said you get a cold from freezing days or from staying in the bath for too long, a number of adults would give the same response. It seemed that many mistakes made by children were due to a lack of information. How many adults might say to their children 'Get out of that bath before you catch cold!'? Indeed, some adults show a remarkable ignorance about health and illness.

Bibace & Walsh (1979) quote the case of the 40-year-old male, with a high school education, who was in hospital in an intensive care unit suffering from a heart attack. He insisted on getting up to go to the toilet, despite repeated medical advice to the contrary. The staff could not understand why he continually ignored their advice. A psychiatrist was consulted and said it was due to 'massive denial'. However, a nurse said that he knew why he was being required to stay in bed but had misconstrued his condition. A paraphrase of his statement to the nurse conveyed the following: 'There are four chambers to the heart. I've had two heart attacks. I've got two more to go. After I've had the third attack, I'll listen to you, but not before.'

Some of our thoughts about illness are wrong because we do not have the correct information, and this is the case for children too. Children make mistakes due to lack of knowledge and because they have a different view of the world. The advantage of the Bibace & Walsh (1979) study is that it points to the sort of mistakes children are likely to make about health and illness at certain ages. The disadvantages lie in assuming that children of specific ages are unable to comprehend details of health and illness because of not possessing the necessary cognitive ability. If the information is presented in an appropriate fashion to children then they can take on quite advanced concepts.

Niven (1986) found evidence of one particular project that involved teaching 8- and 9-year-old children about the body and how it works. The project was initiated by a teacher and a paediatrician who collaborated in the presentation of information to the children. As part of the educational project the children visited a maternity ward, discussed kidney donor cards and viewed items brought into the classroom by the paediatrician. The net result was a conceptual comprehension that far outweighed the expectations of the instructors.

6 months after the project had ended Niven tested the children on such things as functions of the body and the reproductive system and found

their knowledge to be extremely sophisticated. The conclusions of those involved with the project were that it was possible to teach 8- and 9-year-old children about illness as a multifaceted process, but it took a great deal of time and commitment on the part of the instructors, and whether this sort of commitment could be maintained was another matter.

To summarise:

- Studies that are based on a Piagetian framework do give a good indication of some of the mistakes children make at different ages.
- Many misconceptions occur due to lack of knowledge. This is the case for adults as well as children.
- Children are able to comprehend quite sophisticated concepts if one is prepared to 'make sense' to them.

Even the very young child is able to contribute a great deal about the type of illness they've got if the adult is prepared to listen and to watch the child expressing, often non-verbally, the kind of upset that's disturbing them. Also and I think very importantly you must always bear in mind that a child's comprehension is far in advance of their ability to communicate, so whereas they may not be able to be very articulate about the particular problem they've got, they will be much more likely to understand your explanations, reassurances and suchlike about the illness or treatment you are giving for it.

Ward-Platt (1986)

Finally, whilst a number of young children will respond to a question about where babies come from with 'From mummy's tummy', the question of how they got there was put to 5-year-olds by the author with the following responses:

ChiChi (age 5½): 'It's God that puts it there.'

A more down-to-earth solution comes in this exchange with Jane (age 5):

'It comes from me mammy's tummy.'
'And how did it get there?'
'Cause the doctor put it in?'
'And who took it out?'
'The nurse.'

OLD AGE: DETERIORATION AND ISOLATION

Two features of the ageing process that have commanded a great deal of attention during recent years are the extent to which:

- there is a decline in such psychological functions as intellect, memory and problem-solving abilities with age
- old people become more isolated as they grow older.

Intellectual decline

A major factor in the decline in psychological functioning with age is the presence of disease. Therefore one has to separate those changes that are due to disease, and those changes that are a result of the ageing process itself.

Birren et al (1963) examined a sample of 47 men between the ages of 65 and 91 years who were found to be healthy on the basis of clinical examination. They were given a series of lengthy examinations on a wide range of medical, physiological and psychological tests. Two groups emerged from these examinations:

Group 1 Optimal health in every regard (N = 27).
Group 2 No clinical disease, but through intensive examination were found to have mild diseases (N = 20).

These groups differed significantly on a number of factors.

Medical data

Measures of cerebral blood flow and oxygen consumption of old men (71 years) and young men (21 years) showed no significant differences. However, there were differences in cerebral blood flow between young men and members of Group 2. Even a subclinical degree of disease may affect the efficiency of brain functioning.

Physiological data

The electroencephalograph readings were found to change with age, irrespective of group membership. The average frequency spectrum of the older subjects was approximately one cycle slower than that of the younger subjects. Group 2 subjects were even slower still. This means that there is some evidence of a slowing down of electrical activity in the brain with age and of disease increasing this trend.

Psychological data

23 tests of intellectual performance were administered to Groups 1 and 2. The scores of Group 2 were poorer on 21 out of the 23 tests. Group 2 were particularly bad at retrieving stored information. Both groups were slower than younger subjects in the speed with which they solved the tests. Thus it seems that disease can affect the retrieval of stored information, whilst a genuine result of the ageing process is a slowing down of psychomotor speed.

The less healthy group performed consistently less well on several personality tests. Mild disease was found to affect such things as the degree to which they terminated responses appropriately in social intercourse, adhered to a task goal and showed ordered sequences of thought. An important finding was that those persons who had suffered marked social losses tended to perform worse on both the intelligence and personality tests.

Birren et al (1963) attributed their findings to the following factors:

- a slowing down of reaction time on numerous tests, which may be related to an overall decrease in cortical excitation
- the effect of social loss on psychosocial and cognitive performance
- the widespread effects of mild disease.

11 years later, a follow-up study was performed on the same group of subjects by Granick & Patterson (1971). They found:

- one-half of the men had died
- most (70%) of Group 2 had died
- most (63%) of Group 1 had survived.

The factors that were related to survival were higher intelligence, faster reaction time, better personality adaptation and lower social loss. However, there were two factors that, when taken together, correctly predicted 80% of the survivors and nonsurvivors:

- not smoking cigarettes
- greater organisation and planning of daily behaviour.

A technique for improving the planning of daily behaviour, called 'cognitive network analysis', will be described in Chapter 8. Thus the presence of even mild forms of disease results in quite significant changes in behaviour.

Similar findings with respect to the effects of cardiovascular disease on intellectual performance have been found by Wilkie & Eisdorfer (1974). In the absence of disease, intellectual abilities are affected by the general slowing down of psychomotor responses so that old people will perform less well on those tasks that incorporate a time factor. Also there is a tendency towards rigidity of thought. This occurs where individuals find it difficult to change their way of looking at the world. Other cognitive processes that have been said to suffer with ageing are memory and problem solving.

Not all people experience memory impairment with advancing age, but it becomes more common among older people. It seems that memory loss may be a result of difficulty of retrieving memorised events from the memory store and also the difficulty of putting the information to be stored into memory in the first place (Craik 1977).

There has been some discussion as to whether experience of life, obtained through age, is associated with better problem-solving ability. Denney & Palmer (1981) presented a series of very practical problems that people might have to deal with on an everyday basis, to people ranging in age from their 20s to their 70s. The best practical problem solvers were the people in their 40s and 50s, and with each further decade, the older groups performed progressively worse. Thus the experience of solving everyday problems gained with age only helps to a certain degree.

A recent study by Schaie & Willis (1986) reliably demonstrated that there was an element of cognitive decline in a sample of 229 subjects (aged 64–95 years) who had been observed over a 14-year period of time. The main purpose of the study was to investigate whether this decline could be reversed. Subjects' test performances on the Thurstone (1948) Reasoning and Spatial Orientation measures were classified as having remained stable or having declined over the prior 14-year interval (1970–1984). There were 107 (46.7%) subjects who had remained stable on both reasoning and spatial skills; 35 subjects (15%) had declined on reasoning; 37 subjects (16%) had declined on spatial skills; and 50 subjects (21.8%) had declined on both. Decline and stable subjects did not differ significantly on educational level or income.

The subjects were assigned to 5-hour training programmes on both abilities, and their responses were measured. The experimenters found that cognitive training techniques could reverse decline in a substantial number of adults in both reasoning and spatial skills. They also found that the training programmes enhanced the performance of many older persons who had remained stable over the 14-year period.

The results of this study suggest that:

- 46% of the subjects exhibited no decline on two primary mental abilities over a 14-year period.
- Those subjects that had demonstrated a decline in performance were able to reverse the deterioration given appropriate training programmes.
- Those subjects that had not experienced any decline in primary mental abilities also benefited from the training.

Schaie & Willis (1986) state:

Most importantly, our findings lend support to the contentions regarding the plasticity of behaviour into late adulthood. They suggest that for at least a substantial proportion of the community dwelling elderly, observed cognitive decline is not irreversible, is likely to be attributable to disuse, and can be subjected to environmental manipulations involving relatively simple and inexpensive educational training techniques.

Deterioration of intellectual functioning with age is not inevitable. Indeed there are large individual differences in performance. Despite a certain degree of uncertainty as to the causes of any decline in cognitive functioning, the most important point is that the situation is not permanent and can easily be reversed using simple, inexpensive training techniques (Schaie & Willis 1991).

The research data on the intellectual competence of the elderly has important implications for those health professionals who have frequent contact with old people. Firstly, intellectual competence does not necessarily decline with age and there is every chance that if a person has been intellectually 'active' during adulthood, then they will continue to be so during old age. A general feature of the ageing process is the need to take more time to perform various tasks. Therefore, the elderly should not be hurried into making decisions, but should be given time to work things through at their own speed. Where there is some deterioration in cognitive functioning, it may be necessary to provide simple training sessions in such things as planning and organising everyday events. Sometimes there may be problems with memory (encoding and retrieval). In these circumstances it is appropriate to investigate the use of aides-mémoire to facilitate recall. Many elderly people worry and get frustrated with memory dysfunction, so anything the health professional can do to alleviate this worry will prove useful. Overall, it is important to make the elderly feel competent to cope with the stresses and strains of everyday life, by reinforcement, training and understanding.

Social isolation

Old people may become isolated for a number of reasons. Often it is due to members of the family moving away from the area where the elderly person resides. But increasingly, and perhaps more disconcertingly, there is a tendency for old people to uproot, leave their families and long-term friends and move to warmer parts of the country to enjoy their retirement in comfort. If new friendships are not developed, elderly people may experience loneliness, uselessness and lower self-esteem. Also the availability of intimate contacts is positively related to the maintenance of psychological well-being

(Kahana 1982). Lowenthal & Haven (1968) interviewed 280 elderly people aged 60 years or older. They found that life crises, such as bereavement, were a lot easier to deal with if there is someone available in whom to confide.

Some psychologists believe that old people actively seek out isolation. *Disengagement theory* (Cumming & Henry 1961) states that elderly people gradually decrease their social contacts, give up their social roles and slowly fade out of the social scene and are happiest when allowed to do so. In contrast, *activity theory* (Havighurst et al 1968) states that the elderly have the same needs as they had in earlier life. Life circumstances may have brought about limitations in their social interaction but this is not their choosing and they would prefer to maintain their activity patterns for as long as possible.

Initial analysis of a study undertaken in the late 1950s (Neugarten et al 1980) provided support for the disengagement theory. Clearly, social participation declined with age and loss of occupational roles, but some individuals, it seemed, withdrew voluntarily from active involvement in social participation. Further analysis indicated that this interpretation of the data was oversimple. For instance, they found that those individuals who appeared disengaged in later life had been relatively uninvolved throughout adulthood. This represented continuity rather than change. Also, it was found that those with a low level of activity and social involvement did not necessarily enjoy life any more than other people in the study. Disengagement theory and activity theory, whilst describing some patterns of ageing should not be construed as adequate descriptions of normal, universal ageing, rather successful ageing relies on variability in personality and situational factors (Schaie & Willis 1991).

Measurement of social interaction

One of the problems associated with the study of interpersonal relationships in elderly people is the development of an objective measure of social interaction and isolation. Cohen & Sokolovsky (1979) used the technique of 'network analysis', as a descriptive tool, to illustrate the exact nature of the interrelationships between

a sample of elderly people and their friends, family and other acquaintances.

A social network refers to the people with whom one is likely to have some form of contact over a specified period of time. Network analysis was originally used by social anthropologists such as Barnes (1954) and Bott (1957) to aid them in their investigations of a Norwegian parish and a London neighbourhood. A network is similar to a communication diagram and indicates the nature of the relationships between people. As such, an individual's social network can be seen as a support system involving the 'giving and receiving of objects, services, social and emotional supports defined by the receiver and the giver as necessary or at least helpful in maintaining a style of life' (Lopata 1975).

Two sets of criteria are used to define social networks:

- *Interactional criteria*—frequency of interaction, duration of interaction, direction of flow, content of interaction. Some may be described as 'uniplex' relations, where links are represented by only one type of content, such as visiting, loans and health care; others may be described as 'multiplex' relations, which contain more than one content.
- *Morphological criteria*—the size, density and clustering of a network. Density refers to the ratio of actual links to potential ones; clustering refers to areas of high density.

The advantages of constructing social networks for a population of elderly people was demonstrated by Cohen & Sokolovsky (1979). They used network analysis in the investigation of the aged inhabitants of 11 mid-Manhattan 'hotels'. The single-room occupancy hotel houses large numbers of individuals with a wide range of mental, physical and social disorders. One neighbourhood agency serving elderly single-room occupancy residents reported that 31% of its clientele had a history of chronic alcoholism or mental illness, 15% were homebound and approximately 50% were in need of social and health services. There was little doubt that the majority of the residents needed some form of care, but were extremely reluctant to have any form of contact with the community services. Cohen & Sokolovsky (1979) claim that social network analysis can provide a number of useful functions for this particular population:

1. It introduces the community health and social services to the notion that their clients are not always socially isolated, but often have viable support networks. The networks of 96 hotel residents were mapped and it was found that the average number of contacts was 7.5, with more than half of these links involving multiplex relations. Further, 62% of the relationships occurred outside the hotel.

2. It enables staff to view behaviour in terms of an individual's social and physical environment. All too often the focus of community treatment has been seen in terms of the individual in need of help; network analysis helps to focus attention on the behavioural context (see Case History 7.1).

3. It enables resources to be allocated much more effectively. Elderly males who became ill, had fewer links with their families than healthy males. Males tended to have larger networks outside the hotels and women larger networks inside the hotels. Therefore it was important to concentrate on facilitating family links for males and also to concentrate one's efforts with females inside the hotel.

4. They found that the old people would form themselves into small groups often with as many as 6–11 'family members'. Each of these groups tended to have a leader, or mother, who took on the responsibility for providing food, support and a place to meet. These people had considerable influence over the other members of the group and were also found to be more

---

CASE HISTORY 7.2 MR R.

Mr R., a 74-year-old white male, had a history of severe emphysema, heart disease and difficulty walking. His life revolved around a 'stable-five-member beer-drinking quasi-group'. He was dependent on a Mr A. for groceries and cigarettes. Mr J. was another elderly male who was also dependent on Mr A. but had fewer health problems than Mr R. When Mr A. left the hotel, Mr R. still had a fully functioning social support group who were able to take on the responsibility for providing him with necessities. Mr R.'s health was worse than Mr J.'s, yet because he had an intact support group, he was able to remain in a noninstitutionalised environment.

---

receptive to the efforts of the community staff to provide care and information. Since the majority of the residents would have nothing to do with the community staff, it was essential that the staff identified the leaders and furnished them with appropriate resources. In this way it became possible to obtain access to people who otherwise would not have been part of the care system (see Case History 7.2).

5. The final advantage of network analysis refers to the disruption that might occur following a well-intentioned intervention. For example, offering to lend a person some money may result in the discontinuation of ties with neighbours who not only lend the person money, but also provide important conversation and emotional support. Before providing an individual with care it is necessary to assess the degree of social support provided by the network. Inadvertent intervention may result in the disruption of the support network and the consequent dependence of the individual on the care specialist.

In the case of the inner-city elderly hotel population, network analysis can be demonstrated to be an effective clinical tool. However, the same principles can be applied to elderly populations in different environmental contexts with equivalent success. Indeed, the analysis of social networks and social support is useful in a wide variety of contexts as we have already seen. Whether a formal network analysis is used or not, the more information one has about the nature of interpersonal links in the community,

---

CASE HISTORY 7.1 MRS R.

Mrs R., a 66-year-old white female, was consuming increasing amounts of alcohol. Much of the increase in the consumption of drink seemed to be due to the death of her husband. Initially, it was thought that her personality was at fault in some way, but close analysis of her social network revealed that the death of her husband had resulted in her becoming friendly with a group of individuals who used to drink a lot when they met. It became clear that involvement with this group was partially responsible for her increased drinking.

the more this will result in an efficient provision of health care for the elderly.

CONCLUSION

The developmental model presents a unique perspective on health behaviour. It enables us to gain information concerning the process of development, from infancy to old age, and it highlights some of the problems that are associated with child development in particular. Further, it illustrates that people will behave in significantly different ways according to age and stage of development. Unfortunately there is not room to discuss all the features of the developmental approach that are important for health care professionals, but it is hoped that the areas mentioned have indicated the relevance of a developmental analysis of behaviour and that the reader will be encouraged to pursue the topics further.

REFERENCES

Accredolo L P, Hake J L 1982 Infant perception. In: Wolman B B (ed) Handbook of developmental psychology. Prentice-Hall, Englewood Cliffs NJ

Ahrens R 1954 Beitrage zur Entwicklung des Physiognomie und Mimikerkemmers. Zeitschrift für Experimentelle und Angewandte Psychologie 2: 412–494, 599–633

Ainsworth M D S 1967 Infancy in Uganda. Johns Hopkins University Press, Baltimore

Ainsworth M D S, Blehar M, Waters E, Wall S 1978 Patterns of attachment. Erlbaum, Hillsdale NJ

Andrews S R, Blumenthal J B, Johnson D et al 1982 The skills of mothering: a study of parent–child development centers. Monographs of the Society for Research in Child Development 47: (Whole No 198)

Barnard K E, Bee H L, Hammond M A 1984 Developmental changes in maternal interactions with term and preterm infants. Infant Behaviour and Development 7: 101–113

Barnes J 1954 Class and committees in a Norwegian island parish. Human Relations 7: 39–58

Bell R Q 1974 Contributions of human infants to caregiving and social interaction. In: Lewis M, Rosenblum L A (eds) The effect of the infant on its caregiver. Wiley, London

Bibace R, Walsh M E 1979 Developmental stages in children's conception of illness. In: Stone G C, Cohen F, Adler N E (eds) Health psychology. Jossey Bass, New York

Bibace R, Walsh M E 1980 Development of children's concepts of illness. Pediatrics 66: 912–917

Birren J E, Butler R N, Greenhouse S W, Sokoloff L, Yarrow M R 1963 (eds) Human aging: a biological and behavioural study. HSM 71-9051, US Government Printing Office, Washington DC

Boakes R A 1987 Eating habits. Wiley, London

Bohlin G, Hagekull B, Lindhager K 1981 Dimensions of infant behaviour. Infant Behaviour and Development 4: 83–96

Borke H 1975 Piaget's mountains revisited: changes in the egocentric landscape. Developmental Psychology 11: 240–243

Bott E 1957 Family and social networks. Tavistock, London

Bower T G R 1989 The perceptual world of the new-born child. In: Slater A, Bremner G (eds) Infant development. Erlbaum, London

Bowlby J 1951 Maternal care and mental health. World Health Organization, Geneva

Bowlby J 1969 Attachment and loss Vol 1: Attachment. Hogarth Press, London

Bowlby J 1973 Attachment and loss Vol 2: Separation, anxiety, and anger. Hogarth Press, London

Bowlby J 1980 Attachment and loss Vol 3: Loss, sadness and depression. Basic Books, New York

Bremner J G 1988 Infancy. Basil Blackwell, London

Buss A H, Plomin R 1984 Temperament: early developing personality traits. Erlbaum, New Jersey

Clarke A M, Clarke A D B 1976 (eds) Early experience. Open Books, London

Clarke-Stewart K A 1973 Interactions between mothers and their young children: characteristics and consequences. Monographs of the Society for Research in Child Development 38 (Whole No 153)

Cohen C I, Sokolovsky J 1979 Clinical use of network analysis for psychiatric and aged populations. Community Mental Health Journal 15: 203–213

Corso J F 1987 Sensory-perceptual processes and aging. In: Schaie K W (ed) Annual review of gerontology and geriatrics. Springer, New York, vol 7

Cowart B J 1981 Development of taste perception in humans: sensitivity and preference throughout the life span. Psychological Bulletin 90: 43–73

Craik F I M 1977 Age differences in human memory. In: Birren J E, Schaie K W (eds) Handbook of the psychology of aging. Van Nostrand Reinhold, New York

Craik F I M 1986 A functional account of age differences in memory. In: Klix F, Hagendorf H (eds) Human memory and cognitive capabilities. Elsevier, Amsterdam

Cumming E, Henry W E 1961 Growing old: the process of disengagement. Basic Books, New York

Dayton C D Jnr, Jones M H, Giu P et al 1964 Developmental study of coordinated eye movements in the human infant: 1 Visual activity in the newborn human: a study based on induced auto-kinetic nystagmus recorded by electrooculography. Archives of Ophthalmology 71: 856–870

DeCasper A J, Fifer W P 1980 Of human bonding: newborns prefer their mothers' voices. Science 208: 1174–1176

Denney N W, Palmer A P 1981 Adult age differences on traditional and practical problem-solving measures. Journal of Gerontology 36: 323–328

Dollard J, Miller N E 1950 Personality and psychotherapy. McGraw-Hill, New York

Donaldson M 1978 Children's minds. Fontana, London

Douglas J W B 1975 Early hospital admissions and later disturbances of behavior and learning. Developmental Medicine and Child Neurology 17: 456–480

Egeland B, Sroufe L A 1981 Attachment and maltreatment. Child Development 52: 44–52

Engen T 1982 The perception of odors. Academic Press, New York

Engen T, Lipsitt L P, Peck M B 1974 Ability of newborn infants to discriminate sapid substances. Developmental Psychology 10: 741–746

Fielding D 1985 Chronic illness in children. In: Watts F (ed) New directions in clinical psychology. Wiley/BPS, Chichester

Fishbein H D, Lewis S, Keiffer K 1972 Children's understanding of spatial relations: coordination of perspectives. Developmental Psychology 7: 21–33

Flavell J H, Botkin P T, Fry C L, Wright J W, Jarvis P E 1968 The development of role taking and communication skills in children. Wiley, New York

Fogel A 1984 Infancy: infant, family and society. West Publishing, St Paul

Fozard J L, Wolf E, Bell B, McFarland R A, Podoisky S 1977 Visual perception and communication. In: Birren J E, Schaie K W (eds) A handbook of the psychology of aging. Van Nostrand Reinhold, New York

Fozard J L 1990 Vision and hearing in aging. In: Birren J E, Schaie K W (eds) Handbook of the psychology of aging 3rd edn. Academic Press, New York

Ganchrow J R, Steiner J E, Daher M 1983 Neonatal facial expressions in response to different qualities and intensities of gustatory stimuli. Infant Behaviour and Development 6: 189–200

Gardner H 1982 Developmental psychology, 2nd edn. Little Brown, Boston

Gewirtz J L 1965 The course of infant smiling in four child-rearing environments in Israel. In: Foss B M (ed) Determinants of infant behaviour. Methuen, London, vol 3

Goldfarb W 1943 Effects of early institutional care on adolescent personality. Journal of Experimental Education 12: 106–129

Goldsmith H H, Campos J J 1982 Toward a theory of infant temperament. In: Emde R N, Harmon R J (eds) The development of attachment and affiliative systems. Plenum, New York

Granick S, Patterson (eds) 1971 Human aging II: an eleven year follow up biomedical behavioural study. Pub No HSM 71-9037. US Government Printing Office, Washington

Granick W, Kleban M H, Weiss A D 1976 Relationships between hearing loss and cognition in normally hearing aged persons. Journal of Gerontology 31: 434–440

Grossman K, Thane K, Grossman K E 1981 Maternal tactual contact of the newborn after various post-partum conditions of mother–infant contact. Developmental Psychology 17: 158–169

Gustafson G E, Harris K L 1990 Women's responses to young infants' cries. Developmental Psychology 26: 144–152

Harlow H F 1958 The nature of love. American Psychologist 13: 673–685

Havighurst R J, Neugarten B, Tobin S S 1968 Disengagement and patterns of aging. In: Neugarten B (ed) Middle age and aging. University of Chicago Press, Chicago

Haynes H, White B L, Held R 1965 Visual accommodation in human infants. Science 148: 328–330

Hubert N C, Weeks T, Peters-Martin P, Gandour N J 1982 The study of early temperament: measurement and conceptual issues. Child Development 55: 571–600

Hughes M, Donaldson M 1983 The use of hiding games for studying coordination of viewpoints. In: Donaldson M, Grieve R, Pratt C (eds) Early childhood development and education. Blackwell, Oxford

Huyck M H, Hoyer W J 1982 Adult development and aging. Wadsworth, Belmont CA

James W 1961 (originally pub 1892) Psychology: the briefer course. Harper Row, New York

Kagan J 1979 The growth of the child. Methuen, London

Kahana B 1982 Social behaviour and aging. In: Wolman B B (ed) Handbook of developmental psychology. Prentice-Hall, Englewood Cliffs NJ

Keith R W 1975 Middle ear function in neonates. Archives of Otolaryngology 101: 375–379

Kempe R S, Kempe H 1981 Child abuse. Fontana/Open Books, London

Kenshalo D R 1977 Age changes in touch, vibration, temperature, kinesthetics, and pain sensitivity. In: Birren J E, Schaie K W (eds) Handbook of the psychology of aging. Van Nostrand Reinhold, New York

Klaus H M, Kennell J H 1976 Maternal–infant bonding. Mosby, St Louis

Korner A F, Hutchinson C A, Kopeski J A, Kraemer H C, Schneider P A 1981 Stability of individual differences of neonatal motor and crying patterns. Child Development 52: 83–90

Lipsitt L P, Engen T, Kaye H 1963 Developmental changes in the olfactory threshold of the neonate. Child Development 34: 371–376

Lopata H 1975 Support systems of the elderly: Chicago of the 1970s. Gerontologist 15: 35–41

Lowenthal M, Haven C 1968 Interaction and adaptation: intimacy as a critical variable. American Sociological Review 33: 20–30

Macfarlane A 1977 The psychology of childbirth. Open Books, London

Makin J W, Porter R H 1989 Attractiveness of lactating females' breast odors to neonates. Child Development 60: 803–811

Meltzoff A N, Borton R W 1979 Intermodal matching by human neonates. Nature 282: 403–404

Moskowitz H R, Kumaraiah V, Sharma K N, Jacobs H L, Sharma S D 1975 Cross-cultural differences in simple taste preferences. Science 190: 1217–1218

Neugarten N et al 1980 Personality in middle and late life. Arno, New York

Niven N 1986 Children's conception of illness. Paper presented to 'The doctor, the patient, the illness' conference. University of Durham

O'Connor S, Vietze P M, Sandier H M, Sherrod K B, Attemeier W A 1980 Quality of parenting and the mother–infant relationships following rooming-in. In: Taylor P M (ed) Parent–infant relationships. Grune Stratton, New York

Parmelee A H 1986 Children's illnesses: their beneficial effects on behavioural development. Child Development 57: 1–10

Paton D, Craig J A 1974 Cataracts: development, diagnosis, management. CIBA Clinical Symposia 26: 1–32

Perrin E C, Gerrity P S 1981 There's a demon in your belly: children's understanding of illness. Pediatrics 67: 841–849

Piaget J 1953 The origins of intelligence in the child. Routledge Kegan Paul, London

Piaget J 1970 Piaget's theory. In:Mussen P H (ed) Carmichael's manual of child psychology, 3rd edn. Wiley, London

Piaget J, Inhelder B 1956 The child's conception of space. Routledge Kegan Paul, London

Pinneau S 1955 The infantile disorder of hospitalism and anaclitic depression. Psychological Bulletin 52: 429–452

Provence S, Coleman R 1957 Environmental retardation (hospitalism) in infants living in families. Pediatrics 19: 285–292

Quinton D, Rutter M 1976 Early hospital admissions and later disturbances of behaviour: an attempted replication of Douglas's findings. In: Clarke A M, Clarke A D B (eds) Early experience. Open Books, London

Rheingold H L 1956 The modification of social responsiveness in institutional babies. Monographs of the Society for Research in Child Development 21: No 2 (Whole No 63)

Rothbart M K 1981 Measurement of temperament in infancy. Child Development 52: 569–578

Rothbart M K 1986 Longitudinal observation of infant temperament. Developmental Psychology 22: 356–365

Rovee C K, Cohen R Y, Shlapack W 1975 Life-span stability in olfactory sensitivity. Developmental Psychology 11: 311–318

Rutter M 1976 Parent–child separation: psychological effects on the children. In: Clarke A M, Clarke A D B (eds) Early experience. Open Books, London

Rutter M 1978 Early sources of security and competence. In: Bruner J S, Garten A (eds) Human growth and development. Oxford University Press, London

Rutter M 1981 Maternal deprivation reassessed, 2nd edn. Penguin, Harmondsworth

Rutter M 1987 Psychosocial resilience and protective mechanisms. American Journal of Orthopsychiatry 57: 316–331

Salzen E A 1963 Visual stimuli eliciting the smiling response in the human infant. Journal of Genetic Psychology 102: 51–54

Schaffer H R 1971 The growth of sociability. Penguin, Harmondsworth

Schaffer H R 1977 Mothering. Fontana/Open Books, London

Schaffer H R 1991 Early social development. In: Woodhead M, Carr R, Light P (eds) Becoming a person. Open University/Routledge, London

Schaffer H R, Callender W M 1959 Psychologic effects of hospitalisation in infancy. Pediatrics 24: 528–539

Schaffer H R, Emerson P E 1964 The development of social attachments in infancy. Monographs for the Society for Research in Child Development 29: No 3 (Whole No 94)

Schaie K W, Willis S L 1986 Can decline in adult intellectual functioning be reversed? Developmental Psychology 22: 223–232

Schaie K W, Willis S L 1991 Adult development and aging, 3rd edn. Harper Collins, New York

Schumaker S S, Reizenstein J E 1982 Environmental factors affecting impatient stress in acute care hospitals. In: Evans G W (ed) Environmental stress. Cambridge University Press, Cambridge

Smart M S, Smart R C 1982 Children: development and relationships, 4th edn. Macmillan, London

Spitz R A 1945 Hospitalism: an enquiry into the genesis of psychiatric conditions in early childhood. Psychoanalytic Study of the Child 1: 53–74

Steiner J E 1979 Human facial expressions in response to taste and smell stimulation. In: Reese H E, Lipsitt L (eds) Advances in child development and behaviour. Academic Press, New York, vol 13

Strehler B L 1977 Time, cells and aging, 2nd edn. Academic Press, New York

Thomas A, Chess S, Birch H G 1970 The origin of personality. Scientific American 223: 102–109

Thomas A, Chess S 1977 Temperament and development. Brunner/Mazel, New York

Thompson R A, Lamb M R, Estes D 1982 Stability of infant–mother attachment and its relationship to changing life circumstances in an unselected middle class sample. Child Development 52: 1341–1343

Thurstone L L 1948 Primary mental abilities. University of Chicago Press, Chicago

Tizard B 1977 Adoption: a second chance. Open Books, London

Tizard B 1991 Working mothers and the care of young children. In: Woodhead M, Light P, Carr R (eds) Growing up in a changing society. Open University/Routledge, London

Tizard B, Hodges J 1978 The effect of early institutional rearing on the development of eight-year-old children. Journal of Child Psychology and Psychiatry 19: 99–118

Vaughn B E, Egeland B, Sroufe L A, Waters E 1979 Individual differences in infant–mother attachment at twelve and eighteen months: stability and change in families under stress. Child Development 50: 971–975

Vuyk R 1981 Overview and critique of Piaget's genetic epistemology 1965–1980. Academic Press, London

Ward-Platt M 1986 Personal communication

Weber R A, Levitt M I, Clark M C 1986 Individual variation in attachment security and strange situation behaviour: the role of maternal and infant temperament. Child Development 57: 56–65

Wilkie F, Eisdorfer C 1974 Terminal changes in intelligence. In: Palmore, E (ed) Normal aging II. Duke University Press, Durham NC

Wolff P H 1969 The natural history of crying and other vocalisations in early infancy. In: Foss B M (ed) Determinants of infant behaviour. Methuen, London, vol 4

Wright P, Macleod H A, Cooper M J 1983 Waking at night: the effect of early feeding experience. Child Care Health and Development 9: 309–319

RECOMMENDED READING

Eiser C 1985 The psychology of childhood illness. Springer-Verlag, New York
  This is very much a research orientated book. It contains a number of studies investigating many different aspects of childhood illness, but reading through the research is well worth the effort.
Kaplan P S 1991 A child's odyssey: child and adolescent development, 2nd edn. West, St. Paul
  There are many, many texts on child development. I have tried to select one that I think contains good, solid research and yet is easy to read. However, if your library does not have this particular text do not be afraid to consult others.
Paton D, Brown S 1991 Lifespan health psychology, nursing problems and interventions. Harper Collins, London
  As the title suggests this book takes a life span perspective to human development, starting with young children and finishing with old age. Each chapter starts with a case study and then goes on to investigate the relevance of health psychology to each case.

Schaie K W, Willis S 1991 Adult development and aging, 3rd edn. Harper Collins, New York
  This text also includes sections on adulthood. It covers many aspects of ageing such as personality, motivation, learning and memory, death and bereavement. It is written by two people who have contributed a great deal of research to the study of old age.

Bee H 1985 The developing child. Harper Row, New York
Clarke A M, Clarke A D B 1976 (eds) Early experience. Open Books, London
Kimmel D C 1980 Adulthood and aging, 2nd edn. Wiley, New York
Schaffer H R 1977 Mothering. Fontana/Open Books, London
Sugarman L 1986 Life-span development: concepts, theories and interventions. Methuen, London

8

Ecology, environment and culture

Environmental psychology may be defined as the study of human behaviour in its physical setting. This definition encompasses a wide range of topics such as crowding, noise, temperature, pollution and the interplay between the design of buildings and its effect on our psychological well-being. Another neglected area of psychology has been an analysis of culture's influence on human behaviour. The majority of psychological studies have used Western subjects in Western contexts. If the prediction of human behaviour is an important goal of psychology, then it must be the prediction of all human behaviour and not just American and European behaviour.

The interrelationship between environment and health has been a concern of epidemiologists for many years. Until recently, however, psychologists have tended to neglect the role of the environment in determining behaviour. Bronfenbrenner (1979) cites a study by Larson (1975) that examined 902 published papers in the Journals of Child Development, Developmental Psychology and Journal of Genetic Psychology between the years 1972 and 1974. Larson found that 76% of the studies were conducted in the psychological laboratory, whereas only 8% were carried out in 'natural settings'. Within the last decade there has been a shift towards ecological approaches to explaining behaviour. It has manifested itself in cross-cultural psychology (Berry 1976), developmental psychology (Bronfenbrenner 1979), perception (Gibson 1979), animal behaviour (Davey 1990), community psychology (Orford 1992) and also in the field of health psychology (Moos 1979).

The terms environmental psychology and ecological psychology seem to be similar but there are important differences. Environmental psychology may be defined as the study of human behaviour in its physical setting. This definition encompasses a wide range of topics such as: crowding, noise, temperature, pollution and the interplay between the design of buildings and its effect on our psychological well-being. Regardless of the specific context, environmental psychology views behaviour as an interaction between man and his environment, rather than a phenomenon wholly explicable in intrapsychic terms.

The first studies were concerned with the influence of ward design on patient behaviour in mental hospitals (Osmond 1957). During the 1960s the research field expanded to include psycho-architectural studies of people's perceptions of space and design in the inner city (Lynch 1960), crowding and territoriality in rats (Calhoun 1962), and the anthropology of space (proxemics) (Hall 1966). At the end of the 1960s a new journal, Environment and Behaviour, was launched, whose variety of papers reflected the interdisciplinary nature of the field.

Ecological psychology has a different background. It was pioneered by Roger Barker borrowing from the theories of Kurt Lewin and Egon Brunswick. Barker and his colleagues defined ecological psychology as 'dealing with naturalistic studies of a person's everyday behaviour and his or her psychological situation' (Barker et al 1977). The initial focus was upon evaluating children's psychological situations, that is, observers' descriptions of the influences of parents, teachers and other children on the child they were studying. Barker extended his approach to include an analysis of 'behaviour settings'. These were defined as independent behavioural events that occurred at specific times in community life (a lecture, annual general meeting or a football match). This extension of the theory came to be known as eco-behavioural science. Barker views behaviour settings as comprising: physical properties, human components and programmes. For Barker, environmental psychology is concerned with the physical properties of settings and can be described as one aspect of eco-behavioural science.

A neglected area of psychology has been an analysis of culture's influence on human behaviour. The majority of psychological studies have used Western subjects in Western contexts. If the prediction of human behaviour is an important goal of psychology then it must be the prediction of all human behaviour and not just American and European behaviour. In relation to health psychology, it is necessary for health professionals to have some idea of the ways in which culture can affect thinking, perception and communication.

One of the main contributions to health psychology has been the social-ecological model of Moos. The first section of the chapter describes his model, gives an example of how it can explain the interaction between individuals and their environment and finally looks at the practical implications of the model. The second section looks at a different way of approaching the relationship between environment and health behaviour. Instead of developing a model and applying it to specific circumstances, it is also useful to select an area of concern, such as the design of hospitals, and illustrate how the concepts of environmental psychology can be used to promote health care. The third section examines some features of culture's influence on behaviour and attempts to provide health professionals with a guide to the problems of communication and understanding the behaviour of different cultural groups.

SOCIAL ECOLOGY
A model

Moos (1976, 1979) presents a model designed to illustrate the relationship between environmental and physical variables and health status. The model consists of six elements: environmental system, personal system, cognitive appraisal, degree of activation or arousal, efforts at adaptation or coping and finally health status and health-related behaviour.

Environmental system

There are many ways to interpret and categorise the environment. Moos has decided to categorise environmental variables into:

- *Physical setting.* Where you live can affect your health. Temperature, rainfall and pollution, as well as architectural design characteristics, are important variables in health behaviour. Hollander & Yeastros (1963) studied the pain sensations of arthritic patients who were exposed to a controlled experimental climate. They found that a 'stormlike pressure and humidity' produced increasingly negative reports of symptoms. Evans & Jacobs (1984) reviewed the research on the health effects of air pollution. They concluded that photo-chemical oxidants (smog), sulphur oxides, nitrogen oxides and carbon monoxide have all been associated with health disorders, but they point to one or two methodological shortcomings of some of the studies in their review.
- *Organisational factors.* The work setting has an impact upon people's health. Smaller psychiatric hospitals were found to have higher rates of discharge than larger ones, even when such factors as background and personality characteristics and conditions of ward facilities were considered (Linn 1970). Organisational issues are reviewed in considerable detail in the next chapter.
- *Human aggregate.* This factor refers to the various characteristics of the people inhabiting a particular environment, such as age, ability, background etc. Social epidemiology, particularly when it is concerned with the study of a cluster of average background characteristics of an environment, is synonymous with this factor.
- *Social climate.* There are three categories in this area:
  - relationship dimensions assess the extent to which people are involved with each other and support each other
  - personal growth dimensions assess self-actualisation and enhancement
  - system maintenance and change refer to

the degree of structure in a particular environment and the maintenance of control and change.

Personal system

The features that describe this category are such things as age, socioeconomic status, sex, intelligence, cognitive and emotional development, self-esteem and previous coping experiences. These factors affect the meaning of a particular situation for an individual and relate to the psychological resources available to confront such situations. Other personal variables are attitudes, values, expectations and one's 'role' (people who have responsible roles tend to perceive organisations as more beneficial than those who do not have a responsible role). These variables, taken together, influence the individual's perception of the environment. A person with a heart condition, working on the sixth floor with no lift would view this in a different way to a healthy person.

Mediating factors

Appraisal. The role of cognitive appraisal in the experience of stress has been discussed in Chapter 4. In this context, the construct's meaning is essentially the same. Whilst one may measure the direct effects of an environment on health such as air pollution, it is the way an environment is perceived by a person that is critical in determining the extent of the deleterious effects.

Activation. If the environment is perceived as requiring some action, an individual may set in motion a response designed to restructure the environmental threat. An example might be where a person perceives an office environment to be a health threat due to the number of workers smoking. Activation would involve some degree of segregation or a ban on smoking in the presence of non-smokers.

Adaptation. In numerous circumstances, it may prove impossible to activate some change and so the individual may have to adapt to the environmental threat. The person may tend to deny the seriousness of the situation or even seek to discover evidence which minimises the perceived threat. A non-smoker might have no opportunity to change her situation and may have to accept it. Under these circumstances, dissonance is reduced by rehearsing arguments for the limited health consequences of a polluted environment.

Health status and health-related behaviour

Moos (1976) proposes that an individual's health status and health-related behaviour can be indexed according to:

- the onset and subsequent development of an illness
- the course of an illness and the outcome of the treatment programme
- the degree to which the health services are utilised and the degree to which the individual complies with therapeutic regimens
- functional effectiveness
- satisfaction and well-being.

In assessing the overall effectiveness and relevance of Moos's model it has to be said that some elements of the model are vague and difficult to conceptualise. However, to help make the operation of the model clearer, he provides an analysis of how it can organise and help us understand the research in one particular area (population density and crowding). A 'concrete' example will be useful in clarifying the operational effectiveness of the model.

Population density and crowding

It is important to distinguish between density and crowding (Paulus 1980). Population density refers to measures of outside density such as the number of people per acre. Crowding refers to measures of inside density such as the number of people per unit of living space. But there is an important third factor which is the social perception of crowding and refers to an individual's feelings of being crowded. For example a person in a large crowd at a football match or a rock festival may enjoy the experience. In contrast, a person in a crowded shopping mall at Christmas may detest the experience. Density may be equally high in both situations but negative feelings associated with crowding only occur in the latter.

Let us examine how the model of Moos conceptualises the relationships between density, crowding and health.

Environmental factors

Physical setting. Levy & Herzog (1974) found associations between population density and overall age-adjusted death rate, age-adjusted male death rate for heart disease, admissions to general and mental hospitals, illegitimate births and divorce.

Galle et al (1972) studied four components of population density and crowding in Chicago:

- the number of persons per room
- the number of rooms per housing unit
- the number of housing units per residential structure
- the number of residential structures per acre.

They found a relationship between these four components and fertility, delinquency and mental hospital admission rates. Another approach has been to interview the residents themselves.

Booth (1976) investigated crowding at both the dwelling unit and the neighbourhood level in Toronto. He found that indexes of household crowding were related to the extent to which parents hit their children, to the numbers of quarrels reported by mothers and to the quality of the relationship between spouses. They also noted that objectively crowded neighbourhoods were more likely to produce greater incidences of extramarital and incestuous relationships. Care must be taken in interpreting these results as there are other factors which are very likely to be associated with these variables as well as crowding. Evans et al (1989) found that serious residential crowding in inner cities could result in withdrawal and the breakdown of support networks leading to a decline in psychological health.

Epstein (1982) reports that crowded living has widely variable effects on behaviour. He cites a study by Mitchell (1971) relating inside density to measures of stress, entertainment patterns, emotional health and parental supervision. The people in the higher density dwellings rated themselves as less happy and more worried than people in lower density units. Also those individuals who were living on the upper floors of buildings, were more likely to complain of headaches, nervousness and insomnia.

Moos (1979) states that 'crowded conditions can affect health directly (through interpersonal contact) and indirectly (through their effect on emotional resources and coping abilities).' Further, he suggests that the physical setting can be altered to mitigate the effects of density and crowding. Providing gardens, balconies and more open spaces can help; also more pictures, partitions and the shapes of the rooms themselves may influence the perceptual and behavioural effects of crowding.

Some of the problems with the diverse findings on crowding may be a result of cultural differences. Gillis et al (1986) have found that culture affects perceptions of density. British subjects reported more strain than Asian subjects when room density was increased.

Organisational factors. Moos (1979) suggests that social density (the size or number of people in a group) is an important factor in determining the effects of crowding. Paulus et al (1978) found that higher social density led to more illness complaints, higher blood pressure and increased numbers of psychiatric admissions. However, Moos cites the work of Kasl (1977) who illustrated the importance of how the dwelling space was organised; it was not so much the level of dwelling unit density that was important, but the way in which the space was used.

Human aggregate. Social interaction and the level of interpersonal proximity mediate the effects of crowding. MacDonald & Oden (1973) investigated three married couples living together in a room 30 ft square for 12 weeks. The couples were doing this to try to simulate possible hardship conditions that they might experience during their Peace Corps assignment. MacDonald

& Oden found that because the couples developed a high degree of cooperation with each other and experienced a high degree of decisional control over their environment, the couples in fact showed the positive effects of crowding, that is 'they showed enhanced marital relationships, were chosen as socio-emotional leaders by other volunteers, and regretted leaving their accommodation more than those who had been living in hotel accommodation'.

Social climate. Socially cohesive groups have the capacity to mitigate harmful effects of high density. In studies of dormitory crowding by Karlin et al (1978), individuals were found to experience more stress, act more competitively, show poorer performance in exams and feel more helpless. However, Baum et al (1975) noted that cohesive student groups in a crowded dormitory experienced less stress and reported feeling less crowded than colleagues who had not formed themselves into such groups.

These contradictory results may be understood with reference to perceived control and the interpersonal relationships between the residents. Living in a crowded dormitory need not be so bad if people get on well together and determine as a group to try to do something to make the crowded conditions better. One of the reasons why the effects of living in family residences differ from living in dormitories is that there is often more control and cooperation in family residences. In contrast, in dormitories containing young adults, there is usually less control and less cooperation.

Person-related factors

Moos (1979) says that there is evidence for three sets of variables that have considerable influence in mediating the impact of the environment on health:

- *Sociodemographic variables.* Age, sex and socioeconomic status have been found to be related to crowding and health. Kasl (1977) suggested that women and young children are particularly influenced by the effects of crowding. Also people with lower education and income are more affected by population density and other environmental stressors.

• *Stress and impairment factors*. Edwards & Booth (1977) found that family relationships were affected by dwelling unit density and that these relationships were put under even more pressure by the presence of stress.

• *Biological risk factors*. Moos (1979) regards this area as being under-researched but cites a study by Szklo et al (1976) who found that household crowding acted as a risk factor for myocardial infarction among women, only when a history of hypertension, angina pectoris or diabetes was present.

In general people who are disabled, impaired or under stress are more likely to be influenced by environmental conditions. A review of the literature by Cohen et al (1979a) concluded that certain groups in society were more vulnerable to population density and crowding (very young/old, low income/education and those under stress).

ENVIRONMENT

Cognitive appraisal of the environment

There are two main models that have been put forward to account for the ways in which individuals appraise and cope with the environment:

Information overload. Cohen (1978) has proposed that we have a limited capacity to process information. We can only take in so much at a time. When there are too many inputs and our capacity to deal with them is exceeded, information overload occurs. Social density leads to information overload because we are unable to gain a clear image of the situation. Saegert (1985) distinguishes between information overload and decisional overload. The latter concept involves responding to complex, unpredictable tasks in a high density environment. Both information and decisional, load lead to an increase in arousal and stress.

Behavioural constraint. This second model proposed by Altman (1978) emphasises the importance of maintaining personal control over the environment. It states that when individuals feel that they have no control over a particular situation, then they are likely to experience high stress levels. In the context of crowding, the model focuses on reduced freedom of choice and loss of behavioural options. It should be emphasised that it is the individual's perception of the event that is important not the event itself. The importance of perceived control was illustrated by Rodin et al (1979). In a densely packed lift, those people who were standing by the control panel felt less crowded and actually thought the lift was larger than those standing away from the panel.

A way of reducing the deleterious effects of overload and behavioural constraint is to use the technique of cognitive network analysis mentioned in the previous chapter. The realisation that events and actions can be ordered and structured in a parallel fashion not only reduces the overload but also leads to feelings of increased control.

Adaptation and coping

If people are faced with information overload, they are unable to deal with all the inputs at the same time, therefore some of the inputs have to be neglected in order to cope with the situation. Cohen (1978) has suggested that the inputs that tend to be sacrificed are those that refer to other people, that is, we tend to focus our attention on items that are relevant to ourselves first and then go on to respond to other social and non-social cues expressed, often subtly, by others. This means that, under crowded conditions, we pay less attention to such things as helping behaviour and responding to others' needs in a truly empathic fashion.

Other methods of coping and adaptation include withdrawal and isolation, a greater degree of passivity and helplessness and feeling at the mercy of the environment. Saegert (1978) lists six coping mechanisms:

• reducing the number of decisions made
• engaging in more routine activities
• avoiding new situations

- relying on easily observable interpersonal cues
- organising the environment into large, diffuse units
- relying on religious or political groups for information.

There seems to be a tendency to relinquish personal control over the environment and rely increasingly on simple, structured, formal authoritarian routines to reduce cognitive complexity. Moos's model is useful in that it provides a conceptual structure for understanding the rather complex interrelationships between environment, health and behaviour. It enables one to select specific variables, fit them into the model and analyse the results. In this context it is useful for health professionals who wish to gain a better understanding of health behaviour.

There are practical implications that emanate from such an analysis:

- There is a need to analyse environments in terms of their effects on human behaviour. Architects and all those responsible for planning and designing our environment need to consider how their structures affect human behaviour.
- Individuals need to be taught how to exert more control or, as Cohen et al (1979a) put it, 'to enhance people's sense of control over their environment'. People also need to be given information about the psychological consequences of crowded living. Langer (1984) found that providing information that explained people's experiences and feelings resulted in reducing the emotional and behavioural consequences of crowding.
- The main contribution of the work of Moos is to concentrate our attention on changing the social climate. If health professionals are to make significant advances in the area of prevention, then they should recognise the important role of social organisation within the community. There is a need to develop cohesion and support so that communities become more competent at dealing with the pressures of everyday life. Empowering community groups to take more

control over their health care needs a careful analysis of the relationships between the individuals themselves and their environmental circumstances. The advantage of Moos's model is that it enables such an analysis to be made, but it is only the first step in a process designed to facilitate health and well-being. Having identified the problems the next stage is to do something about them. Methods of accomplishing problem resolution are discussed in the next chapter.

Applied environmental psychology

A contrasting approach to developing a model of social ecology and investigating how it may be applied to specific health concerns is to take a particular health environment, such as a hospital and determine how the research of environmental psychology can be applied to bring about a more enlightened understanding of the effects of that environment on health, physical comfort, stress and pain.

The hospital environment

DiMatteo & Friedman (1982) state that hospitals have always had a negative reputation and that this largely stems from them not being particularly hospitable places. They suggest that the problem is not just their association with disease but the nature of the hospital environment itself.

The hospital is one of the few places where people forfeit almost all control over their life . . . Patients must operate according to the schedule of the hospital and follow its rules, with little chance for individuality.

DiMatteo & Friedman (1982)

Another source of negative feelings towards hospitals can stem from their past associations. Wainwright (1985) states '. . . any nurse who has worked in older English hospitals situated in buildings which once housed the local workhouse will be familiar with the reluctance (and occasionally utter refusal) of elderly patients to be admitted to what was once a place of disgrace and social stigma'.

On the basis of these two quotations, it appears

that, even before people are admitted to hospitals, their perceptions of the institutions are negative. It is very important, therefore, to examine how the hospital environment can be altered to improve its standing in the eyes of the general population and to investigate the effects of the environment on the psychological correlates of health. Some of the issues that have generated concern are privacy, physical comfort and the symbolic meaning of the environment.

Privacy

Wainwright (1985) suggests that the issues of individuality and control are brought together by the concept of privacy and that the extent to which it is possible to maintain a sense of privacy is largely determined by the nature of the architectural environment. The main features of the architectural environment that affect privacy are size of rooms, number of occupants, whether there is a door that can be closed, sound insulation, the provision of screens, bathroom and toilet facilities, control of heating, lighting and ventilation. Lack of privacy, apart from causing patients to become irritable, can be a cause of anxiety and contribute to the perception of pain (Wainwright 1985).

Altman (1975) has argued that the provision of privacy is critical to an individual's health and well-being. Hospital settings limit patient privacy and thereby increase levels of stress. In some instances it is difficult to reconcile the needs of medical staff with the needs of patients. Jaco (1979) found that patients in radially designed wards complained about lack of privacy, although this design was congruent with nurses' needs for easy access and monitoring of patients. Duffy et al (1986) said that those who design facilities for others often ignore the importance of privacy and territoriality. Similarly, patients may feel that having to expose their bodies to a myriad of strangers is particularly stressful, yet this is difficult to avoid if appropriate care is to be provided.

Proshansky (1971) itemises the psychological benefits of a single-bedded room: more social activity, greater choice of privacy of social inter-action and a greater range of activities. Fagerhaugh & Strauss (1977), on the other hand, highlight the advantages of multiple-bedded rooms in a burns unit. They suggest that patients can learn about the course of their illness from the observation of others. Patients are able to 'rehearse and interpret their own illnesses and pain trajectories and compare them with those of others'. Further there are individual differences in the degree of privacy needed by people. Some individuals are happy with, and indeed used to, little or no privacy and would dislike what they might perceive as isolation.

Despite these conflicting research findings, there are a number of courses of action open to architects and health professionals alike:

- Hospitals should be designed with the aim of providing the patient with as much choice as is possible over the privacy issue.
- Perceived control is just as important as privacy. Screens or curtains placed around a patient's bed do afford a certain degree of visual privacy, but the patient usually is not in direct control over operating the curtains and has to ask for them to be opened or closed. Under certain circumstances people might be reluctant to ask for assistance because they do not want to appear fussy or difficult. They might even fear becoming labelled 'a difficult patient'. Thus patients should have a certain degree of control over screening.
- The cost, both in financial and medical terms, of giving patients more control over their environment must be measured against the psychological benefits, which are substantial.
- Medical staff must be able to empathise with patients' need for privacy and where possible make patients feel in more control over their environment.

Another environmental issue related to privacy is territoriality. Edney (1974) argues that territory provides people with security and stimulation and can enhance their personal identities. People feel more comfortable when they are on 'home ground'. Territory may be classified according to degree of control. There are primary territories where people exercise complete control (e.g. one's own home); secondary territories are semipublic (e.g. a front lawn or backyard); and there are public territories (e.g. libraries, public houses and buses).

Hospitalised patients leave their own homes (primary territory) and are placed in an ambiguous situation. Whilst in some circumstances they might be allocated their 'own room', it is by no means the same as the room in their own house. They have no choice about the furnishings and only limited control over who comes into the room. In addition, they are expected to perform behaviours in this environment that previously they would only perform in their primary territory.

Shumaker & Reizenstein (1984) say that there are a number of strategies that can be adopted to help patients personalise their environment: '... allowing patients to personalise their setting enables them to establish their own territory within a hospital and thereby decreases the negative impact of the discontinuity that occurs between home and hospital'. They put forward the hospital design decision maker as the individual with a critical role in the personalisation of space. They specifically recommend such things as a bulletin board viewable from the patient's bed, a locker for clothes with shelves for grooming materials and a table within easy reach of the patient. However, the specific details of personalisation would differ from one hospital environment to another. The function of the designer would be to try to view the hospital from the patient's point of view and personalise the space accordingly.

Schumaker & Reizenstein (1984) point to a number of obstacles relating to the implementation of personalised patient space:

- space in hospitals is a valued commodity and the inclusion of more space for the patient's personal items would reduce the space available for other needs
- the personalisation process is costly and must therefore compete with high-priority technical equipment
- highly personalised space disrupts the

rhythm of medical staff and makes housekeeping duties difficult
- personal objects can be stolen.

These obstacles must be balanced against the positive psychological benefits of personalising the hospital environment such as increased sense of security, reduced stress and the promotion of other coping strategies (rest and relaxation).

Physical comfort

There are a number of features of the hospital environment that directly relate to patients' physical comfort. Some of these are noise, temperature, lighting, ergonomics and smells.

Noise. Certain sounds in the hospital may not be loud but can still cause irritation, anxiety and stress. Patients are usually more susceptible to noise because of their illness or because lying in bed with little or no stimulation accentuates even the slightest sounds. Sounds which seem unimportant to some are of greater significance to others and can often cause reactions that seem oversensitive. Some sounds in the hospital cause anxiety because they are unfamiliar, others, such as moaning or crying, cause distress due to their emotional nature. Whilst some investigators have suggested the greater use of sound-attenuating surfaces (carpets) to reduce noise (Simmons et al 1982), the main problem lies with the lack of awareness on the part of staff, visitors and other patients of the need for quiet. Topf (1992) investigated the effects of personal control over hospital noise on sleep. Subjects in the experimental condition heard audiotape-recorded critical care unit night-time sounds while attempting to sleep. Instructions in how to deal with sound seemed to have no effect; however, there was a strong relationship between CCU sounds and sleep. Subjects in the noise condition had poorer sleep efficiency, more difficulty in falling and staying asleep, more difficulty in progressing from one stage of sleep to the next and had more intrasleep awakenings than the control group who had quiet conditions.

Temperature. A frequent complaint from staff and patients alike refers to the hospital either being too hot or too cold, and it is difficult to see how this can be remedied without a major restructuring of design. That people respond in negative ways to the vagaries of temperature variation there is no doubt and the nature of these responses has been documented in some detail by Bell & Greene (1984). In the hospital, different people have varying needs according to their condition. Those who are immobile or feverish and have a need for heat are in the same environment as those who are mobile and have a reduced need for increases in temperature. Similar problems are posed with heating systems that go on and off in response to the time of year rather than the weather. Also the orientation of wards and patient rooms may cause problems according to the direction in which they are facing. Designers have a clear role to play in creating hospital environments that provide temperatures conducive to the comfort of the staff who have to work in them as well as the patients who have to live in them.

Lighting. The provision of appropriate lighting in the hospital environment is complicated by the need to satisfy the demands of different groups of people. In numerous circumstances medical staff require high levels of illumination, whereas some patients will require low levels of illumination.

Barnaby (1980) conducted a study of workers performing a difficult task under different levels of illumination. The results suggested that productivity and accuracy increased at higher levels of illumination. Workers evaluated the higher illumination levels as more satisfying, less stressful and making them feel more motivated towards the task in hand. This need for high illumination by staff when they are working can be at odds with patients who need to rest and sleep. Despite this problem there are many instances where different client groups are not in conflict for appropriate lighting systems. In these instances architects and designers can have a significant impact on the design of a 'user friendly' hospital lighting system. Thus it is proposed that:

- There should be a desire on the part of the designers to speak to staff and patients about the problems they have experienced in the past with lighting and the sorts of lighting system they would like in the future.

- The lighting system should be integrated with other design features (e.g. highly polished floors and fluorescent lighting can result in a large amount of glare.)

- There should be a willingness to take notice of recent advances in environmental psychology which can give information on such things as window size and placement, type of glass and curtains used, how to integrate natural and artificial lighting, the quality of artificial lighting, particularly whether high-pressure sodium lighting is more acceptable than its fluorescent counterpart, and finally the specific problems posed by video display units (Wineman 1984).

- Resources to finance a good hospital lighting system should not be viewed as a luxury; good lighting can increase staff motivation and decrease patient discomfort, both of which are cost effective in the long term.

Ergonomics. The science of ergonomics is concerned with the relationship between men/women and the design of their workplace. The adequacy and arrangement of the work surface, chair and storage space have been shown to affect comfort and health (Tichauer 1973). A comfortable chair and good lighting were identified by 70% of workers as factors that affected their personal comfort a great deal (Harris 1980).

In the same study the majority of workers reported problems with their backs, some of which they felt were directly related to the nature of their work. Lifting patients incorrectly may be a source of back pain, but the majority of the individuals in the Harris study were office workers. It seems that back pains suffered by many health professionals are not purely due to inadequate lifting skills. The hospital environment provides a wide range of problems for the ergonomic scientist since the workplaces within the hospital are so varied. Each one needs to be examined from the point of view of the health professional's experience and the ergonomist's expertise to devise workplaces that are congruent with individual needs.

Similarly, the ability of the patient to be able to manipulate various furnishings and equipment is essential to his physical comfort. Chairs may not give proper back support, televisions might be too high up and far away to see, the location of equipment sometimes makes its operation difficult and finally, whilst some of the difficulties might seem relatively minor, when added together they represent a large source of irritation that could easily be eliminated.

Smells. From the point of view of medical staff within the hospital, the source of irritating odours can come from their colleagues (e.g. cigarette smoke for non-smokers) and from the patients (e.g. urine soaked carpets in a geriatric hospital). From the patients' point of view, irritating odours come from other patients (e.g. vomitus and urine) and staff (e.g. disinfectants). Some of the problems can be circumvented by the allocation of specific areas for smoking and non-smoking; some odour problems are unavoidable and everybody concerned must rely on an efficient system of ventilation.

It is very difficult for architects and designers to be aware of all the factors that contribute to the physical comfort of staff and patients within the hospital environment. Apart from the myriad of different settings within the hospital there are many different sorts of patient, the old, the young, the very ill, the very healthy. A way forward is for the designers to consult more with health professionals who can contribute their knowledge and experience of working in a hospital environment to the design skills of the planners.

Symbolic meaning

To some individuals who work in a hospital environment a solution to many problems would be to provide more finance. If more money were spent improving the environment many of the problems would disappear. Finance is a problem, but it does not explain why some institutions that are extremely well financed are not very nice places in which to live and work. Similarly, some institutions not so well financed do not experience 'staff burnout' (a discussion of the problems facing health professionals form the basis of the next chapter). Why should this be the case?

Firstly, hospitals convey a 'hidden' meaning or 'message'. This message is related to the physical design, the structure of the rooms, provision of plants, suitable furnishings, attention to little details and items of physical comfort and privacy discussed above. In some instances, a hospital may be perceived as warm and friendly but too loose and unprofessional. Another hospital may be perceived as cold and depersonalised but highly competent and professional. It might be decided that the image that one wants to portray to the patient is one of competence, professionalism, warmth and personal control. The problem lies with how to portray these 'symbolic meanings'. We have already discussed the role of the designer in meeting the psychological needs of the people who use hospitals. Precisely how do designers get information on an environment that conveys the symbolic meanings above? Indeed how do we know that it is these factors that contribute to a positive view of the hospital?

One approach is to ask for patients' reactions to hospitals. Kenny & Canter (1979) quote studies which refer to the problems posed by multiple-bedded wards, environmental noise and lack of privacy. Patients have difficulty with the control of information about themselves when others are able to overhear conversations. They also complain about the heating and lighting and frequently complain about the lack of privacy when using the bathroom and toilet. Most of the factors mentioned relate to the patient's inability to control his immediate environment and as such represent a common complaint that designers can act upon. However, exactly how does one convey to patients and staff alike such things as warmth and friendliness by way of features of design? We have to look for some reliable means of interpreting environmental symbols and predicting their effect on the individual, then we can come to some form of prescription for a built environment that is low in terms of stress and anxiety, high in terms of factors relating to the recovery of the patient.

Martyniuk et al (1973) placed groups of 12 subjects in a room with six different lighting systems. The subjects were required to rate the lighting systems in three areas of perception: evaluative, perceptual clarity and spaciousness. The evaluative scale contained a series of word pairs. Subjects were required to rate the lighting systems on a scale between the following pairs:

friendly	hostile
pleasant	unpleasant
like	dislike
harmony	discord
satisfying	frustrating
beautiful	ugly
sociable	unsociable
relaxed	tense
interested	monotonous

There were 96 subjects in the experiment. The results indicated that the most popular lighting configuration was a combination of overhead downlighting, peripheral and overhead diffuse lighting. This technique can be used to good effect when designing appropriate lighting systems in hospitals. The subjects, patients and staff are given the opportunity to sample numerous lighting systems in situ and the most popular lighting arrangement is selected.

The isolation of those physical elements of a design that constitute a therapeutic environment is at the moment very difficult and this aspect of environmental psychology is still in its infancy. We are unable to determine exactly what constitutes a warm friendly environment, but if there is cooperation between designers and the people who live and work in hospitals to produce a physical environment that pays attention, not just to major elements of design, but to the small details as well, then the hidden message emanating from the hospital environment is 'you are important'.

The community environment

Health professionals who work in the community are aware that there are certain features of the environment that can affect people's health and their behaviour. It is proposed to examine four of these features: noise, pollution, temperature and architectural design.

Noise

The presence of noise in the community has been found to affect health and behaviour in different ways. Firstly, there seems to be a direct relationship between noise levels and health disorders themselves. Secondly, noise levels seem to play a crucial role in children's development. Thirdly, noise affects how we feel about others and reduces the extent to which we are likely to engage in prosocial behaviour.

Noise has been associated with a wide range of health disorders. Knipschild (1977) found there was more heart trouble, pregnancy complications, and higher blood pressure in people who lived in neighbourhoods close to Amsterdam airport than people who lived in other parts of the country. In America, Meecham & Shaw (1979) reported that an increase in noise levels from aircraft was associated with increased death rates due to strokes and cirrhosis of the liver. In Russia, Karagodina et al (1969) found noise-associated increases in nervous and gastrointestinal diseases, cardiac insufficiency and blood pressure abnormalities in children 9–13 years old in a survey of areas around nine airports. London's Heathrow airport has come under some criticism for producing higher incidences of psychiatric admission rates (Abbey-Wickrama et al 1969), though admission to hospital represents only the severest of cases; most people go to their GP first, hence we are unable to quantify the exact effects of noise on mental health.

A considerable amount of attention has been focused upon the effects of noise on children's development. It has been found that behaviour can be affected during noise. Cohen et al (1973) conducted a study investigating the effects of noise on children living in a high-rise housing development in New York City. The development was built over a 'motorway', and as a result, the noise was higher on the lower floors than on the upper ones. Tests of ability to read and to tell one sound from another showed that children living on the lower floors had greater reading and hearing deficits.

Another study by Cohen et al (1986) investigated noise in the classrooms of four primary schools situated under the flight path of Los Angeles airport. There were 300 flights per day, one flight every 2½ minutes during school hours. The children in the noisy schools were matched with children in other schools on such variables as grade, ethnic background, education and parents' occupation. They were tested in a quiet environment on a number of variables. Firstly children from noisy schools were found to have higher blood pressure than children from quiet schools. Secondly when given a problem-solving task, those children who succeeded in solving the problem took longer to do so if they had spent more than 3½ years in a noisy school. Lastly the children from the noisy schools were more likely to give up when faced with a difficult problem to solve. Cohen et al (1981) also found that after a year of exposure to the planes, the same effects were observed, indicating that children do not adapt to the noise over periods of time.

Mathews & Cannon (1975) found that noise diminishes the degree to which individuals will engage in helping or prosocial behaviour. One would suspect that when somebody dropped a pile of books we might help them pick the books up, but if he had a plaster cast around one arm then we would be much more likely to help him. In a field experiment they found that when a man was observed to get out of a car and drop a pile of books, 20% of the passers-by helped him. When the same man wore a cast, 80% of the passers-by helped him.

They then investigated the effects of noise on this helping behaviour. In the background they produced a noisy lawnmower (87 dB) and looked at what effects this could have on whether the passers-by would help the man. When there was noise and nothing 'wrong' with the man, 10% helped him, a reduction of 10%. However, when there was noise and the man was wearing a cast, only 15% of the passers-by helped him, a reduction of 65%. It was as if the presence of noise served to distract or reduce the importance

of the cast in some way leading to a reduction in a desire to help others.

Pollution

There is a large body of research that has established the negative effects of pollution on health. For instance, Blot et al (1977) discovered that those people who lived close to oil refineries where there were airborne hydrocarbons had significantly higher rates of lung cancer and cancer of the nose, sinuses and skin than people who lived elsewhere. Photochemical oxidants (smog) have also been linked with nausea, headache, anorexia and pulmonary oedema. Sulphur oxides (principal source is combustion of fossil fuels) produce irritation of the upper respiratory passages, reduced mucociliary clearance and reduced pulmonary functioning. Nitrogen oxides (sources are fossil fuels, cars and power stations) have been associated with reduced pulmonary functioning, reduced host resistance to disease, diminished weight gain, general bronchial inflammation and lipid peroxidation of haemoglobin. Carbon monoxide (sources are cars and smoking) affects birth weight, cardiovascular disease and impaired liver function. Finally, asbestos, lead, mercury, other heavy metals and halogens can prove particularly lethal: asbestos—pulmonary lesions and carcinoma and mesothelial tissue damage; lead—gastrointestinal cramping, anaemia and impaired neural functioning; mercury—neural dysfunction, upper respiratory inflammation and thyroid disturbance (Coffin & Stokinger 1977). However, pollution also affects psychiatric admission rates, social behaviour, performance and stressful life events.

Atmospheric pollution has been correlated with psychiatric disturbance. Rotton & Frey (1981) recorded the calls received at Dayton, Ohio police and fire stations over a 2 year period. They were able to link high levels of pollution with domestic disturbances, obscene phone calls and psychiatric cases.

Lewis et al (1970) compared the performance of subjects who had breathed polluted air with subjects who had not on four information-processing tasks. Polluted air was obtained from a not particularly busy road in England. The subjects who had breathed the polluted air performed worse on three out of the four tasks. This effect of pollution on people's ability to pay attention to tasks and their ability to perform tasks may be a significant contributory factor in road accidents.

Social behaviour is also affected by polluted atmosphere. Rotton et al (1978) found that pollution produced negative feelings towards both people and objects. With respect to aggression, the effects are similar to those of heat; moderately bad smells produce more aggression, whereas really bad smells actually decrease aggression (Rotton et al 1979), presumably because the odour is so bad that people just cannot stand it and move away. Baron (1990) found that the presence of pleasant smells from air fresheners led subjects to engage in more agreeable interpersonal behaviour than those whose room did not contain air freshener.

Evans & Jacobs (1984) cite a study that measured such things as depression, hostility, anxiety, use of physical and mental facilities over a 3-year period. They also looked at stressful life events, social support, illness reporting biases and sociodemographic data. The study was carried out in the city district of Los Angeles and they found a number of interesting details. First of all, they established that those people who had experienced high levels of stress were more susceptible to the negative effects of high photochemical oxidants. Second, the people who had recently moved into the area had different perceptions about the nature of the pollution than the long-term residents. It seemed to be the case that those people who had resided in Los Angeles for 5 years or more tended to view the smog as less of a problem, exaggerated their health and had a high external locus of control. Thus people tend to adapt to the adverse effects of pollution by altering their frame of reference or tending to view the environment in a different way to people not so familiar with the habitat. (This latter point is particularly relevant to the discussion on health behaviour in Chapter 6.) Pollution affects our health directly but it is also an important factor in determining the way

we react to, and perceive, the environment in which we work and live.

Temperature

There is a general feeling that temperature affects our mood, indeed the weather is one of the most common topics of conversation, certainly in the UK. But there are two main behavioural phenomena that are subject to the vagaries of changes in temperature: performance and aggression. Whilst temperature as an environmental stressor does not command the same amount of attention as crowding or noise, it is nevertheless important.

Heat like other environmental stressors causes us to feel annoyed but does it lead to more aggression? An examination of the incidences of riots during the summer months would lead one at first to suppose that there was in fact a direct relationship between the two. However, a series of experiments by Baron & Bell (1975) and Bell & Baron (1976) have shown that aggression increases with moderate amounts of heat, but when temperatures get too hot, aggressive behaviour is actually reduced.

Baron & Ransberger (1978) looked at weather records to get the temperatures where 102 riots had taken place in the US between 1967 and 1971. The most dangerous outbreaks of violence occurred when temperatures reached the mid-80s, but when the temperature climbed higher, aggressive crowd behaviour decreased. Carlsmith & Anderson (1979) have questioned these results pointing out that there are more riots in temperatures of the mid-80s because there are simply more days in the summer when temperatures are in the mid-80s. Also other factors might be responsible for crowd disturbance in the summer such as increased alcohol consumption. However, recent studies by Cohn (1990) and Simpson & Perry (1990) have found a positive relationship between temperature and interpersonal aggression.

Given the opportunity, what sort of community environment do people want? Balling & Falk (1982) found that children preferred flat grassy scenes with a scattering of trees. The authors suggest that this preference stems from our long evolutionary history originating in the savannas of East Africa. They suggest that with age we can learn to like other settings to an equal degree. This is fortunate for those who do not have a choice of where to live. Whether people chose to or not, over 60% remain in the environment where they were born. It seems quite remarkable that when people are asked what they feel about a dirty, polluted, cold environment, many respond positively towards it. The answer to the question 'Why?', lies in the quality of the social environment that makes it bearable and sometimes rewarding.

A central feature of Sarason's (1981) community psychology is the development of competence in the community. This may be achieved through greater control and what Rappaport (1981) and Gibson (1991) call 'empowerment'. Control of the physical environment is one manifestation of control over one's life and this includes control over one's health. This means that when designers, architects and planners take the trouble to involve the community residents in designing the sorts of dwellings that they want, it leads to more involvement in other areas of community life such as health care. Health professionals can play a significant role in facilitating the growth of 'community empowerment' by setting up community health groups and self-health projects on a formal and informal basis (Milner 1994).

CULTURE

Membership of a particular culture can influence health directly, but culture also influences health behaviour as well. From a psychological point of view, it is important to consider how culture can affect such things as communication, the perception of pain and whether people from different cultures think in totally different ways. Knowing a culture's language does not necessarily guarantee fluent communication. For example, a situation may arise where a woman from a totally different culture is having a baby in Britain. As she does not speak English an interpreter is used. The problem lies not with the

language itself but the communication of concepts, actions and objects that the woman has not experienced before. A second area of interest concerns the perceptions of illness of health professionals from different cultures. Does an Indian nurse attending an Indian patient with severe burns assess the person's pain and distress in the same way as a British nurse caring for a British patient with the same condition? The third area of concern relates to the area of medical anthropology and examines the distinctions between cross-cultural health psychology and medical anthropology.

Communication

The problems of communication between people of different cultures has been illustrated by Cole & Scribner (1974). They describe a communication experiment designed to illustrate the ways in which simple instructions can easily be misinterpreted. Two people from the Kpelle tribe of West Africa were sitting side by side at a table. They were separated from each other by a partition. On the table in front of each of them was a pile of sticks. The experimenter sat in front of the table. He was a fluent speaker of the Kpelle language. The experimenter instructed the subjects to select certain sticks (the long, thin one; the short, fat one) and place them in a line in front of them on the table. After they had done this, the partition was removed and the sticks that had been selected by the subjects were compared.

Cole & Scribner (1974) found that the sticks that had been selected by the Kpelle subjects were, in many instances, not the same. The subjects had responded to the experimenter's requests by selecting different sticks. This seemed surprising considering that the task was quite straightforward and the experimenter spoke the language fluently. Cole & Scribner (1974) explain their results by pointing to the different conceptual realities of both experimenter and subject. What seemed to be a perfectly straightforward experimental situation to the experimenter was totally alien to the subjects. They had never experienced anything like it before and were thus unsure of what to do and what was going on. Also the authors suggest that, whilst the experimenter was fluent in the language, he might not have been able to communicate the meaning of his requests adequately.

The implications of this study for health professionals are:

- speaking the language of people from a different culture does not necessarily mean that they will always be able to understand what is being said
- even when using an interpreter to convey requests to patients in their language, they still may not understand what is happening due to the strangeness of the whole situation.

For instance if one took a Kpelle woman who was about to give birth and placed her in a delivery suite in one of our Western hospitals there would be considerable communication difficulties, even if there was a person present who could speak the Kpelle language. Because the situation is totally alien to the woman she is unable to comprehend what is happening. The Kpelle language cannot adequately describe the strange circumstances in a way that the woman can understand.

Pain

Davitz & Davitz (1985) conducted a large-scale survey of 1400 nurses' attitudes to pain in 13 countries. Each nurse was given a series of 60 'vignettes' describing a patient with a particular illness or condition. For each patient, the nurses were required to give an indication of the degree of psychological distress and the amount of physical pain and discomfort on a scale from 1 to 7. The countries were: Korea, Puerto Rico, Japan, Uganda, India, Nigeria, United States, Thailand, England, Israel, Belgium, Taiwan and Nepal. The results (Table 8.1) indicated that nurses from different countries varied in their inferences of both physical pain and psychological distress.

Davitz & Davitz (1985) make the following points about their research findings:

Table 8.1 Mean ratings of nurses for each country

Country	Psychological distress	Physical Pain
Korea	4.84	3.80
Puerto Rico	4.80	3.06
Japan	4.63	3.72
Uganda	4.60	3.60
India	4.54	3.68
Nigeria	4.53	3.39
United States	4.43	3.00
Thailand	4.39	3.20
England	4.36	2.81
Israel	4.29	3.25
Belgium	4.16	3.00
Taiwan	4.06	3.53
Nepal	3.60	3.56

- Many Westerners have a stereotype of Oriental people as forming one group. This study shows that Oriental groups differ among themselves just as Western societies differ.
- Nepalese and Chinese nurses gave the lowest responses to the psychological distress factor. This did not mean that these nurses were unfeeling, merely that their cultures rewarded a certain inner peace. Chinese nurses working with Western patients are often astounded by the level of turmoil evidenced by the patients.
- Puerto Rican nurses rated psychological distress very high and physical pain very low. The nurses explained this finding by saying that they knew that their people were very emotional and dramatic but this did not necessarily mean that they were in great pain.
- In an earlier study by Davitz & Davitz (1980) American nurses judged Jewish patients as suffering the most of any ethnic group. The present study shows that Israeli nurses did not share this judgement, they inferred relatively low levels of pain and psychological distress.
- Finally, English nurses had the lowest rating of physical pain. They were noted to find patients from other cultures to overreact to pain; they were astonished to find patients complaining about 'small matters'. This led to English nurses being labelled as efficient but

unsympathetic. The nurses were not unsympathetic, but found it difficult to comprehend the dramatic expression of pain. Thus in hospitals with a wide diversity of cultures, conflicts can occur between nurses and patients due to cultural misperceptions.

A solution does not involve giving up one's cultural norms and values, it involves an appreciation of the differences between cultures in the expression of psychological distress and pain. Further, it should be realised that there are vast individual differences within any one culture. A recognition of these differences can lead to an avoidance of misunderstandings between health professionals and patients alike.

Cross-cultural health psychology and medical anthropology

In the psychological literature there has been a traditional distinction between cross-cultural psychology and psychological anthropology. Cross-cultural psychology has sought to determine whether theories of human behaviour, constructed in the West, are applicable to all cultures throughout the world. Psychological anthropology has attempted to try to understand the behaviour of a particular culture using fieldwork techniques. Of course some of the differences between the two represent the distinction between a psychological approach and an anthropological approach. The methodology adopted reflects this distinction with the former relying extensively on experimentation and testing and the latter using culture-based methods such as ethnomethodological research.

Arising from these distinctions are two questions for health psychology:

- Can one make similar distinctions between cross-cultural health psychology and medical anthropology?
- Are theories of health behaviour (developed in the West) applicable to people throughout the world?

The answer to both these questions can be provided, in part, with reference to an analysis of 'magical death' provided by McElroy & Townsend (1985). They cite an account of the acute terror experienced by an Aborigine who believed he was the victim of an attack by a 'sorcerer' and that death was inevitable.

The man who discovers that he is being boned by an enemy is indeed a pitiable sight. He stands aghast, with his eyes staring at the treacherous pointer, and with his hands lifted as though to ward off the lethal medium, which he imagines is pouring into his body. His body begins to tremble and the muscles twist involuntarily. He sways backward and falls to the ground, and after a short time appears to be in a swoon; but soon after he writhes as if in mortal agony. From this time onwards he sickens and frets, refusing to eat and keeping aloof from the daily affairs of the tribe. Unless help is forthcoming in the shape of a countercharm, his death is only a matter of a comparatively short time.

The man is neither poisoned nor shamming. McElroy & Townsend (1985) say that when such patients are admitted to hospital they do not respond well to treatment. In one case of 'boning', a man refused to eat and drink until he died. The doctors decided that his death was suicide through voluntary rejection of fluids. His tribe, however, believed he had died because he had broken a taboo. Another explanation of his behaviour is provided by the reformulated learned helplessness theory discussed in Chapter 6. The faulty cognitions of the man have led him to believe that there is no way out of the spell and he must die. It does not matter what he does, the outcome is death. These negative cognitions are thus responsible for an individual's demise, just as positive beliefs have been found to contribute to the efficacy of hypnosis and acupuncture.

Whether theories of health behaviour can help to explain medical phenomena in different cultures depends on the degree of ethnocentric bias involved, that is, the focus of attention should be the culture or society rather than the health theory. Cole et al (1971) have laid great emphasis on living with a specific culture before conducting any psychological examination. In this way one is able to gain a better idea of a culture's behaviour. When this perspective has been achieved the psychological experimentation can begin. A similar approach is recommended for the cross-cultural health professional; through living and working with people from specific cultures one gains an idea of norms, values, beliefs and behaviour. After this has been achieved we can apply our knowledge of health psychology to further our knowledge of a culture's health behaviour. Thus the 'anthropological method' can be combined with the 'psychological' theory to produce a more meaningful analysis of any particular culture's health problems.

Two examples may serve to illustrate the ways in which cultures think in different ways. Gladwin (1970) spent a number of years living with the Puluwat Islanders in the South Pacific. He was concerned with examining a widely held view that people from such cultures were disadvantaged because they thought in an inferior way; they were unable to think in abstract terms and were confined to 'concrete' thought.

Gladwin (1970) administered a problem-solving task to the islanders designed to test heuristic thought. They did not do particularly well; indeed much worse than the performance of many Western schoolchildren under similar circumstances. If one were to take these test results at their face value then one might conclude that the islanders were indeed disadvantaged. However, Gladwin noted that the islanders who navigated the 'canoes' were able to navigate hundreds of miles without using any instruments. They did this postulating abstract islands and estimating the speed of the boat by listening to the sound of the waves on the hull. He argues that these skills are extremely sophisticated and require a high degree of intellectual reasoning. Thus, the islanders are not disadvantaged in their thought but different. Environmental circumstances have shaped the direction of their thought processes along specific lines that are relevant to their existence, just as Western thought develops in different culture-specific ways.

Labov (1970) was concerned at the poor performance of Philadelphia black ghetto children on standard measures of linguistic skills. Many thought that their poor performance was either due to a genetic inferiority or some form of cultural deprivation (Jensen 1973; Bereiter & Engleman 1966). Labov (1970) found that when he talked to the teenagers in an informal environment with their peers present they produced powerful reasoning and debating skills, but they spoke in a way that would be understood in the ghetto and not in a way that would have pleased their teachers. Labov (1970) argues that these children do not have a deficit at all, but have channelled their intellect into the ghetto environment. They see formal education as largely irrelevant and thus do not try to succeed. Again a cultural, or in this case a sub-cultural, difference is proposed rather than a lack of competence.

These studies, and others like them, have considerable implications for health professionals working at home and abroad. When dealing with people from different cultures, it is all too easy to assume that inability to comprehend the instructions of the health professional is due to stupidity or lack of intellectual capacity to understand. The studies mentioned above illustrate that this is not the case and that people from different cultures have equivalent levels of intellectual competence. The breakdown in communication arises from the way culture, via both social and physical environment, has directed thought along different paths.

This latter point presents a large problem for cross-cultural psychologists wishing to investigate the effects of culture on thought. How can the Western psychologist understand the thought processes of another culture if they think in totally different ways to her? Segall et al (1990) suggest that there are no easy solutions but indicate two ways out of the dilemma. The first is for the psychologist to spend considerable time with the culture to 'throw off' her ethnocentric bias and view the world through the 'eyes of the culture'. Secondly, there may be considerable value in training people from the culture in question to become psychologists. In these ways a better understanding of the culture may be obtained.

This advice also pertains to health professionals. For those who are working in parts of the world where communication seems to be a problem, it is important to try to understand health from the perspective of the indigenous culture and to avoid transposing 'foreign' ideas without a good deal of thought (Hellman 1990). Also, from a 'home-based perspective' it is necessary to provide the opportunity for people from different cultural groups within the community to train as health professionals in order to reduce the barriers that can occur due to different ways of seeing the world.

CONCLUSION

There are certain common features of ecology, environment and culture that are based on taking the science of health psychology out of the laboratory and into the 'real world'. Bronfenbrenner (1979) argues that psychology in general, and child psychology in particular, has become '... the science of the strange behaviour of children in strange situations with strange adults for the briefest possible periods of time'. Health psychology does not have to be confined to laboratories. Indeed, by its very nature, it requires us to examine the health behaviour of individuals within the contexts of their ecology, environment and culture. The advantage of experimentation in the laboratory is the ability to control and manipulate all the variables. Many of the early studies on such areas as pain attempted to do this. But simulating pain in the laboratory and examining people's reactions to it is a far cry from the problems of chronic pain patients in the hospital and in the community. Strict experimental rigour has to give way to relevance. This does not mean that studies should be sloppily designed, but it is only by examining behaviour within its environmental and cultural context that we can obtain a less contrived view of human health behaviour.

REFERENCES

Abbey-Wickrama I, a'Brook M F, Gattoni F W G, Herridge C F 1969 Mental hospital admissions and aircraft noise. Lancet 2: 1275–1277

Altman I 1975 The environment and social behaviour: privacy, personal space, territory, and crowding. Brooks Cole, Monterey California

Altman I 1978 Crowding: historical and contemporary trends in crowding research. In: Baum A, Epstein Y (eds) Human responses to crowding. Eribaum, Hillsdale NJ

Balling J D, Falk J H 1982 Development of visual preference for natural environments. Environment and Behaviour 14: 5–28

Barker R G, Wright H F, Schoggen P et al 1977 Habitats, environments, and human behaviour. Jossey Bass, New York

Barnaby J F 1980 Lighting for productivity gains. Lighting Design and Application. Feb 2–28

Baron R A 1990 Environmentally induced positive affect: its impact on self-efficacy, task performance, negotiation and conflict. Journal of Applied Social Psychology 20: 368–384

Baron R A, Bell P A 1975 Aggression and heat: mediating effects of prior provocation and exposure to an aggressive model. Journal of Personality and Social Research 31: 825–832

Baron R A, Ransberger V M 1978 Ambient temperature at the occurrence of collective violence: the 'long, hot summer' revisited. Journal of Personality and Social Psychology 36: 357–360

Baum A, Harpin R, Valins S 1975 The role of group phenomena in the experience of crowding. Environment and Behaviour 7: 185–198

Bell P A, Baron R A 1976 Aggression and heat: the mediating role of negative affect. Journal of Applied Social Psychology 6: 18–30

Bell P A, Greene T C 1984 Thermal stress: physiological, comfort, performance, and social effects of hot and cold environments. In: Evans G W (ed) Environmental stress. Cambridge University Press, Cambridge

Bereiter C, Engleman S 1966 Teaching disadvantaged children in the preschool. Prentice-Hall, Englewood Cliffs NJ

Berry J W 1976 Human ecology and cognitive style. Wiley, New York

Blot W J, Brinton L A, Fraument J F, Stone B J 1977 Cancer mortality in US counties with petroleum industries. Science 198: 52–53

Booth A 1976 Urban crowding and its consequences. Praeger. New York

Bronfenbrenner U 1979 The ecology of human development. Harvard University Press, Cambridge Mass

Calhoun J B 1962 Population density and social pathology. Scientific American 206: 139–148

Carlsmith J M, Anderson C A 1979 Ambient temperature and the occurrence of collective violence: a new analysis. Journal of Personality and Social Research 37: 337–344

Coffin D, Stokinger H 1977 Biological effects of air pollutants. In: Stern A C (ed) Air pollution, 3rd edn. Academic Press, New York, vol 3

Cohen S 1978 Environmental load and the allocation of attention. In: Baum A, Singer J E, Valins S (eds) Advances in environmental psychology. Eribaum, Hillsdale NJ, vol 1

Cohen S, Glass D C, Singer J E 1973 Apartment noise, auditory discrimination, and reading ability in children. Journal of Experimental Social Psychology 9: 407–422

Cohen S, Glass D C, Phillips S 1979a Environment and health. In: Freeman H E, Levine S, Reeder C G (eds) Handbook of medical sociology. Prentice Hall, Englewood Cliffs NJ

Cohen S, Evans G W, Krantz D S, Stokols D, 1979b Physiological, motivational and cognitive effects of aircraft noise on children: moving from laboratory to field. American Psychologist 35: 231–243

Cohen S, Evans G W, Krantz D S, Stokols D, Kelly S 1981 Aircraft noise and children: longitudinal and cross-sectional evidence on adaptation to noise and the effectiveness of noise abatement. Journal of Personality and Social Psychology 40: 331–345

Cohen S, Evans G W, Stokols D, Krantz D 1986 Behaviour, health and environmental stress. Plenum, New York

Cohn E G 1990 Weather and violent crime: a reply to Perry and Simpson 1987. Environment and Behavior 22: 280–294

Cole M, Bruner J S 1971 Cultural differences and inferences about psychological processes. American Psychologist 26: 867–876

Cole M, Scribner S 1974 Culture and thought. Wiley, New York

Cole M, Gay J, Glick I, Sharp D W 1971 The cultural context of learning and thinking. Basic Books, New York

Davey, G 1990 Ecological learning theory. Methuen, London

Davitz L L, Davitz R 1980 Nurses' responses to patient suffering. Springer, New York

Davitz L L, Davitz R 1985 Culture and nurses' inferences of suffering. In: Copp L A (ed) Perspectives on pain. Churchill Livingstone, Edinburgh

DiMatteo M R, Friedman H 1982 Social psychology and medicine. Oelgeschlager Gunn Hain, Cambridge Mass

Duffy M, Bailey S, Beck B, Barker D G 1986 Preferences in nursing home design: a comparison of residents, administrators and designers. Environment and Behaviour 18: 246–257

Edney J J 1974 Human territoriality. Psychological Bulletin 81: 959–975

Edwards J, Booth A 1977 Crowding and human sexual behaviour. Social Forces 55: 791–808

Epstein Y 1982 Crowding stress and human behaviour. In: Evans G W (ed) Environmental stress. Cambridge University Press, Cambridge

Evans G W, Jacobs S V 1984 Air pollution and human behaviour. In: Evans G W (ed) Environmental stress. Cambridge University Press, Cambridge

Evans G W, Palsane M N, Lepore S J, Martin J 1989 Residential density and psychological health: the mediating effects of social support. Journal of Personality and Social Psychology 57: 994–999

Fagerhaugh S Y, Strauss A 1977 Politics of pain management: staff–patient interaction. Addison-Wesley, California

Galle O, Gove W, McPherson J 1972 Population density and pathology: what are the relations for man? Science 176: 23–30

Gibson C H 1991 A concept analysis of empowerment. Journal of Advanced Nursing 16: 354–361

Gibson J J 1979 The ecological approach to visual perception. Houghton Mifflin, New York

Gillis A R, Richard M A, Hagan J 1986 Ethnic susceptibility to crowding: an empirical analysis. Environment and Behavior 18: 683–706

Gladwin T 1970 East is a big bird: navigation and logic on Puluwat Atoll. Harvard University Press, Cambridge Mass

Hall E T 1966 The hidden dimension. Doubleday, New York

Harris L 1980 The Steelcase national study of office environments, No 11 Comfort and productivity in the office of the 80s. Steelcase Incorporated, Michigan

Hellman C H 1990 Culture, health and illness: an introduction for health professionals, 2nd edn. Wright, Bristol

Hollander J, Yeastros S 1963 The effects of simultaneous variations of humidity and barometric pressure on arthritis. Bulletin of the American Meteorological Society 44: 489–494

Jaco E C 1979 Ecological aspects of patient care: an experimental study. In: Jaco E G (ed) Patients, physicians and illness: a sourcebook in behavioural science and health, 3rd edn. Free Press, New York

Jensen A R 1973 Educability and group differences. Methuen. London

Karagodina I L, Soldatkina S A, Vinokur I L, Klimukhin A A 1969 Effect of aircraft noise on the population near airports. Hygiene and Sanitation 34: 182–187

Karlin R A, Epstein Y M, Aiello J R 1978 Strategies for the investigation of crowding. In: Esser A, Greenbie B (eds) Design for community and privacy. Plenum, New York

Kasl S V 1977 The effects of the residential environment on health behaviour: a review. In: Hinkle L E, Loring R E (eds) The effects of the man-made environment on health and behaviour. US Government Printing Office, Washington

Kelly I G 1968 Towards an ecological conception of preventive interventions. In: Carter J W (ed) Research contributions from psychology to community mental health. Behavioural Publications, New York

Kenny C, Canter D 1979 Evaluating acute general hospitals. In: Canter D, Canter S (eds) Designing for therapeutic environments. Wiley, Chichester

Knipschild P 1977 Medical effects of aircraft noise. International Archives of Occupational and Environmental Health 40: 185–204

Labov W 1970 The logical non-standard English. In: Williams F (ed) Language and parents. Markham Press, Chicago

Langer E J 1984 The psychology of control. Sage, Beverley Hills

Larson M T 1975 Current trends in child development research. Unpublished manuscript. School of Home Economics, University of Michigan

Levy L, Herzog A 1974 Effects of population density and crowding on health and social adaptation in the Netherlands. Journal of Health and Social Behaviour 15: 228–240

Lewis J, Baddeley K, Banham K, Lovitt D 1970 Traffic, pollution and mental efficiency. Nature 225: 95–97

Linn L 1970 State hospital environment and rates of patient discharge. Archives of General Psychiatry 23: 346–351

Lynch K 1960 Image of the city. MIT Press, Cambridge Mass

MacDonald W S, Oden C N V 1973 Effects of extreme crowding on the performance of five married couples during twelve weeks intensive training. Proceedings of the 81st Annual Convention of the American Psychological Association 8: 209–210

McElroy A, Townsend P K 1985 Medical anthropology in ecological perspective. Westview Press, Boulder Colorado

Martyniuk O P, Flynn J E, Spencer T J, Kendrick C 1973 Effects of environmental lighting on impression and behaviour. In: Kuller R (ed) Architectural psychology: Proceedings of the Lund conference. Dowden Hutchinson Ross, Pennsylvania

Mathews K E, Cannon L K 1975 Environmental noise level as a determinant of helping behaviour. Journal of Personality and Social Psychology 32: 571–577

Meecham W C, Shaw N 1979 Effects of jet noise on mortality rates. British Journal of Audiology 13: 77–80

Milner S 1994 Evaluation of a drop-in health centre. Unpublished PhD Thesis, University of Northumbria

Mitchell R E 1971 Some implications of high density housing. American Sociological Review 36: 18–29

Moos R H 1976 The human context: environmental determinants of behaviour. Wiley, New York

Moos R H 1979 Social-ecological perspectives on health. In: Stone G C, Cohen S, Adler N E (eds) Health psychology. Jossey Bass, New York

Orford 1992 Community psychology: theory and practice. Wiley, Chichester

Osmond H 1957 Function as the basis of psychiatric ward design. Mental Hospitals 8: 23–30

Paulus P B 1980 Crowding. In: Paulus P B (ed) Psychology of group influence. Erlbaum, New York

Paulus P B, McCain G, Cox V C 1978 Death rates, psychiatric commitments, blood pressure and perceived crowding as a function of institutional crowding. Environmental Psychology and Nonverbal Behaviour 3: 107–116

Proshansky H M 1971 Environmental psychology and the design professions. In: Architecture for human behaviour: collected papers from a mini-conference. Philadelphia Chapter. The American Institute of Architects

Rappaport J 1981 In praise of paradox: a social policy of empowerment over prevention. American Journal of Community Psychology 9: 1–27

Rodin J, Solomon S K, Metcaff J 1979 Role of control in mediating perceptions of population density. Journal of Personality and Social Psychology 36: 988–999

Rotton J, Frey J 1981 Weather, air pollution and social pathology: first approximations. Unpublished manuscript, Florida International University

Rotton J, Barry T, Frey J, Soler E 1978 Air pollution and interpersonal attraction. Journal of Applied Social Psychology 8: 57–71

Rotton J, Frey J, Barry T, Milligan M, Fitzpatrick M 1979 The air pollution experience and physical aggression. Journal of Applied Social Psychology 9: 397–412

Saegert S 1978 High density environments: their personal and social consequences. In: Baum A, Epstein W (eds) Human responses to crowding. Erlbaum, Hillsdale NJ

Saegert S 1985 The role of housing in the experience of dwelling. In: Altman I, Werner C (eds) Home environments: human behavior and environment. Plenum, New York

Sarason S B 1981 Psychology misdirected. Free Press, New York

Schumaker S A, Reizenstein J E 1984 Inpatient stress in acute care hospitals. In: Evans G W (ed) Environmental stress. Cambridge University Press, Cambridge

Segall M H, Dasen P, Berry J W, Poortinga Y H 1990 Human behaviour in global perspective: an introduction to cross-cultural psychology. Allyn & Bacon, Boston

Simmons D, Reizenstein J E, Grant M A 1982 Considering carpets in hospital use. Dimensions in Health Services 59: 18–21

Simpson M, Perry J D 1990 Crime and climate: a reconsideration. Environment and Behaviour 22: 295–300

Szklo M, Tonascia I, Gordis L 1976 Psychosocial factors and the risk of myocardial infarction in white women. American Journal of Epidemiology 103: 312–320

Tichauer E R 1973 Ergonomic aspects of biomechanics. The industrial environment: its evaluation and control. US Government Printing Office, Washington

Topf M 1992 Effects of personal control over hospital noise on sleep. Research in Nursing and Health 15: 19–28

Wainwright P 1985 Impact of hospital architecture on the patient in pain. In: Copp L A (ed) Perspectives on pain. Churchill Livingstone, Edinburgh

Wineman J D 1984 The office environment as a source of stress. In: Evans G W (ed) Environmental stress. Cambridge University Press, Cambridge

RECOMMENDED READING

Evans G W 1984 (ed) Environmental stress. Cambridge University Press, Cambridge
This is still one of the most comprehensive accounts of the relationship between psychology, environment and stress. The book examines the psychological components of a wide range of environments.

Hellman C 1990 Culture, health and illness: an introduction for health professionals. Wright, Bristol
This is essentially a book on medical anthropology. However, it gives readers a sound theoretical background to the topic providing case studies and practical examples to illustrate the cultural dimensions of health and illness.

Orford J 1992 Community psychology: theory and practice. Wiley, Chichester
Community psychology was in the doldrums for a number of years but seems to have returned with a vengeance. This book reports the recent developments in the field as well as giving an introduction to some basic concepts.

Segall M H, Dasen P, Berry J W, Poortinga Y H 1990 Human behaviour in global perspective: an introduction to cross-cultural psychology. Allyn & Bacon, Boston
By far the majority of studies in health psychology, and psychology in general for that matter, have been conducted in the West. Health psychology should be concerned with the health behaviour of everyone everywhere. This book, written by experts in the field, provides an introduction for those wishing to spread their health psychology interests and thus become less ethnocentric.

Dasen P R, Berry J W, Sartorius N 1988 (eds) Health and cross-cultural psychology. Sage, New York

Moos R H 1976 The human context: environmental determinants of behaviour. Wiley, New York

Rappaport J 1977 Community psychology: values, research, and action. Holt Rinehart Winston, New York

9

Organisational model

Organisations need to be healthy as well as individuals. This chapter discusses some of the problems associated with working in large organisations such as staff burnout. Restructuring the work setting can improve motivation as well as job satisfaction. Health professionals involved in the prevention of illness and disease get little reinforcement, for if they are successful nobody knows about it. Finally, methods of organisational change are examined.

Just as we refer to some individuals as being in good health, so too can we refer to organisations as being in good health. Bennis (1962) proposes that we view organisational health in the same way as we view individual health and borrows from Jahoda's (1958) attempt to characterise the constituents of positive mental health in his analysis. He proposes the following criteria of a healthy organisation:

- *Adaptability.* The ability to solve problems and to react with flexibility to changing environmental demands.
- *A sense of identity.* Knowledge and insight on the part of the organisation of what it is, what its goals are, and what it is to do.
- *Capacity to test reality.* The ability to search out, accurately perceive, and correctly interpret the real properties of the environment, particularly those which have relevance for the functioning of the organisation.
- *Integration.* A state of integration among the subparts of the total organisation, such that the parts are not working at cross-purposes.

Whilst these criteria apply to all organisations, some systems are prone to particular types of problem. One which has received considerable attention over the past few years is the problem of staff burnout.

BURNOUT

Burnout may be defined as 'the process where professional attitudes and behaviour change in negative ways in response to some form of job stress'. Recently, there have been many articles on burnout in a wide range of health care journals, from the stress symptoms, burnout and suicidal thoughts of Finnish physicians (Olkinuora et al 1992) to the coping strategies used by Canadian ward nurses to deal with job stress (Ogus 1992). This illustrates the concern of health professionals about the problem and also provides us with a number of different interpretations of the phenomena.

Some of the characteristics that have been put forward to describe the burnout syndrome are:

1. labelling patients
2. feeling unappreciated and guilty
3. a sense of failure
4. intolerance of colleagues and patients
5. hating going to work every day
6. cynicism and dislike of patients
7. illness and absenteeism
8. clock-watching
9. exhaustion
10. isolation and withdrawal
11. 'going by the book' all the time
12. lack of concentration
13. boredom
14. sleep difficulties
15. depersonalisation.

Dewe (1989) examined a sample of 1801 general nurses for evidence and frequency of tension and tiredness at work. There were five main sources of stress:

1. *Work overload.* Problems of staff shortage and dealing with too many patients were the most stressful experiences, allied to trying to maintain high standards at the same time.
2. *Difficulties in relating to other staff.* Arguments and conflict with colleagues were found to be the next stressful events.

3. *Problems with nursing critically ill patients.* Some of the reported difficulties were having to respond to demands for instant action, operating unfamiliar equipment and working with new procedures or treatments.
4. *Anxiety and concern over patient treatment.* Not knowing when and how much to tell patients about their condition comes fourth in the list of stress factors. Also in this category was working with doctors who did not appear to understand the needs of the patients.
5. *Patients' condition.* Finally, the least stressful events were related to nursing patients who failed to improve, such as patients with chronic pain and the terminally ill.

A positive feature of this piece of research is that, whilst it is probably impossible to eradicate chronic pain and terminal illness, it is not impossible to develop ways to improve relationships between staff, reduce role ambiguity and address work overloads. Indeed, Llewelyn (1989) says that this is exactly what should occur but organisational and political changes need to take place before the imbalance between perceived demands and perceived resources can be achieved. 'Hence, nurses need to be taught about how organisations function, and why change is difficult and threatening to those who work in organisations. Only then will nurses be able to reduce their feelings of powerlessness and hence their experience of stress.'

Problems of definition

Many people would agree that burnout involves some form of change in attitude towards one's job, but many would also disagree on the nature of how this change occurs. For Edelwich & Brodsky (1980) burnout consists of four stages of disillusionment:

- enthusiasm, over-identification with patients and inefficient expenditure of one's energy
- stagnation, where one merely conducts the work
- frustration with the work
- apathy used as a defence against the frustration.

Maslach & Pines (1979) propose phases of fatigue:

- *Phase 1*
  — emotional exhaustion (feeling tired when thinking about going to work)
  — physical exhaustion (sleeping poorly, prone to colds, headaches, aches and pains)
- *Phase 2*
  — develop negative cynical, dehumanised attitudes about coworkers
  — feel negative about patients/clients
  — dislike themselves for these negative feelings
  — withdraw into a shell and do a minimum of work
- *Phase 3*
  — total disgust for self, everything and everyone.

It is important to point out that burnout is not just a response to work overload, for individuals can also become disillusioned as a result of having too little to do. Burnout is essentially a response to any factor that changes a person's attitude to his or her job in a negative way.

A transactional model

Cherniss (1980, 1992) wants us to view burnout as a transactional process. By this he means that burnout is a process consisting of three stages. The first stage is characterised by resources not meeting demand. The second stage is the emotional response to this deficit—anxiety, tension, tiredness and finally exhaustion. The third stage is a change in attitude and behaviour such as becoming detached and increasingly cynical.

Thus a person who is experiencing high levels of job stress will utilise appropriate coping mechanisms and change her attitude or behaviour to provide a psychological escape. This often manifests itself in a detachment from the situation and can lead to an impersonal attitude toward patients and their problems. Probably the most damaging feature of the syndrome is the degree to which it reinforces itself. Once the process of negative attitude change is initiated it

not only destroys that individual's commitment, but it is also extremely infectious and can lead to other members of the organisation developing similar attitudes. It is therefore very important to set up mechanisms whereby the early detection of any disaffection is a priority rather than an option to be incorporated if one has the time.

Therefore not only are patients treated in a detached and mechanical fashion but colleagues will also suffer the consequences of the 'burnout' individual in the form of lack of cooperation, criticism of attitudes toward care and an inability to construct a positive approach toward problem solving.

Unfortunately, due to the differences in the way burnout has been defined, and as a result of its popularity, it has become a catch-all phrase to describe a variety of conditions. Jones & Klarr (1985) compared a number of community mental health departments and, not surprisingly, found incidences of burnout. But in one department they noted that:

the staff worked with an even more difficult and demanding population. The staff in this department worked with equal intensity and for longer hours. Management in this department had less interest and concern for the problems of burnout. Few precautionary or intervention measures were implemented. Despite this, there was little or no evidence of staff burnout. A staff member who had been with the department for twelve years commented, 'We don't have time for burnout.' In the face of bureaucratic pressure and patient demands, this department manifested a minimal amount of burnout.

Herein lies the problem with the concept of burnout; how do we explain its absence in circumstances ideal for its growth? The plethora of definitions give little help in explaining away these findings. Maslach (1982) recognises some of the difficulties and proposes that the fascination with burnout has increased the number of phenomena to which it refers. This can impair our understanding of the concept and be a major reason why some people have become so cynical and reject it altogether.

The answer lies not in rejecting the concept altogether, but in seeking to delve deeper into specific features of the relationship between individuals and their workplace. Negative changes in attitude can result from a number of factors and occur at a number of different levels. So in order to get a better idea of burnout we must examine its growth at four different levels: individual, group, organisation and institution. In other words, people can become 'burnt-out' because of themselves, because of the people they work with, because of the work setting itself and finally because of the way the institution is organised. Unfortunately in some cases individuals may be suffering at not just one level, but a combination of all four at the same time. Let us start by examining how individual factors contribute to the ways in which people view their work.

INDIVIDUAL FACTORS
Realistic expectations

Many of the underlying causes of job stress and burnout can be examined in terms of inadequate staff development programmes. A great deal of stress is caused by the excessive demands that workers impose on themselves. For instance, new workers can bring unrealistically high goals to a job, such as thinking that they can cure, or at least help in some way, all the people that they come into contact with. Norris (1982) feels that it is a delusion or myth that nurses can significantly influence patients' lives. She considers it irrational to think that change is possible for a patient during a 3- to 5-day hospital spell. When staff fail to achieve their goals they often abandon them, adopting the most minimal of custodial roles. However, through constructing carefully designed staff development programmes, workers can be helped to become more aware of what their personal goals are in order to alleviate the problems of unrealistically high or low expectations.

Rewards

It is also important to help people to adopt new goals, as well as providing alternative sources of gratification. They may be helped to see the potential dangers of becoming too dependent on

work for need-fulfilment and encouraged to develop other sources of gratification outside the job. This process is best accomplished during the training phase. Weitz, as long ago as 1956, reported how one company successfully reduced 'reality shock' and turnover in its sales personnel by providing new trainees with a booklet that described typical examples of the kinds of frustrations and disappointments that they might encounter in the job. The company had previously used a booklet that emphasised the positive features of the job in the hope that prospective employees would not be scared away by mentioning difficulties and problems right at the beginning. They found that those who had received the realistic booklet were much more likely to remain in their job than those who had received the positive booklet.

It is heartening to note that this careful attention to initial orientation is in fact present in many of the training programmes in operation at the moment. For instance, a number of community nursing and health visiting courses try to give their trainees a realistic idea of what their job is going to be like at the beginning of the course. In addition to attending various lectures and seminars, students are encouraged to accompany experienced staff on their rounds 'in the field'. Gradually the students begin to assume more responsibility, working with the patients themselves whilst being observed by their supervisors. Inevitably at some stage there is bound to be some form of assessment of the trainees' practical skills. It is useful if the practical work teachers and supervisors do not have to provide these assessments until late on in the training programme. In this way one can avoid certain amounts of ambiguity, concern about performance and feelings of being ill at ease in the training environment.

Sometimes the problems have not so much to do with individuals having excessively ambitious goals, but relate to difficulty in realising that they have had any positive effect. How many times does a patient provide her GP with positive reinforcement by going back after treatment and saying thanks? It seems that the people who do tend to keep returning are the unsuccessful cases. Thus in behavioural terms there is little positive reinforcement. When levels of reinforcement become critically low, people will become increasingly disenchanted by lack of apparent progress. So it is very important to construct a system which is able to monitor small gains in treatment and feed these back at frequent intervals to the health professionals involved.

Pines & Aronson (1988) have highlighted the importance of positive conditions in the work place: 'Stress research has concentrated on the presence of negative conditions in the environment as a source of stress and has virtually ignored stress reactions that result from the lack of positive conditions.' They conclude that the absence of positive conditions constitutes a unique source of stress that is independent of the presence of negative conditions.

Problem solving

Durlak (1983) provides a model of professional frustration which has, as a central theme, the inability to pinpoint problems and identify the necessary information and organise it in a problem-solving manner. An obvious way to increase psychological success is to help staff develop their skill and ability in their work by providing opportunities to learn new techniques for working with patient problems, to refine old techniques or to develop greater theoretical sophistication in diagnosis and treatment.

One particularly useful focus for training is conflict resolution and organisational problem solving. Much of the frustration and stress that occurs is a response to conflict between the needs and goals of staff on the one hand and the demands of the profession on the other. When these conflicts occur, people often feel helpless because they know little about how the system works and have not acquired the skills for negotiating it. Conflicts with supervisors, colleagues and people from other professions are a common source of job stress and it is the knowledge and skill involved in handling these conflicts that could help staff feel more confident and competent.

Kramer (1974) has developed a successful training programme in organisational problem solving and conflict resolution for nurses. She designed the programme by collecting examples of typical organisational conflicts and frustrations from experienced nurses. She also asked the most organisationally adept and successful nurses how they would handle those incidents. These problems and solutions then formed the basis of a training programme for novices. Kramer (1974) found that new nurses who were exposed to this programme experienced less role strain and maintained their initial enthusiasm and commitment to a greater extent than did a control group. Planned in-service training programmes that are designed to give staff the ability to confront their problems can significantly decrease dissatisfaction.

Developmental counselling

Another way to influence job satisfaction is to have periodical counselling sessions with individuals who have been trained in staff development and who do not have any supervisory role. In such a way, current sources of frustration, stress and dissatisfaction may be discussed in a confidential manner without fear of the contents of any discussion being used by other people. Staff are helped to assess how job pressures might be affecting attitudes and performance and some form of action plan can then be discussed.

Schwartz & Will (1961) dealt with what they termed 'an epidemic' of burnout on a ward of a psychiatric hospital through a series of counselling interviews with one of the nurses. The nurse was encouraged to ventilate her feelings and to adopt an 'attitude of enquiry' toward her negative reactions to patients and colleagues. Although initially resistant, the nurse gradually opened up, and within six sessions her attitudes had dramatically changed. They found that this form of developmental counselling not only helped the nurse, but also other nurses seemed to respond positively through a 'chain reaction' effect.

The power of groups can also be utilised to great effect. Many staff believe that their problems, feelings and reactions are unique. They rarely have the opportunity to discuss these work-related difficulties with others in a setting that encourages both emotional support and positive problem solving. Through carefully planned and skilfully run support groups, staff in these settings can be helped to cope adaptively with the stress associated with their jobs.

Exchanging resources

An important feature of community psychology in recent years has been the establishment of resource exchange networks. Sarason (1977) has indicated that the exchange of ideas and experiences in such contexts as conferences, interdisciplinary seminars and task-oriented action programmes can help all concerned in furthering their interests and ability to cope with problems in their work. Staff can receive concrete help that reduces the burdens of their jobs, and horizons are broadened as they come to know people involved in different settings working with different types of problems. Just the process of sharing information and exchanging resources reduces the sense of isolation that so often characterises work in the health services. Sarason (1977) says that individuals who participate in such networks experience a sense of community and participation that increases their sense of efficacy, renews hope and optimism, and counteracts the sense of helplessness that all too often contributes to a negative attitude change. Thus the formation of resource exchange networks within and across organisations represents another useful way of promoting a healthy working environment.

SOCIAL FACTORS

The approach of Maslach, Pines and Jackson has been to emphasise the social nature of difficulties at work. In a series of studies over the 1970s and '80s they found that the most useful analysis of job stress was provided by a social psychological perspective. Maslach & Jackson (1982) say that:

It is an approach that identifies the crux of the problem not as psychological stress per se, but as a particular type of stress arising from the social relationship between providers and recipients. It

directs attention to certain classes of variables, such as perceptual biases, attributional inferences, and group processes, which provide many insights into possible solutions for burnout.

They point to a number of variables that affect the development of burnout:

Degree of contact

Maslach & Jackson (1982) found a direct relationship between the amount of time spent in direct care of patients and emotional exhaustion. They administered the MBI (Maslach Burnout Inventory) to a number of staff physicians at a health maintenance organisation and then got them to give estimates of the amount of time they spent in various professional activities. They found that the greater the amount of time spent in direct contact with patients, the higher the physicians' scores on the MBI subscale of emotional exhaustion. Scores were lower for those who spent some time in teaching and administration. Patient care is emotionally demanding in a number of ways, sometimes it can be due to the feelings and behaviours of the patients themselves, sometimes it is the nature of the patients' health problem and sometimes it is due to communications problems, on the part of health professional and patient alike. Also, dealing with members of the patients' families can prove stressful in its own right.

Control

In health care settings, many aspects of the professional's environment are beyond his or her control and, as we have seen in Chapter 4, the ability to be able to predict and control events in one's environment is extremely important in reducing the effects of stress. Frustration is produced by the inability of modern medicine to control the diseases of all the patients and by the reluctance of some patients to cooperate with prescribed treatments. However, it is coping with lack of control over decisions made by doctors and administrators that formed the basis of nurses' feelings of exhaustion in the Maslach & Jackson (1982) study. Emotional exhaustion was higher for nurses who felt that they were unable to influence decisions of doctors and the policies of administrators. There were frequent complaints about (a) having no opportunity to be creative, and (b) doctors who failed to turn up for appointments, or disappeared without leaving word where they could be contacted. Similar relationships between perceptions of control and burnout have been found in a recent study of hospital nurses in the USA (Glass et al 1993).

The nurses were found to have one advantage over the doctors, and this was their freedom to have more time off and their ability to reschedule patients. Nurses were much more likely to report taking time off as a way of coping (61% of nurses, 12% of doctors). When asked whether they rescheduled their work in order to spend more time with those patients with whom they felt they were being more successful, 83% of nurses said 'yes' as compared to 48% of doctors. The authors suggest that time off and rescheduling are effective methods of coping with the strains and stresses of patient care.

Role ambiguity

This is a major cause of poor performance and job stress (Abraham & Shanley 1992). Therefore to what extent does role ambiguity exist among health professionals? Stein (1967) says there is a 'doctor–nurse game'. The rules are not out in the open and the game must be learnt through trial and error. The nurse's objective is to 'be bold, have initiative, and be responsible for making significant recommendations, while at the same time she must appear passive. This must be done in a manner so as to make her recommendations appear to be initiated by the physician.' There are no 'points' awarded for playing the game well, but penalty 'points' are gained for playing the game badly. The nurse is thus placed in the invidious position of uncertainty and ambiguity about the quality of her performance. This lack of positive feedback in an ambiguous situation, not surprisingly, produces emotional exhaustion. Although nursing has changed considerably since 1967, the extent

to which the game is still played will be left for the reader to judge.

Attribution errors or 'it is the patient's fault'

This item needs little introduction since attribution errors were discussed in detail in Chapter 2. Maslach & Jackson (1982) suggest that the fundamental attribution error is made worse by the utilisation of the medical model. That is, there is a tendency to see individuals in isolation about their problems and thus concentrate on what it is about that person that is causing the difficulty rather than investigating situational factors. The way patient records are kept also contributes to an emphasis on person-centred evaluations of problems, and there is little room for noting the circumstances in which the illness developed.

If the process of blaming the patient continues then the health professional gradually develops a depersonalised, detached and often cynical view of patients. The general impression develops that no matter what one does or how hard one works, patients will continue to disregard medical advice and abuse themselves. This attitude inevitably affects helping behaviour and the quality of patient care. It represents an important shift in the practitioner's view of health care; from a positive, humanised orientation to a negative and depersonalised one.

Social support

Different people adopt different ways of coping with the stresses and strains of work, but two methods that have been found to be effective are isolation and social support. It might seem at first that those who use isolation as a means of coping are a different group from those who use social support, but this need not be the case. In fact, both techniques can be used to advantage by the same person.

Firth & Britton (1989) conducted a long-term analysis of the relationship between role ambiguity, perceived support and factors related to burnout such as absence and turnover amongst

British nurses. They concluded that emotional exhaustion and lack of perceived support both influenced motivation. Further, ambiguity about the limits of authority led nurses to avoid some situations. If emotional exhaustion has resulted from the continuous close contact with people, then it is not surprising that one way of coping with this is to get away from them completely. This can be achieved by physically distancing oneself from the 'interpersonal mêlée' such as taking more time off or, if this proves impracticable, to at least have a period of time after work to unwind. Some of the distancing techniques include going for a run, listening to music, meditation or relaxing in a hot bath. Equally important as physical isolation is psychological isolation, for it is no good separating yourself physically from the job if one is going to think about it all the time.

Many psychologists would argue that isolating oneself is only an appropriate coping strategy as long as it is used in conjunction with social support (Duck 1992). Putting a certain amount of distance between us and the job is similar to what Lazarus & Launier (1978) term a palliative coping style. Coping in this fashion helps because it changes our internal response to the stress though it does little actively to reduce the stress stimulus itself. Social support, in the form of organised, peer-group discussion meetings, can go a long way to actually changing the individual's perception of the stressful stimuli.

Sharing one's feelings with other people who are in the same position serves a number of functions:

- It can make one realise that certain problems are not necessarily unique to one individual.
- The meetings can serve as a reference point, that is they can give information about what may be a normal reaction to a particular situation.
- Peers can provide the positive feedback that is so often absent from work with patients.
- They serve to save individuals from thinking that everything is their fault and highlight the situational nature of problems.
- They can act as an outlet for simply talking about similar difficulties.

Dewe (1987) found that expressing feelings and frustrations was one of six strategies that nurses in New Zealand used to cope with job stress.

Maslach & Jackson (1982) report that those doctors and nurses who scored low on their scale of emotional exhaustion and depersonalisation were actively involved in peer support groups. They were also more likely to seek advice from other staff, discuss with patients the limitations of their professional relationship and try to view circumstances from the patients' point of view.

Thus the social approach emphasises the interpersonal side of job stress and suggests that we look towards an analysis of our relationships with others if we want to come to a clearer understanding of the dynamics of job stress.

THE WORK SETTING

Although reducing role conflict and role ambiguity are important strategies for preventing job dissatisfaction, there are a number of other features of the work setting that may be manipulated to facilitate a positive working environment. Just as important as reducing overload is the concept of increasing interest and involvement in the job. Merely eliminating the nasty and distasteful elements of the job is not good enough, for under these circumstances employees may lack a sense of purpose and direction, which can be equally destructive in organisational terms. However, the way in which a person's job is organised can have a significant impact on his attitude towards it (Hawkins 1987). Role structure is as important as role ambiguity and role conflict.

Overload

Maslach & Pines (1977) found that they could significantly reduce the effects of overload by manipulating responsibility. Suppose four staff share the responsibility for 20 patients. They can share the responsibility for all of them or they can each be responsible for five patients. Maslach & Pines (1977) found that when the load was divided so that each member of staff was responsible for a small group of patients, then there was less stress and fewer reported feelings of being overloaded. Even though the actual ratio of patients to staff was exactly the same in both circumstances, when the responsibility was divided into small groups, it resulted in less stress. Some of the reasons put forward for this result were that the role structure probably contributed to a closer and more meaningful relationship with the patients, and the staff probably felt a greater sense of personal responsibility, autonomy and control when they were solely responsible for a small group of patients. Limiting the number of people for whom staff are responsible appears to be an effective method of combating overload.

Not all patients require the same amount of care. There are some who may be labelled 'difficult' to work with and exercise more mental and physical energy than others. Therefore it makes sense to share the load amongst all members of staff even though there may be some people who openly express a desire to work with 'problem patients', for it is often these individuals that subsequently experience high levels of burnout. Similarly, it is important to try to balance the rewarding and unrewarding activities throughout the day, for concentrating all the 'dirty jobs' either at the beginning or at the end of the day can increase stress. There are always going to be aspects of jobs that are distasteful and unrewarding but spreading and balancing the load throughout the day reduces the amount of strain that they may cause any one individual.

Taking a break

No matter what the job, whether it be health professional or bringing up children, if one does not get a rest every now and then, pressure and strain will mount up till the burden reaches a critical level. Opportunities for taking some time off, no matter how brief, should be built in to any job programme. Apart from giving staff a rest from their work, time-off can also provide an opportunity to reflect on one's position. However, in times of limited resources, there is a problem finding the time to give personnel a rest.

It might seem strange to say that sometimes it is necessary to encourage people to take a break, but this is in fact the case. Allowing holiday or vacation time to accumulate is regarded by some individuals as a status symbol that they can parade around work. Also there are some workers who take great pride in announcing that they have worked 10 or 12 hours that day. It might illustrate dedication but the long-term consequences of such actions are detrimental to both staff and patient alike and should be discouraged.

Staff development

Much lip service is paid to this concept in many organisations, but often the opportunities open to staff for development are limited. The words 'personal and professional growth' are sometimes used to refer to staff development and it is important to realise that development is important in both the professional and personal spheres. The main issue is how to gauge individuals' needs in this particular domain. One method often used is the 'developmental interview' sometimes known as developmental counselling. Here staff are invited from time to time to discuss, usually with their superiors, issues relating to their development. The success of these sessions almost entirely depends on the attitude of the person conducting the interview, for if members of staff feel inhibited in discussing important matters relating to their job, then the usefulness of the session is limited. Therefore it is incumbent on supervisory staff to create an atmosphere of mutual trust and confidentiality in order to reduce the amount of suspicion that is often created by the very nature of the unequal status of the participants.

An important factor to consider in creating a feeling of active involvement is establishing the opportunity for individuals to become involved in developing ideas, projects and programmes of their own. This serves the dual purpose of providing a creative outlet for members of staff and also hopefully leads to some form of improvement in the functioning of the organisation itself.

In similar vein, the provision of some form of career ladder that is directed towards both professional and academic development provides a necessary form of reinforcement. As Schein (1980) points out, financial and verbal rewards are not good enough in themselves for generating appropriate levels of motivation. Therefore there needs to be a clear programme by which people can see how they might progress from one stage to the next. Individuals should be encouraged to take time off to attend academic courses relevant to their particular discipline in order that they may progress up the career ladder and bring new knowledge to their professional practice. It is equally important for those institutions that provide the courses to construct a programme that is available to all, no matter what the initial qualification, so that individuals may progress from certificate level right the way through to degree and masters level.

Management development

One consequence of progressing up the career ladder is that eventually one is more likely than not to find oneself in some form of managerial role, often with little experience of management itself. Good health practitioners may not make the best managers. In-service management training programmes can help develop those skills and attitudes necessary for managing people. In this way managers can be helped to develop their awareness of their own operational philosophy and alternative philosophies and the consequences of adopting such alternatives. They may not even know about ways of preventing staff burnout.

Feedback is just as important for managers and administrators as it is for their subordinates. Hegarty (1974) found that when anonymous feedback was provided to managers, their managerial style improved. Staff were provided with questionnaires which asked them to evaluate their superiors on a number of criteria. They were also asked to provide information about the qualities they most valued in a superior. The information was anonymous and only the managers saw the results. Some months later the survey was repeated with the same group; the evaluation scores on this occasion had risen. Managers are not immune to the effects of job stress; there is often ambiguity and role conflict in their position.

Conflict resolution

Problems with interpersonal and organisational conflict at their core will always occur, no matter what the management structure. However, mechanisms may be built in to organisations to alleviate conflicts. Filley (1975) recommends three courses of action:

• The creation of a formal mechanism for group problem solving and conflict resolution.
• Staff training in the skills of interpersonal problem solving and conflict resolution.
• The determination of an optimal level of staff participation in decision making.

Building into programmes formal group problem-solving mechanisms means that there should be times during the week when all staff can meet to discuss any problems. These meetings should be organised so as to encourage staff and supervisors alike to take part and promote an atmosphere of mutual support.

Developing training programmes for staff in the area of interpersonal problem solving and conflict resolution serves to benefit individuals themselves in the handling of their everyday problems and conflicts as well as to facilitate the process of group problem-solving sessions.

The third recommendation concerns the extent to which staff should be allowed to take part in the decision-making activities of the organisation. Whilst there is evidence to suggest that more staff participation leads to less conflict and higher morale (Cherniss & Egnatios 1978), it is often difficult to put this into practice. Therefore each situation must be organised so as to accommodate an optimum level of staff participation. This need not necessarily mean more committees, more meetings, for if it is organised properly, it can actually lead to less work. It is also wise to take note of the findings of the experiments on group decision making that were discussed earlier in the book.

A sense of direction

Clear, consistent and, most of all, realistic goals can provide the focus that staff need to overcome the negative effects of vague, inconsistent or even conflicting institutional philosophies. Where an organisation refuses to give its members a clear sense of purpose, then staff are bound to ask questions about what they are meant to be doing, or even what they are doing there. Reppucci (1973) states that the development of a guiding philosophy of treatment or service is a particularly effective method for creating a sense of purpose. It should not be left up to individuals themselves to try to develop their own philosophy or approach in the absence of direction from the institution. In such cases people can become very quickly disillusioned.

Finally, it may be necessary under certain circumstances to redefine the aims and goals of organisations. For instance, Seymour Sarason, a leading figure in community psychology, has said repeatedly that we set our goals too high and that organisations must redefine their goals specifically when scarce resources are in demand. Rather than assume responsibility for a whole population's health, it is more practical to offset some of this load onto the individuals themselves. By sharing the responsibility for health one redefines a number of roles, hopefully to the benefit of all concerned.

In practice this means that people should be encouraged to be less dependent on health professionals, to think and do more for themselves and ultimately to be able to engage in a mutual decision-making process about their own health care. Many self-health centres see this as one of their fundamental aims. According to Sarason (1977) one of the key features of community psychology is to produce 'the competent community'. It seems reasonable that this competence should encompass health as well as other areas of psychological well-being.

ORGANISATIONAL CHANGE

It should be apparent by now that there are a number of changes that could be made in organisations to make them healthier. However, a typical comment is that 'it is all very well discussing the best approach to this and that, but you try getting it adopted'. Organisations, and people, are remarkably resistant to change.

Attitudes

In numerous instances organisational change is dependent upon attitude change and, as we have seen earlier, changing people's attitudes can prove very difficult indeed. One of the main pitfalls in persuading people to change their attitude is the presence of reactance. This occurs in situations where, because you feel that someone is trying to exert undue influence on you, you lean over backwards to do the opposite of what he or she wanted. These negative reactions tend to occur when we feel someone is trying to limit our personal freedom and can be strong enough to get us to resist the change even when we would have accepted it under normal circumstances (Chapter 2).

Brehm & Brehm (1981) said that this negative attitude change was the result of the desire of most persons to believe that they are masters of their own fate, that they are able to think and act for themselves. This means in management terms that an effective method of reducing reactance to change is to involve people in the decision-making process itself so that they can have some say in the nature and direction of the change and thus feel that they have an important contribution to make. However, Baer et al (1980) say that the reactance effect is due to a desire for other people to see us as autonomous individuals able to make up our own minds. It is not so much whether we are given the opportunity to have our say or not that is important but that other people are able to see that we can think for ourselves. If Baer et al (1980) are correct, then it is merely necessary for management to give its personnel the illusion that they are contributing to the decision-making process so that individuals can see each other expressing their own points of view. It is not necessary to give them actual decision-making powers.

The father, or perhaps grandfather, of organisational change theory is Kurt Lewin. His two famous maxims were:

- If you want to understand an organisation, try to change it.
- There is nothing so practical as a good theory.

Lewin felt that the only way to study organisations was to intervene in some way in their inner workings or dynamics, but that one should not 'fiddle about' in a random fashion. Interventions had to be guided by an appropriate theory. He wasted no time in putting forward what he thought was an appropriate theory which, despite having been modified in many different ways over the years, still remains one of the most relevant guidelines to organisational change. Schein (1980) is one of those people who have elaborated on Lewin's original model and starts with the following assumptions:

- Any change process involves not only learning something new, but unlearning something that is already present and possibly well integrated into the personality and social relationships of the individual.
- No change will occur unless there is motivation to change, and if such motivation to change is not already there, the induction of that motivation is the most difficult part of the change process.
- Organisational changes such as new structures, processes, reward systems and so on occur only through key members of the organisation; hence organisational change is always mediated through individual changes.
- Most adult change involves attitudes, values, and self-images, and the unlearning of present responses in these areas is inherently painful and threatening.
- Change is a process that involves a number of stages, all of which have to be negotiated before a stable change can be said to have taken place.

These assumptions underlie a model comprising three stages. Let us first look at the model itself and then see how it has been applied in the health context:

A model

Stage 1: Unfreezing

The first stage, referred to as unfreezing, is concerned with creating the motivation to change and depends upon the operation of three specific mechanisms:

- Here individuals come to realise that what they thought about themselves or their job is incorrect and therefore want to change. It could be that their behaviour is not producing desired or expected outcomes and they experience a certain amount of discomfort at this imbalance, which in turn leads to a desire to change, or it could be that individuals are unaware that anything is wrong and need to be informed. This latter course raises ethical considerations of whether it is right to create motivation by inducing discomfort in people.
- The discomfort must be a real motivator. If discomfort is low, then no action will be taken, the person utilising some defence mechanism to deny or avoid the situation. However, if the person realises that there really is a problem, then he will feel motivated to do something about it.
- It is no good going from the 'frying pan into the fire'. In other words people must have an assurance that everything will be all right if they do take the recommended course of action and change. Schein (1980) says: 'Probably the single most difficult aspect of initiating change is the balancing of painful disconfirming messages with reassurance that change is possible and can be embarked upon with some sense of personal safety.' Once a person has accepted the need to change, and feels that it is safe, new learning can take place.

Stage 2: Changing

Changing may be defined as 'developing new attitudes and behaviours on the basis of new information and cognitive redefinition'. The effect of creating a motivation to change is to open up people to new ideas or new ways of looking at existing practices (cognitive redefinition). Changing occurs in two main ways:

- The social learning approach. A key concept in social learning theory is imitation. One of the most powerful ways of learning new ideas, attitudes or behaviour is to be 'exposed' to a significant role model. This can be a friend or a colleague. The important point is that one is able to see a new way of doing things in action and if this person commands a certain degree of respect from everyone, so much the better. However, identification with a role model does have its drawbacks in that it tends to focus on a single source of information which in some circumstances can prove counterproductive. A way of getting around this drawback is to adopt the next method.
- Searching the environment for new information that fits our particular case is more difficult to do but more relevant since the role model's approach may not always fit our situation. Thus searching the environment for information that specifically relates to one's particular problem is relevant and enables individuals to remain in control of the information they use. It is extremely important to note that change will not occur unless a real motivation to change is present. So often, programmes fail by skipping Stage 1 and start by presenting new ideas and work practices. This new information will fall on deaf ears unless there is a genuine motivation to change.

Stage 3: Re-freezing

The process of re-freezing is concerned with stabilising the changes. Often the programmes designed to induce attitude change have observable effects during the training phase but these effects do not last once the person is back in his normal routine. This may be due to the fact that the learned behaviour does not fit properly into the person's total personality or it may be due to the inability of an individual's colleagues to accept the new attitudes and put resultant pres-

sure on the person to revert back to what they regard as more comfortable ways of operating. There are two mechanisms by which the process of re-freezing may be accomplished:

- Individuals should have the opportunity of testing whether the new attitudes or behaviours really fit his or her self-concept. One advantage of adopting a 'searching' approach as opposed to an 'imitation' approach is that people are able to select the behaviour that suits them, rather than having to imitate the behaviour of a model, which may prove to be inappropriate later.
- The person should have the opportunity to test whether his other colleagues will accept the change in behaviour. Where there is difficulty in operationalising this course of action, the change programme should be targeted at sets of people or groups who will be able to reinforce the behaviours in each other. Team training may be more effective in this context than individual training.

Health implications

Olsen (1979) has illustrated how Lewin's change techniques may be utilised within the context of the health system. With regard to the first stage of unfreezing, she warns that the person initiating the change must be prepared for the ramifications or consequences of any individual strategy used. She gives an example of a health professional taking a group to another institution to view the change he or she wants to implement. The reaction to the visit may be: 'That change is fine for that organisation, but not for ours.' A way of avoiding these sorts of comments is to emphasise the selective nature of the visit. Rather than imitating another process, the group should be encouraged to select the sorts of practices that would fit into their organisational structure. Also when volunteers are asked to change on a trial basis, care must be taken to avoid alienating non-volunteers by giving them less attention.

She calls Lewin's second stage 'moving' and says that the health professional may find that the system does not provide rewards to facilitate moving. In other words it is important to identify and provide meaningful rewards, either external or internal, that are conducive to behavioural change. The environment should be supportive, non-threatening, and educational.

The final phase ought to involve positive feedback and constructive criticism. A plan for evaluating the new process should be constructed. However, there may be problems relating to setting up a support system and preventing future change before the initial one is stabilised.

Other approaches to organisational change within the health system are adopted by Reinkemeyer (1970) and Smoyak (1974). Reinkemeyer (1970) proposes seven stages of planned change:

1. Development of a felt need and desire for change.
2. Development of a change relationship between the agent and the client system.
3. Clarification or diagnosis of the client system's problem, need, or objective.
4. Examination of alternative routes and tentative goals and intentions of actions.
5. Transformations of intentions into actual change behaviour.
6. Stabilisation.
7. Termination of the relationship between the change agent and the client system.

These phases need not necessarily proceed in this order.

Smoyak (1974), on the other hand, employs a confrontation model similar to that of Alinsky (1971), which has three phases of confrontation:

1. *Planning the confrontation*. In the initial phase, strategies are planned for confronting 'the opposition'. Such things as who will confront who, the level of confrontation and time scales are worked out.
2. *Confronting the system*. The next phase involves the processes of initiation, progress review, evaluation, and sharing with others. Regular meetings are held.
3. *Strengthening new images and relationships*

following the confrontation. After successful use of this model and resolution of the issue, people have insight into new roles and relationships.

Before the implementation of such a model, extreme care should be taken to make sure that all group members are at ease with the technique and that there is a consensus in favour of using confrontation.

No matter what model of change is used, there will always be a certain degree of resistance. Bennis et al (1969) state that people tend to resist change under the following conditions:

- When the nature of the change and its effects are not clearly explained to those involved. However, merely giving full information may not by itself eliminate resistance.
- When information is distorted, especially if people have felt uncomfortable and threatened in past work situations.
- When the change is made on personal grounds rather than according to the impersonal requirements of the group or organisation.
- When change ignores the established norms or customs of the group
- When excessive work pressure is involved in the change.
- When the planning of change fails to consider in detail exactly how the change will be brought about.
- When there is little consideration given to problems that are likely to arise and how to deal with them.
- When there is fear of failure, or when the change is seen as inadequate or ineptly managed.
- When no provision is made for adequate two-way communications.

Some common reasons for resistance to change include clinging to existing satisfactions, cost, time investment, threat (from either the change or the change agent), selective perception and retention, vested interests, and fear of failure or disorganisation.

If people want to implement change, then it is

hoped that the information provided above will be of some practical use and that individuals will delve deeper into the theories and the models themselves in order to obtain the most appropriate course of action that will suit their particular circumstances.

At the start of this chapter there was reference to the criteria that characterise a healthy organisation. To finish this section here are Schein's (1980) internal organisational conditions that are necessary for effective coping:

- Successful coping requires the ability to take in and communicate information reliably.
- Successful coping requires internal flexibility and creativity to make the changes which are demanded by the information obtained.
- Successful coping requires integration of and commitment to the multiple goals of the organisation, from which comes the willingness to change when necessary.
- Successful coping requires an internal climate of support and freedom from threat, since being threatened undermines good communications, reduces flexibility, and stimulates self-preservation rather than concern for the total system.
- Successful coping requires the ability to continuously redesign the organisation's structure to be congruent with its goals and tasks.

SOCIAL INNOVATION

So far, in the main, the focus of attention has been on attempts at social change from within the organisation. There are, however, many people who prefer to adopt an approach from without, that is individuals who are not employees and bound by the existing set-up can present experimental evidence to show the benefits of a different form of organisation. This strategy has been termed 'experimental social innovation' by Fairweather and his colleagues (Fairweather 1967, 1972; Fairweather & Tornatzky 1977; Fairweather et al 1969, 1974).

Fairweather (1972) suggests that historically the two most popular ways to create social change have been violent action or non-violent protest. He finds violent actions to be ineffective in creating genuine solutions to problems of social well-being for several reasons, including the fact that violence creates roles for people that are not functional once the violence is ended, and that such a means of creating social change is not compatible with the goals of human well-being. On the other hand, he views most non-violent protest methods, such as demonstrations, as an ineffective solution to social problems. Non-violence also does not necessarily lead one to the best solutions. Fairweather favours the systematic development of innovations and argues that the development of an atmosphere of continuous problem solving and change is required. By innovation, he means new ways of doing things that have been demonstrated to work better than present ways.

Unlike technical innovations, social innovations often constitute a change in the role relationships between members of society and therefore are more difficult to implement. For example, if providing a group of chronic mental patients with a place to live and the means to operate a small business, as well as autonomy from mental health professionals, were shown to be more effective and less expensive as a means to rehabilitation than current confinement and control, this would be more difficult to implement than if a pill were discovered to have the same results.

Implementation of such changes requires more than their invention. If it is to be adopted, a social innovation needs to be met by a receptive society and requires an advocate or a salesperson who may or may not be the same person as the inventor. It is how to create this atmosphere of acceptance and what to do when advocating an innovation that concerns Fairweather.

The kinds of social innovations that Fairweather is suggesting are considerably different from those suggested by organisational psychology. He is clearly interested in changing the priorities and goals of social institutions on which organisations are based, rather than with enhancing their ability to do the job more efficiently, or to keep their employees satisfied. That is what is meant by a social innovation.

Mental health change

Fairweather's research focused on the mental health system. He found that the creation of small group homes with work facilities over which chronic mental patients had autonomous control was a far more effective means of keeping patients living productively in the community, than keeping them in a hospital. He also found that this system of 'community lodges' was cost effective and much cheaper than the hospital alternatives.

Armed with this information, he set out to disseminate the data in the hope that he might create change in mental health organisations. He started with the institution in which he had developed the original innovation. He found it extremely difficult to convince them to adopt his programme, even on a trial basis. Apparently it was one thing to develop a social treatment programme; incorporating it into the hospital was another.

Strategies for change

Fairweather began to ask what techniques, strategies, and tactics could be used to incorporate new programmes into existing organisations, and conducted an experiment to find out. The experiment was designed to investigate how autonomous living units for chronic patients could be incorporated into mental hospitals throughout the USA. Fairweather and his colleagues decided to contact, by a personal phone call, almost every mental hospital in the USA. During this telephone conversation the researchers discussed the results of their early studies which had demonstrated the effectiveness of their plan for treating chronic patients, and offered to a representative of the hospital the opportunity to explore its possible value to that hospital in one of three ways:

- *Brochure.* One group of hospitals was offered a brochure detailing the ideas and outcomes of previous work.

- *Workshop.* With the second group, one of the research team offered to visit the hospital and run a workshop.
- *Demonstration unit.* For the third group, the team offered to set up a demonstration unit in the hospital in order to try out, in a pilot study, the programme's feasibility.

The phone calls were arranged so that the initial contact was with someone from one of the five levels of 'status hierarchy' including hospital superintendents, chiefs of psychiatry, psychology, social work, and nursing.

To those hospitals that accepted the offer, the brochure, workshops or demonstration units were supplied. The team assessed how many of the hospitals in each group were then willing actually to try to set up the new treatment programme.

The next step was the 'adopting phase'. Each hospital that expressed a willingness to adopt the programme was matched with another hospital. One of the pair was given a detailed manual explaining, step by step, how to do it, and the second was provided with an 'action consultant' who would aid them in carrying out the programme. Each hospital was observed over a 2-year period.

The overall results are summarised in Table 9.1. Far more hospitals agreed to allow entry when the entry itself was low cost in terms of commitment (a brochure or a workshop). More than two-thirds of the hospitals that were offered these services agreed to accept them; however, less than one-quarter of the hospitals that were asked to set up a demonstration ward

Table 9.1 Results of different modes of presentation of data

	Mode of presentation					
	Brochure		Workshop		Ward	
	(N)	(%)	(N)	(%)	(N)	(%)
Total contacted by telephone	85	100	85	100	85	100
Rejection of entry	26	30	17	20	64	75
Permitted entry only	55	65	58	68	12	14
Agreed to attempt adoption	4	5	10	12	9	11

agreed to entry. Of the 59 hospitals agreeing to be sent the brochure, only 4 (7%) later agreed to adopt the new programme; and of the 68 agreeing to the new workshop only 10 (15%) later agreed to adopt. Although only 21 hospitals agreed to a demonstration ward, 9, or 43%, later decided to adopt the actual project. This seems to indicate that, although an initial request for a substantial active commitment will be rejected by about 75% of the organisations contacted, of those that do make the commitment, a substantial proportion is likely to adopt the innovation. Although a passive commitment to reading material and workshops allows entry to more organisations, the potential for change by these means is limited.

Other findings were that none of the demographic variables of the hospitals (e.g. urban versus rural, state versus federally funded) predicted acceptance or rejection of the innovation; nor did the status of the person contacted have any effect either. Nor were the financial resources available to the hospital predictive of adoption. Finally, of those hospitals that did agree to try adoption, those that were given an action consultant, who met with them and helped them to implement the project, were found to be significantly more successful in implementation of the programme than those hospitals that were provided with a detailed manual.

This last finding has implications for the dissemination of research findings in general. If Fairweather's work is correct, then publishing the details of research in a journal or in a report may bring them to the attention of one's target group, but will be unlikely to lead to that group taking action on them.

There are two other disappointing findings. Those hospitals that adopted the innovation did so because of the small, committed action group. There was little evidence of a generalisation to the entire hospital. Secondly, to the extent that total organisational change is the goal, this experiment failed to produce it. Of the 255 hospitals contacted in this study, less than 10% ultimately agreed to even try the innovation, despite the fact of research evidence demonstrating its effectiveness.

Fairweather and his colleagues recognise the difficulties and some of the shortcomings of their research, but nevertheless feel that they have learnt from the experience. They suggest several principles to be followed by experimental social innovators as guidelines for action and say that they represent the first steps toward a psychology of social change.

Guidelines for action

Principle of perseverance

The reality is that a great deal of constant effort *is* required to obtain even the smallest movement. Fairweather, in his book, shows how to 'stick to it'.

Principle of discontinuity and independence

The results of the study found little relationship between resources and acceptance of the innovation. Fairweather, therefore, encourages us to 'Forget the problem of scarce resources and instead find someone in the institution with the will, and help that person to organize and create a group for change based on action.'

Principle of outside intervention

Fairweather suggests that the role of the intervener must be to serve as an active, personally involved worker who encourages others on the one hand to view the project as their own, but on the other hand who keeps it consistent with its major ingredients. The actual style of the outside change agent is less important than the ability to keep up the morale of the change group.

Principle of action-oriented intervention

Strategies based on tasks to be accomplished and behaviours to be completed work better than those aimed at attitude change.

'Foot-in-the-door' principle

A strategy of gradually moving from discussion to behavioural commitment is to be encouraged.

For example, the researchers hypothesise that they might have been successful if they had gone back to those who refused a demonstration unit and offered them a workshop, followed by a new request for a demonstration unit.

Do not be constrained by the power structure

Those in higher positions are no more essential to change than those at lower levels. Find whoever is willing to change and start there. Change can start from the bottom as well as the top.

Principle of participation

Get as many groups as possible involved; the innovation will not automatically diffuse.

Principle of group action

A group that is cohesive and committed must be developed. The members can come from any status level.

Most of these suggestions are based on a combination of empirical data and observation and are similar to the suggestions of others who have adopted a non-empirical approach.

CONCLUSION

An important function of health care programmes is the prevention of illness and disease by concentrating on developing healthy lifestyles in the target population. In this way, primary prevention can achieve significant savings in time, cost and effort due to the competence of individuals to deal with the strains and stresses of everyday life. Organisations can benefit in a similar way. If organisations can become healthy enough to cope with the pressures of change and adaptation, then they, too, can become competent to achieve the aims and objectives they set for themselves.

REFERENCES

Abraham C, Shanley E 1992 Social psychology for nurses. Edward Arnold, London

Alinsky S D 1971 Rules for radicals. Random House, New York

Baer R, Hinkle S, Smith K, Fenton M 1980 Reactance as a function of actual versus projected autonomy. Journal of Personality and Social Psychology 38: 416–422

Bennis W G 1962 Toward a truly scientific management: the concept of organisational health. General Systems Yearbook 7: 269–283

Bennis W G, Benne K, De Chin R 1969 The planning of change, 2nd edn. Holt Rinehart Winston, New York

Brehm S, Brehm Y W 1981 Psychological reactance: a theory of freedom and control. Academic Press, New York

Cherniss C 1980 Staff burnout: job stress in the human services. Sage, Beverly Hills

Cherniss C 1992 Long term consequences of burnout—an exploratory study. Journal of Organizational Behaviour 13: 1–11

Cherniss C, Egnatios E 1978 Clinical supervision in community mental health. Social Work 23: 219–223

Dewe P J 1987 Identifying strategies nurses use to cope with work stress. Journal of Advanced Nursing 12: 489–497

Dewe P J 1989 Stressor frequency, tension, tiredness and coping. Some measurement issues and a comparison across nursing groups. Journal of Advanced Nursing 14: 308–320

Duck S 1992 Human relationships, 2nd edn. Sage, London

Durlak J A 1983 Social problem-solving as a primary prevention strategy. In: Felner R D, Jason L A, Moritsugu J N, Farber S S (eds) Preventive psychology: theory, research and practice. Pergamon, New York

Firth H, Britton P 1989 'Burnout', absence and turnover amongst British nursing staff. Journal of Ocupational Psychology 62: 55–59

Edelwich J, Brodsky A 1980 Burnout: stages of disillusionment in the helping professions. Human Sciences Press, New York

Fairweather G W 1967 Methods for experimental social innovation. Wiley, New York

Fairweather G W 1972 Social change: the challenge to survival. General Learning Press, Morristown NJ

Fairweather G W & Tornatzky L G 1977 Experimental methods for social policy research. Pergamon, Oxford

Fairweather G W, Sanders D H, Cressier D L, Maynard H 1969 Community life for the mentally ill: an alternative to institutional care. Aldine, Chicago

Fairweather G W, Sanders D H, Tornatzky L G 1974 Creating change in mental health organisations. Pergamon, New York

Filley A C 1975 Interpersonal conflict-resolution. Scott Foresman. Glencoe IL

Glass D C, McKnight J D, Valdimarsdottir H 1993 Depression, burnout and perceptions of control in hospital nurses. Journal of Consulting and Clinical Psychology 61: 147–155

Gottlieb B H 1981 Social networks and social support. Sage, Beverly Hills

Hawkins L 1987 An ergonomic approach to stress. International Journal of Nursing Studies 24: 307–318

Hegarty W H 1974 Using subordinate ratings to elicit behavioural changes in supervisors. Journal of Applied Psychology 59: 764–766

Jahoda M 1958 Current concepts of positive mental health. Basic Books, New York

Jones P, Klarr A C 1985 A comparison of burnout in eight mental health departments. Paper presented to 'Burnout in health care' conference. University of Newcastle

Kramer M 1974 Reality shock: why nurses leave nursing. Mosby, St Louis

Lazarus R S, Launier R 1978 Stress-related transactions between person and environment. In: Pervin L A, Lewis M (eds) Perspectives in interactional psychology. Plenum, New York

Lewin K 1952 Group decision and social change. In: Swanson G E, Newcomb T N, Hartley E L (eds) Readings in social psychology. Holt, New York

Llewelyn S 1989 Caring: the costs to nurses and relatives: In: Broome A (ed) Health psychology: processes and applications. Chapman & Hall, London

Maslach C 1982 Job burnout: how people cope. In: McConnell E A (ed) Burnout in the nursing profession. Mosby, St Louis

Maslach C, Jackson S E 1982 Burnout in health professions: a social psychological analysis. In: Saunders G S, Suis J (eds) The social psychology of health and illness. Erlbaum, Hillsdale NJ

Maslach C, Pines A 1977 The burn-out syndrome in the day-care setting. Child Care Quarterly 6: 100–113

Maslach C, Pines A 1979 Burn-out: the loss of human caring. In: Pines A, Maslach C (eds) Experiencing social psychology. Knopf, New York

Norris C M 1982 Delusions that trap nurses . . . into dead end alleyways away from growth, relevance, and impact on health care. In: McConnell (ed) Burnout in the nursing profession. Mosby, St Louis

Ogus E D 1992 Burnout and coping strategies: a comparative study of ward nurses. Journal of Social Behaviour and Personality 7: 111–124

Olkinuora M, Asp S, Juntunen J, Kauttu K, Strid L, Aarimaa M 1992 Scandinavian Journal of Work Environment and Health 18: 110–112

Olsen E M 1979 Strategies and techniques for the nurse change agent. In: McConnell E A (ed) Burnout in the nursing profession. Mosby, St Louis

Pines A M, Kanner A D 1982 Nurses' burnout: lack of positive conditions and presence of negative conditions as two independent sources of stress. In: McConnell E A (ed) Burnout in the nursing profession. Mosby, St Louis

Pines A, Aronson E 1988 Career burnout: causes and cures. Collier Macmillan, London

Reinkemeyer A 1970 Nursing's need: a commitment to an ideology of change. Nursing Forum 9: 341–355

Reppucci N D 1973 Social psychology of institutional change: general principles for intervention. American journal of Community Psychology 1: 330–341

Sarason S 1977 Community psychology, networks, and Mr Everyman. American Psychologist 31: 317–328

Schein E H 1980 Organisational psychology, 3rd edn. Prentice Hall, Englewood Cliffs NJ

Schuler R S 1980 Definition and conceptualisation of stress in organisations. Organisational Behaviour and Human Performance 25: 184–215

Schwartz M S, Will G 1961 Intervention and change in a mental hospital ward. In: Bennis W G, Benne K, Chin R (eds) The planning of change. Holt Rinehart Winston, New York

Smoyak S 1974 The confrontation process. American Journal of Nursing 74: Sept. 1632–1635

Stein L I 1967 The doctor–nurse game. Archives of General Psychiatry 16: 699–703

Weitz J 1956 Job expectancy and survival. Journal of Applied Psychology 40: 245–247

RECOMMENDED READING

Bailey R, Clarke M 1989 Stress and coping in nursing. Chapman & Hall, London
This book contains a number of chapters on the nature of stress as well as an analysis of the stress of nursing. It also examines the types of coping strategies that are typically deployed to deal with stress.

Baron R A, Greenberg J 1990 Behaviour in organisations: understanding and managing the human side of work, 3rd edn. Allyn & Bacon, Boston
Provides a broad introduction to the field of organisational psychology. There are chapters on work motivation, leadership, influence and behaviour in work settings.

McConnell E A 1982 (ed) Burnout in the nursing profession. Mosby, St Louis
Many of the issues regarding burnout in the nursing profession are still here even after a decade of research. Thus this book is still a good source of information on job stress and change in a wide range of nursing areas.

Filley A C 1975 Interpersonal conflict-resolution. Scott Foresman, Glencoe IL

Schein E H 1980 Organisational psychology, 3rd edn. Prentice Hall, Englewood Cliffs NJ

Index